Adults with Developmental Disabilities: Current Approaches

in

Occupational Therapy

Edited by

Mildred Ross, OTR/L, FAOTA

Susan Bachner, MA, OTR/L, FAOTA

The American Occupational Therapy Association, Inc.

The American Occupational Therapy Association, Inc., Mission Statement

The mission of the American Occupational Therapy Association is to support a professional community for members, and to develop and preserve the viability and relevance of the profession. The organization serves the interest of its members, represents the profession to the public, and promotes access to occupational therapy services.

Disclaimers

"This publication is designed to provide accurate and authoritative information in regard to the subject matter covered. It is sold or distributed with the understanding that the publisher is not engaged in rendering legal, accounting, or other professional services. If legal advice or other expert assistance is required, the services of a competent professional person should be sought."

  —*From the Declaration of Principles jointly adopted by the American Bar Association and a Committee of Publishers and Associations*

It is the objective of the American Occupational Therapy Association to be a forum for free expression and interchange of ideas. The opinions expressed by the contributors to this work are their own and not necessarily those of either the editors or the American Occupational Therapy Association.

AOTA Director of Nonperiodical Publications: Frances E. McCarrey

AOTA Managing Editor of Nonperiodical Publications: Mary C. Fisk

Text design by World Composition Services, Inc.

Cover design by Irene Z Designs

ISBN 1-56900-084-0

Printed in the United States of America

To

Valnere McLean, MS, OTR/L, FAOTA

&

In Loving Memory of Nicole McLean

Contents

Contributors

Susan Bachner, MA, OTR/L, FAOTA, brings to this book 34 years of clinical practice with individuals who have developmental disabilities. Her experiences from private practice, consultation services, teaching, workshop presentations, and prior publications converge for the readers of *Adults with Developmental Disabilities: Current Approaches in Occupational Therapy.* Evidence of her graduate work in sociology and anthropology is found in "Let's Do Lunch." Susan writes, "It is illustrative of my strong belief that the planning, assessment, assimilation, and execution of occupational therapy practice, if it is to lead to a functional client-centered outcome, must incorporate a clear understanding of the participant's culture, values, and symbols."

Bonnie Hanschu, OTR, had 25 years of experience as an occupational therapist and was directing habilitation services at Cambridge Regional Center, a state of Minnesota ICF-MR facility for adults, when she began devoting her full attention to sensory approaches for people with severe disabilities. Her subsequent work directing the Center for Neurodevelopmental Studies in Phoenix, Arizona, solidified her thinking that disordered sensory processing is, for many individuals, a fundamental and primary barrier to their ability to benefit from other services and treatment approaches. Since 1995, she has worked as a consultant and trainer for therapists, psychologists, teachers, and others interested in sensory approaches. Her courses have been presented throughout the United States, and she has served as a consultant to major organizations, including school districts, hospitals, county and state agencies, and private programs for persons with developmental disabilities. She coauthored with Judith Reisman the popular *Sensory Integration Inventory for Individuals with Developmental Disabilities* and the companion *User's Guide.*

Maria Hinds, JD, MS, OTR/L, is an Assistant Professor at Florida A&M University, Tallahassee, Florida. As an occupational therapist, she has been a private practitioner and an administrator. She provided services in a wide variety of settings. However, whether serving in her capactiy as an attorney or a lecturer, she has been an avid advocate of the rights of individuals with developmental disabilities. In 1994, she founded Care Giving Services, an oranization established to develop and manage residential facilities and community-based programs for people with developmental disabilities. In addition, she has monitored state and private residential facilities established for children and adults with developmental disabilities, and she has served on committees to establish federal and state licensing regulations for allied health professionals. She is interested in participating in a variety of forums, inclusive of research, to increase community awareness and to promote the increase of the quality of life of individuals with developmental disabilities.

Hollis A. Kellogg, OTR/L, received his associate degree as an occupational therapy assistant at Orange County Community College, New York, and worked in nursing homes and at the Burke Rehabilitation Center, New York. He received his BA in occupational therapy from Dominican College, Blauvelt, New York. He has worked in the Orange County Association for the Help of Retarded Citizens, New York, for 10 years. He also has worked in home care and as a nursing home consultant.

Barbara Kornblau, JD, OTR, FAOTA, is a Professor of Occupational Therapy and Public Health at Nova Southeastern University. She is a practicing attorney, a certified case manager, a disability management specialist, and a rehabilitation specialist. She assists businesses, hospitals, insurance companies, local governments, and universities in complying with the Americans with Disabilities Act (ADA) and implementing injury prevention programs. Her current law practice focuses on disability discrimination litigation. She has presented papers, workshops, and training sessions across the country in the area of work rehabilitation and authored more than 60 publications. She is Chairperson of the American Occupational Therapy Association's (AOTA) Standards and Ethics Commission and a former Chair of AOTA's Work Programs Special Interest Section.

Ann T. Neulicht, PhD, CRC, earned her doctorate in rehabilitation research and maintains credentials as a Certified Rehabilitation Counselor, Certified Vocational Evaluator, Certified Disability Management Specialist, Licensed Professional Counselor, and Diplomate of the American Board of Vocational Experts. She was the principal investigator for Project COMPUTE and is the marketing coordinator for Project *TechWork*. Her consulting practice focuses on case management, employability assessment, job placement, life care planning, and career development facilitator curriculum development/

training. She has extensive experience as a rehabilitation/career counselor, marketing manager, and counselor educator. She is the recipient of the 1995 Harley B. Reger Award and the 1996 Distinguished Service Award for her contributions in the areas of research and creative activity, dedication to consumers, and commitment to professional organizations.

Rebecca Renwick, PhD, OT(C), is an Associate Professor in the Graduate Department of Rehabilitation Science and the Department of Occupational Therapy, University of Toronto (Ontario, Canada). She is Co-Director of the Quality of Life Research Unit at the Centre for Health Promotion, University of Toronto. She has a PhD from the University of Lancaster in England and is a graduate of the program in occupational therapy and physiotherapy at the University of Toronto. Her research and publications focus on the quality of life for persons with and without disabilities as well as related issues such as coping, social suppport, and inclusion in community life.

Mildred Ross, OTR/L, FAOTA, an occupational therapist since 1951, has been responding to changes and developments in occupational therapy study and practice with pleasure, inspiration, and the view that it is a consummate challenge. She has been in private practice for the past 13 years. For 12 of these years, she has worked with adults with developmental disabilities. Mildred writes, "This population helped me to improve all my professional skills and this book helps me give back to them a little of what I received. I also take great pride in three caring adult children, Susan, Eric, and Sara-Ann, my nephew Lionel, and my niece Esther Baren, who also chose to be an occupational therapist."

Lynn D. Simpson, OTR/L, graduated from Quinnipiac College in 1981 with a BS in occupational therapy. She worked for the Capitol Region Educational Commission and for Northwest Village School, Plainville, Connecticut, with children with developmental disabilities, behavioral problems, and hearing impairments. For the past 10 years, she has worked for the state of Connecticut, Department of Mental Retardation, providing services to group homes for adults with developmental disabilities. In addition, she has a private practice in which she treats adults and children with acute and chronic pain problems and focuses on the structural component of behavioral and movement problems.

T. Ann Williams, OTR/L, is a graduate of the University of Central Arkansas. She has practiced occupational therapy for 10 years and has worked with people with various diagnoses, including those with developmental disabilities. She is a staff therapist at the Eye Foundation of Kansas City. At this facility, she assists those with vision loss to regain their independence at home and in the community. Her interest in computers and their uses for those individuals who have vision loss has led her to specialize in this area at the Eye Foundation and to pursue certification as a programmer and analyst.

David J. Wysocki, MS, OTR/L, ATP, is Co-Director of Project *TechWork* and a therapist at Murdoch Center, a facility for people with developmental disabilities in North Carolina, where he also serves on the Community Outreach Assistive Technology Team and on the ADA Committee. He is a RESNA-certified Assistive Technology Practitioner (ATP), has served on the Passing-Score Committee for the RESNA certification exam, and chairs a RESNA committee to develop protocol for computer access assessments. David is a recent NOVA award winner for outstanding contributions to the practice of occupational therapy in the first 5 years of practice from NCOTA, where he will serve as the first Technology-SIS Chair on the NCOTA Executive Board.

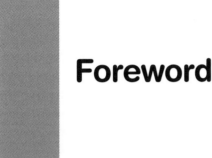

Foreword

Adults with developmental disabilities constitute a substantial proportion of those who benefit from the services of occupational therapists. *Adults with Developmental Disabilities: Current Approaches in Occupational Therapy* offers occupational therapists and other health professionals practice strategies that focus on needs of clients, applications for functional performance, and potential outcomes of those applications.

Many authors have proposed evaluation and programming for adults with developmental disabilities according to conditions such as autism, cerebral palsy, and feeding disorders. In contrast to a disability-specific approach to therapy and rehabilitation for adults with developmental disabilities, this book treats the population as a whole. By so doing, it provides the therapist with a holistic perspective for approaching the person with developmental disabilities regardless of primary condition or diagnosis. The focus of the work is on assisting the individual as he or she strives to move from disability to ability and from dysfunction to function.

The Americans with Disabilities Act (ADA) has opened the door to many previously unavailable options for adults with developmental disabilities. However, it is incumbent upon therapists who work with this population to assist these adults to utilize the new opportunities. The advocacy mode described in this volume provides an avenue for this support and education. To implement this approach, education for caregivers, other professionals, and clients must become a part of the rehabilitation of adults with developmental disabilities.

Frames for reference are described through which to determine and understand the needs of adults with developmental disabilities. These are based on listening to clients' stories and helping them to create a reality that is commensurate with their abilities. Community practice is essential to the fulfillment of the expectations held by adults with developmental disabilities and allows them to partake of all that the community has to offer. These community opportunities include work and leisure and recreational activities. Quality of life issues, herein presented conceptually, provide an excellent backdrop for the key components of work and leisure pursuits.

Mildred Ross and Susan Bachner, as contributors and editors, have brought together applications that have stood the test of time in occupational therapy. As community-oriented services, these applications lend themselves to fundable product lines in the form of:

▎adapted sports and recreation programs
▎caregiver training programs
▎community education programs
▎exercise and fitness programs
▎injury prevention programs
▎vocational readiness programs
▎living skills training programs

as described by Baum (1991). Such programs provide opportunities for therapists to provide needed services for adults with developmental disabilities and can form the foundation for viable community practice for occupational therapists who work with this population.

Lela A. Llorens, PhD, OTR, FAOTA
Professor Emeritus, San Jose State University
Consultant in Occupational Therapy and Gerontology

REFERENCE

Baum, C. (1991). Identification and use of environmental resources. In Christiansen, C., & Baum, C. *Occupational therapy: Overcoming human performance deficits.* Thorofare, NJ: Slack.

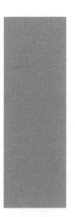

Preface

The intent of *Adults with Developmental Disabilities: Current Approaches in Occupational Therapy* is to provide clinicians with a working guide for practice when delivering services to adults with developmental disabilities. This guide concerns itself with a broad range of contemporary issues within the changing healthcare arena. A new vocabulary makes it imperative to examine how such terms as *client centered treatment, functional outcomes,* and a *managed care environment* affect this population. If we are to continue to have a place in the dialogue that brings about positive change for this often-underserved population, then therapists, as advocates, must be informed about the present status and future direction of this issue.

The authors, chosen for their proactive and significant practice-based contributions, provide information that deals with all aspects of the delivery of occupational therapy services. In Part I, "The Foundation Issues," clients' legal rights and a comprehensive discussion of what constitutes quality of life and how it can be measured position the therapist for all that comes thereafter.

Part II, "A Profile of Needs," enables the reader to gain a critical understanding of the importance of the visual impact on all aspects of functioning; the current clinical environment, in which many adults with profound disabilities and therapists find themselves; the complexity of group therapy as it enlists physical, social, and emotional components; and finally, a template ready for customization to enable low-cost and time-efficient assessments.

Part III, "Specific Applications," moves the clinician to the treatment arena: sensory-processing disorders, structurally based manual therapy, sessions using the Five-Stage Model with its associated group dynamics, occupations of work within a continuum of environments—all are described in depth and illustrate concepts and techniques available for reproduction.

This text is scholarly in its preparation and user-friendly in its presentation. In each chapter, there are narratives and case examples with which all clinicians can identify and which all clinicians can use. *Adults with Developmental Disabilities: Current Approaches in Occupational Therapy* has a universal appeal: any occupational therapist working with adults challenged by functional deficits will find this book to be of enormous practical value in today's healthcare marketplace.

The Editors

PART 1

The Foundational Issues

Advocating for Clients and Legal Issues

Barbara L. Kornblau, JD, OTR, FAOTA
Maria Hinds, JD, MS, OTR/L

INTRODUCTION

One of the earliest efforts to address the needs of individuals with developmental disabilities occurred in 1945, when President Harry S. Truman organized the "Committee on Employment of the Physically Handicapped and Mentally Retarded." However, it is over the last decade that substantial changes have occurred in the lives of adults with developmental disabilities. Quality of life issues changed from a purely medical model to a quasi-political model. This model reflects correctness of terminology and availability of government funding to provide services for children and adults with developmental disabilities.

The effort, which started as early as 1922 with the establishment of "The International Society of Crippled Children," was still in its infancy in 1945. Most individuals with developmental disabilities lived in large institutions or hospitals. During the 1950s and 1960s, the parents' movement came into fruition spearheaded by John F. Kennedy's visit to Willowbrook. Deplorable conditions at that institution embarrassed the nation into change. President Kennedy's sister, Eunice Kennedy Shriver, became a visible advocate for the rights of individuals with mental retardation. An effective national movement resulted in changes, such as the closing of Willowbrook. Further, support of training programs for special education teachers by the Office of Education resulted from a study, which showed that children with severe forms of mental retardation benefited significantly from "early intervention" pro-grams.

The 1960s and 1970s were times of great social change and unrest. People with disabilities, their families, and their advocates discovered that their common interests far outweighed their differences. A united "disability com-munity" emerged, and the concept of empowerment of this community replaced the institutionalized charity/medical model of ministering to passive victims. Disability took on a quasi-minority status, deserving some of the rights and protections granted other minority groups. This new activism spawned the birth of the disability rights movement and promoted the passage of the Rehabilitation Act of 1973 (29 U.S.C. §791) the Bill of Rights of the 1970s, and the Americans with Disabilities Act of 1990 (Public Law 101-336), considered by many the world's most comprehensive legislation on disability rights.

As the civil rights of individuals with developmental disabilities expanded, the role of the occupational therapist changed accordingly. In the 1950s, occupational therapists provided services to children and adults with devel-opmental disabilities within a recreational, activity-oriented model. Like other professionals, occupational therapy practitioners provided these ser-vices primarily within large institutions, nursing homes, and hospitals.

Today, the role of the occupational therapist is fundamental. Clinicians provide a variety of services that affect the lives of individuals with develop-mental disabilities. Their involvement includes, though is not limited to, research, diagnosis, early intervention, employment, and community integra-tion. Occupational therapy takes a total person-centered approach. As such, case management and advocacy are natural parts of the intricate role that occupational therapy clinicians play in the lives of persons with develop-mental disabilities.

LEGAL RIGHTS IN HOUSING

Laws exist to promote integration of adults with developmental disabilities into the mainstream of society, including housing. Traditionally, society placed individuals with "mental retardation" in large institutions where "people could live protected lives and pose no risk to society" (Mangan, Blake, Prouty, & Lakin, 1994). By the 1960s and early 1970s, advocates for this group realized that people who resided in large institutions missed exposure to a variety of community experiences. Hence, the aggressive movement for deinstitutionalization that resulted in the development of group homes and a variety of residential programs to serve adults and children with developmental disabilities.

However, the 1980s, advocates still criticized these community residential programs as "small institutions," which merely transferred institutional practices to the community. Individuals remained isolated, segregated, dependent on paid staff, and without opportunities to become active participants in their communities. Consumer self-advocacy efforts of the mid-1980s and the Fair Housing Amendments Act of 1988 (42 U.S.C. §2601, *et seq.*) affected the lives of individuals with developmental disabilities (Shea & Forrest, 1993). Individuals expressed their opinions about their living environment and level of support services, either themselves or through their families, friends, or advocates. By the end of the 1980s, voices of concern and advocacy influenced policy and practice at the federal, state, and local levels, resulting in legislation and funding for the development of a variety of creative community residential options (Mangan, Blake, Prouty, & Lakin, 1993):

▌*Group homes*: Supervision and training is provided by staff, serving one to eight nonrelated people with developmental disabilities.

▌*Supervised home or apartment*: Individuals live alone or with roommates in semiindependent units or apartments. Staff may live in a separate apartment at the same location.

▌*Adult foster care*: One or more individuals live with a family who provides care as needed.

▌*Personal care home*: Staff provides assistance with personal care but provides no training to residents.

▌*Board and care home*: Room and board is provided without training or assistance for personal care.

The move into these community-based settings opened a door for the provision of occupational therapy services. Occupational therapists may serve as subcontracted service providers, clinical coordinators, qualified mental retardation professionals, legal guardians, or advocates for persons who reside in the community residential facilities referenced above. Clinicians provide individualized services and programs, such as choice making, functional living skills, adaptive equipment, and purposeful activities that facilitate the individual's integration into and participation in their communities. Increase of independence and choice-making skills facilitate a shift in power from professionals to adults with developmental disabilities.

However, this process of integration into communities was not without opposition. In 1989, the Penhurst longitudinal study identified the "NIMBY" Syndrome—"Not In My Backyard." (Scheffer, 1994). The respondents agreed with the necessity of a transition out of large institutions for the developmentally disabled population. However, most also agreed that those in charge should establish community living options anywhere but in their own neighborhoods. This attitude was common throughout America.

Community concerns included an increase in crime and a decrease in property values. Interviews of neighbors, real estate agents, and fire, police, and health officials took place before and after organizers opened the homes. Virtually everyone interviewed agreed that group homes did not negatively affect the community. Property values and crime rate remained unaffected (Scheffer, 1994). Despite community opposition, over the last decade the development and expansion of community residential options for those with developmental disabilities increased the quality of life for many individuals, thanks in large part to the Fair Housing Amendments Act (FHAA) of 1988.

The FHAA opened opportunities for individuals with developmental disabilities in the area of housing opportunities. The Act defines an individual with a *handicap* as one who has a physical or mental impairment that substantially limits one or more major life activities, has a record of having such an impairment, or is regarded as having an impairment. (Unfortunately, Congress has not seen fit to amend this law to substitute the current politically-correct term *disability* for *handicap*.)

The FHAA makes it illegal to discriminate in the sale or rental of dwellings because the buyer, renter, or prospective resident has a handicap (42 U.S.C. §3604{f}{1}). Further, one may not make unavailable or deny a dwelling to a buyer, renter, or prospective resident because of a handicap. Unlawful discrimination includes a refusal to make reasonable accommodations in rules, policies, practices, or services, when such accommodations may be necessary to afford a handicapped person equal use and enjoyment of a dwelling (42 U.S.C. §3604{f}{3}{B}).

In passing the FHAA, Congress recognized that the right to be free from housing discrimination is essential to the goal of independent living (House Report at 18, 1985). The FHAA represents

> a clear pronouncement of a national commitment to end the unnecessary exclusion of persons with handicaps from the American mainstream. It repudiates the use of stereotypes and ignorance, and mandates

that persons with handicaps be considered as individuals. Generalized perception about disabilities and unfounded speculations about threats to safety are specifically rejected as grounds to justify exclusion.

(House Report at 18, 1985).

In light of the FHAA's broad mandate, many Court decisions have broadly construed its antidiscrimination prescription (*City of Edmonds v. Oxford House, Inc.* 1995). Courts have consistently invalidated a wide range of municipal licensing, zoning, and other regulatory practices affecting persons with disabilities (*Potomac Group Homes Corp. v. Montgomery County* 1983).

In many of these cases, individuals with developmental disabilities found themselves either intentionally discriminated against or in situations where the government or dwelling owner failed to make a reasonable accommodation. These incidents happen particularly with group homes for adults with developmental disabilities. For example, a town may have an ordinance that requires that "group homes for the mentally or physically handicapped" obtain a special permit. Courts would find this type of ordinance intentionally discriminatory and therefore illegal and in violation of the FHAA (*Bangertner v. Orem City Corp.*, 1995).

The mandate to make reasonable accommodations for individuals with disabilities can affect adults with developmental disabilities in several ways. First, suppose Bridgette, a developmentally disabled adult, wished to use the swimming pool in her apartment complex on a Sunday. Further suppose, the complex had a policy of "no guests on weekends" and the only way Bridgette could use the pool was with the assistance of her "best buddy." The apartment complex would be guilty of failing to reasonably accommodate, if it did not make a reasonable accommodation to its rules by allowing the "best buddy" in the pool. Only with this accommodation could Bridgette have equal enjoyment of the pool facilities. Making a reasonable accommodation "means changing some rule that is generally applicable to everyone to make it less onerous to the handicapped individual" (*Oxford House, Inc., v. Township of Cherry Hill,* 1992).

Another way the reasonable accommodation issue may affect adults with developmental disabilities relates to group homes issues. In one case, for example, a city's fire code required that a group home install a fire-warning system and a sprinkler system. The group representing the potential residents asked for a waiver of this requirement as a reasonable accommodation. The city offered no proof that waiving the requirement would threaten the safety of the residents. The residents asserted that the waiver would allow five additional residents to live in the group home. The court found that the city's failure to issue a waiver of the fire code constituted a failure to make a reasonable accommodation under the FHAA (*Alliance for the Mentally Ill, et al., v. City of Naperville*, 1996).

There are many similar situations where city and county regulations place restrictions on group homes for adults with developmental disabilities. For example, cities use local zoning and regulatory restrictions to bar development of community residences for individuals with developmental disabilities. However, court decisions invalidate regulatory and zoning restrictions as discriminatory under the FHAA and a deprivation of the individuals' equal protection under the law.

The FHAA does give cities an exemption for any "reasonable" restriction on the number of individuals permitted to occupy a dwelling. In a suit brought by Oxford House against the City of Edmonds, Washington, the U.S. Supreme Court held: "the exemption did not permit cities to close their single family zones to group homes." The restrictions the FHAA exempted were only those that "apply uniformly to all residents of all dwelling units" (*City of Edmonds v. Oxford House, Inc.*, 1995).

In a suit brought by the Cleburne Living Center against the City of Cleburne, Texas, after being denied a special use permit for the operation of a group home for the mentally retarded, the court held that requiring the permit deprived the mentally retarded of equal protection under the law. The court said "there was no rational basis for believing that the proposed home would pose a threat to the city (*City of Cleburne, TX v. Cleburne Living Center*, 1985).

Occupational therapists may ease these community tensions. Clinicians may facilitate the increase of community awareness to promote the total integration and inclusion of individuals with developmental disabilities into communities by coordinating programs and activities that include residents, family, friends, and neighbors.

LEGAL ISSUES IN EMPLOYMENT

Minimum Wage

Prior to the enactment of the minimum wage laws of the Fair Labor Standards Act of 1938 as amended, (29 U.S.C. §201 *et seq.*), many institutions required developmentally disabled adults to participate in habilitative labor "therapeutic" program plans, which conferred economic benefits on the institutions without compensation, in accordance with the law (Hasazi, Collins, & Cobb, 1988). In other words, institutions required residents to work under the guise of a therapeutic purpose without being paid. Patient-workers of nonfederal hospitals, homes, and institutions for the "mentally retarded" brought suit to compel the Secretary of Labor to undertake enforcement of the minimum wage and overtime provisions of the Fair Labor Standards Act (FLSA) to protect the interests of these adults. The court held that the patient-workers were "employees" within the meaning of the Act and had to be paid based on the minimum wage and overtime provisions of the FLSA, notwithstanding the claim that the work was "therapeutic" (*Nelson Souder, et al., v. Secretary of Labor*, 1973).

Therapists should take careful note of the implications of this decision. Therapists cannot engage their clients in activities labeled "therapeutic" or simulated work, which in reality confer an economic benefit on the institution or agency. Should the work activity include something for which one would normally receive compensation, the law could view this individual as an employee entitled to pay within the meaning of the minimum wage law.

Currently a variety of employment options remain available to developmentally-disabled adults. These include:

- *Sheltered workshops and work activity centers:* These are segregated work and vocational skills development programs.
- *Supported Employment:* These are paid positions for people with disabilities who need special assistance in learning job requirements and performing the associated tasks. A job coach or a supervisor who oversees a crew or enclave of people with disabilities working together at a job site provides support for the clients.
- *Competitive Employment:* Developmentally disabled individuals participate in competitive employment opportunities within the community (Hasazi, Collins, & Cobb, 1988).

Title I Americans With Disabilities Act

While many view the passage of the Americans With Disabilities Act (ADA) as the first real piece of civil rights legislation for individuals with disabilities, in reality, its predecessor, the Rehabilitation Act of 1973 (Rehab Act) holds this distinction. The Rehab Act put into place a system of legal protection meant to give individuals with disabilities including those with developmental disabilities the tools they needed to move further into the mainstream of society. As grandfather of the ADA, the Rehab Act prohibited discrimination against individuals with disabilities in employment and programs by agencies of the federal government, nonfederal government entities under contract with the federal government, and nonfederal government concerns that receive or benefit from federal government funds.

The ADA extended the Rehab Act's protections to private entities, whether or not they received federal funds or were under contract with the federal government (29 CFR §1630.2{b}). Like the FHAA, both the Rehab Act and the ADA define a person with a disability as one who has a physical or mental impairment that substantially limits one or more major life activities, has a record of having such an impairment, or is regarded as having an impairment (29 CFR §1630{2}{g}). Three key areas expand the world for individuals with developmental disabilities, thanks to the ADA:

- employment
- access to state and local government services
- access to places of public accommodations that are privately owned.

The employment provisions of the ADA can facilitate job placement for an individual with developmental disabilities. The following example illustrates this point. Peter, an individual with developmental disabilities, finishes his training program where he learned to work as a janitor. He applies for a job as a janitor with a school system. In order to do the job, Peter will need an on-site job coach, which the training program will provide at the school until Peter performs to the job standards. The school requires Peter to read all of the cleaning products' labels prior to their use and to check off a chart in the bathroom to indicate which tasks he has done. One problem: Peter does not read well enough to read the labels or the chart.

The ADA introduces into the work area new concepts, such as reasonable accommodations, that can expand opportunities for Peter. Further, the ADA prevents an employer from not hiring individuals who can do the job, merely because they have developmental disabilities. However, occupational therapists need to work with Peter and other individuals to teach them how to exercise their rights under the law.

Under the ADA, employers cannot discriminate against individuals like Peter who can perform a job with or without reasonable accommodations. The ADA further mandates that employers provide, at their own expense, reasonable accommodations for their employees. However, employers must only provide these reasonable accommodations if they know the applicant or worker is a qualified individual with a disability *and* if the applicant or worker requests the accommodation. This means clinicians must work with clients toward a goal of being able to tell employers about their disability and the type of reasonable accommodation they may require to enable their performance.

In Peter's situation, he would need to tell the prospective employer that he has a developmental disability and he needs specific reasonable accommodations to do the job. A representative from Peter's training program could assist him with this. Peter then would need to request the specific accommodations he needs.

The occupational therapist's skills with adaptations come into play here. As part of any training or therapeutic program, occupational therapists need to help clients identify needed reasonable accommodations. Unable to read, Peter needs another way to review the information on the cleaning fluid labels prior to using them.

Instead of reading the labels, the employer could set up, on the cleaning cart, color-coded tape recorders matching the color of the cleaning product labels. Peter could play the tape by color for each cleaning product prior to its use. The chart in the bathrooms could be adapted using pictures instead of words. Peter could use a date stamp to indicate the task he has completed. Though the ADA does not require an employer to provide a job coach at its own expense, the employer could allow the program to provide a job coach as an accommodation. Occupational therapy clinicians, with their training in task analysis and adaptations, will find themselves masters in identifying literally hundreds of other possible reasonable accommodations for Peter and other clients in similar work situations.

Clinicians should provide individualized programs with goals that facilitate choice making, job training and/or advancement and retention, and job-site visits to evaluate the need for assistive technology and/or retraining. Occupational therapists should also be involved in the ongoing assessment of functional skills as related to the work environment inclusive of ongoing communication with employers to facilitate increased job performance.

ACCESS TO PLACES OF PUBLIC ACCOMMODATIONS

Title III of the ADA protects individuals with disabilities from discrimination in access to places of public accommodation that are privately owned (28

CFR 36 §102). These include doctors' offices, funeral homes, movie theaters, bus stations, amusement parks, museums, restaurants, and just about any other place where the public goes to eat, bank, shop, or engage in commerce or transact business (28 CFR 36 §104).

Though physical barriers often prevent access, some of the most significant barriers that adults with developmental disabilities face do not involve physical access. Rather, attitudinal barriers often prevent access and inclusion for those with developmental disabilities and their families. While most look at Title III as a building code, in recognition of these nonphysical barriers, Title III also prevents the type of discrimination caused by attitudinal barriers that often result from fear, ignorance, stereotypes, and misconceptions about individuals with disabilities.

Before Congress made the ADA the law of the land, business owners could treat adults with developmental disabilities differently from other adults without disabilities. For example, a movie theater could require a wheelchair user to transfer into a regular theater seat in order to watch a movie or not allow wheelchairs in the theater at all. Congress intended the ADA to rid society of these kinds of barriers.

In addition to a plethora of architectural barrier-removal mandates, the ADA includes certain rules that theaters, malls, doctors' offices, and other places of public accommodation must follow to make it easier for individuals with disabilities, including developmental disabilities, to include themselves and participate in normal life activities. For example, suppose an adult with a developmental disability finds himself unable to read information on a menu at a restaurant. The ADA requires that the restaurant provide a reasonable accommodation to enable access to the menu which, in this case, might include the server reading the menu to the customer (29 CFR §36.303).

Other ADA rules prevent places of public accommodation from segregating individuals with disabilities in the provision of goods and services (29 CFR §36.202). For example, a theater cannot require someone in a wheelchair to sit in the front of the theater just because he or she has a developmental disability and uses a wheelchair. As an accommodation, the theater must remove some of the seats to allow room for people using wheelchairs.

Under the ADA, places of public accommodation cannot treat people differently, like charge them more money or not allow them in at all, just because they have a developmental disability (29 CFR §36.301). Just because a family member is in a wheelchair does not mean that "those in charge" can force him or her to pay more money to sit in the "handicapped section" in the end zone at the football stadium. A restaurant manger cannot tell a family member who drools that he or she cannot eat in the restaurant, just because he or she drools.

The ADA also prevents people from treating family members differently. A restaurant manager can not refuse to allow individuals to eat in a restaurant just because their family member had a head injury. The concert stadium can not make family members bring their own chairs to set next to their family members' wheelchairs at a rock concert. If everyone else is given a chair, they have to give family members or other attendants a chair, too.

The ADA's rules also make it easier for family members and others to care for adults with developmental disabilities (29 CFR §36.205). If family members travel and stop at a rest area on the interstate, they usually have two choices: a men's or women's restroom. What happens if a woman needs to help an adult son with a developmental disability into the bathroom? She must ask a worker at the rest stop to help clear people out or close the restroom. He or she will have to stand outside the bathroom and guard the door so the woman can help her son in either the men's or women's restroom. This is another type of "reasonable accommodation" that places of public accommodation must make (29 CFR §36.302). Newer facilities include "unisex" facilities.

There are many different types of accommodations, depending on the type of barrier one encounters and the type and extent of limitations found in the individual with a developmental disability.

Many places of public accommodation do not know about the ADA. They do not know about the rules they are supposed to follow. Sometimes, even if they know about these rules, they do not know anything about developmental disabilities, so they do not know what accommodations to make or how to make them.

As with the employment provisions of the ADA, to obtain reasonable accommodations under Title III's access provisions, one must request them. Occupational therapy clinicians can assist adults with developmental disabilities and their family members in identifying needed accommodations that enable inclusion in everyday life.

Some accommodations may be very difficult to make. For example, it may not be possible to install a wheelchair ramp to the door of a doctor's office in an old house. The ramp may cost too much money, or it may make it dangerous for other people to walk in the area. The doctor probably would not have to make this accommodation, because it is not a reasonable accommodation. The law only requires that places of public accommodation make reasonable accommodations.

Even though the law says places of public accommodation must make reasonable accommodations, many do not comply with the law, either out of ignorance or by intent. Occupational therapy clinicians may find their efforts to integrate adults with developmental disabilities into the community impaired by the physical and attitudinal barriers their clients face.

Clinicians must be aware of current laws that govern structural barriers and accessibility to community resources, which may include state and local ordinances as well as the ADA. Occupational therapists, as advocates, can increase the successful integration of developmentally disabled individuals into their communities. Some physical barriers often encountered include unreachable store merchandise, inaccessible post offices, and inadequate or nonexistent access signs to buildings within the community. The following provisions within the Americans with Disabilities Act address these problem areas:

1. The law requires that merchants not display their products too high (more than 54") or too low (less than 9").
2. The law considers post offices with only exterior and interior steps, high counters, and untrained personnel inaccessible under the ADA.
3. The ADA requires display of an international symbol indicating accessible entrances.

Ironically, Congress did not apply the ADA to itself until 1995. Senator Max Cleland, an individual with a physical disability, encountered severe obstacles to serving in the Senate. According to the *New York Times* November 8, 1996, he found bathrooms inaccessible, floors of the Senate chamber tiered, and no ramps in most hearing rooms. Developmentally-disabled persons with physical limitations also would find the House inaccessible.

Clinicians should serve as active advocates regarding these issues. This advocacy includes, among other things, bringing access issues to the attention of team members, agency officials, and community officials. Occupational therapy clinicians should make all efforts to encourage the removal of structural barriers that inhibit integration into the community (Parry, 1990).

Without "ADA police" to enforce this law, the ADA becomes a "complaint-driven" law. Where a barrier is found in a place of public accommodation, which the owner will not eliminate once notified, there are several methods for seeking a remedy. The U.S. Department of Justice maintains a complaint line to call to register a complaint: (202) 514-0301(Voice) (202) 514-0381 (TDD). Another alternative is to contact an attorney experienced with ADA litigation.

THE HUMAN RIGHTS OF INDIVIDUALS WITH DEVELOPMENTAL DISABILITIES

The U.S. Constitution specifically guarantees fundamental rights, and *human rights* refers to the basic respect and dignity that should be afforded each individual. Congress can expand Constitutional rights by passing federal laws. The Americans with Disabilities Act is an example of a federal law that expanded the rights of citizens.

In 1948, the General Assembly of the United Nations adopted the Universal Declaration of Human Rights. The Universal Declaration establishes uniform standards for the treatment of all persons. In 1971, the United Nations adopted the "Declaration of Rights of Mentally Retarded Persons" (ARC, 1992).

Individuals with developmental disabilities, like all other citizens, have a vast array of protections under the law inclusive of the Universal Declaration of Human Rights that proclaims that all human beings are entitled to, among other rights, freedom of thought, conscience, and religion; freedom of opinion and expression; the right to work and choose one's work freely; the right to receive equal pay for equal work; and the right to an adequate standard of living.

Service providers, families, and advocates must be especially vigilant of their autonomy and right to equal protection under the law. Because of the long history of oppression, devaluation, and callous disregard for the rights of individuals with developmental disabilities, advocates must carefully monitor issues, such as the right to refuse and/or receive medical treatment or programming, to remain free from harm, and to marry and make informed decisions regarding sexuality and parenthood. Therefore, professionals and advocates involved in the provision of support services must maintain awareness of the ongoing risks and dangers that these individuals face on a daily basis.

Guardianship/Conservatorship

The law provides protection for individuals whom it considers unable to care for their own affairs or property or to meet some of their own essential health and safety needs. While specific grounds and definitions vary from state to state, there are several commonalities. States appoint guardians or conservators to make financial and personal decisions for adults with developmental disabilities whom courts adjudge in need of this assistance.

When a client has a guardian or conservator, this individual makes decisions with regard to where the client will reside and what program the client will attend. In many of these situations, the clinician must look to the guardian or conservator for informed consent prior to initiating occupational therapy treatment since, once adjudicated incompetent, the client lacks the legal capacity to give consent and sign documents on his or her own. Occupational therapy clinicians may find themselves facing ethical dilemmas where the guardian or conservator refuses to consent to treatment that the ward desires or needs.

THE OCCUPATIONAL THERAPIST AS ADVOCATE

As the team member professionally devoted to promoting independence in daily living, occupational therapy clinicians often will find barriers to this goal. Agencies, individuals, institutions, among others, may cause these barriers by failing to comply with laws designed to guarantee certain rights. Failure to comply may result from intentional conduct as well as ignorance. Faced with barriers to achieving goals, occupational therapy clinicians may find that the most effective means of promoting their client's independence is to act as advocates. To effectively advocate for clients, occupational therapy clinicians should follow the Eight Rules of Advocacy.

Eight Rules of Advocacy

1. Know the Laws

Occupational therapists can familiarize themselves with laws that give rights to adults with developmental disabilities without the necessity of a law degree. Many laws provide rights for adults with developmental disabilities. Knowledge of these laws affects the goals therapists set with their clients, as shown in the example of Peter's employment. Occupational therapy practitioners should ensure that they prepare their clients to protect themselves and ask for their rights under the law. In many cases, this may require that clinicians take on the role of educator, to teach clients their rights and how to assert themselves appropriately. Clinicians will find role playing very useful.

Knowledge of the pertinent laws also provides the basis for acting as an advocate for clients with developmental disabilities. One cannot take on an advocate role without having at least a rudimentary grounding in the rights for which one advocates. Without this basic foundation, the therapist runs the risk of looking rather foolish and the client loses.

Occupational therapists advocating for clients with developmental disabilities cannot do their clients justice without an understanding of the Developmental Disabilities Act (42 U.S.C. §6000, *et seq.*) and the protections it affords. Congress passed the Developmental Disabilities Act (DD Act) to ensure that individuals with developmental disabilities and their families could participate in appropriate programs, services, and opportunities that would promote independence, productivity, and integration and inclusion into the community (42 U.S.C. §6000 {b}). The DD Act provides federal funding to support programs that work towards these goals. In order for states to receive this federal funding, each state participating in the program must create a protection and advocacy system empowered to do the following:

■ "pursue legal, administrative, and other appropriate remedies or approaches to ensure the protection of, and advocacy for" persons within the programs

■ "provide information on and referral to programs" addressing the need of persons with developmental disabilities

■ "investigate incidents of abuse and neglect of [persons with developmental disabilities] if the incidents are reported to the [protection and advocacy system] or if there is probable cause to believe that the incidents occurred" (42 U.S.C. §6042{a}{2}).

The DD Act also requires that the protection and advocacy system annually provide the public with an opportunity to comment on the priorities it establishes as well as its activities (42 U.S.C. §6042{C}). Further, the protection and advocacy system must establish a grievance procedure for clients or prospective clients of the system, to ensure that persons with developmental disabilities have full access to the system's services (42 U.S.C. §6042{D}).

The law requires the advocacy and protection agency to exist independent of agencies that provide treatment, services, and habilitation under the DD Act. The advocacy and protection agency must have reasonable access to individuals with developmental disabilities in facilities that provide services under the DD Act, as well as access to their records (42 U.S.C. §6042{H}).

Occupational therapy practitioners may contact many sources to obtain additional information about relevant laws. They may contact directly the government agency charged with enforcing a particular law. For example, if there is a concern about a fair housing issue, they can call the Department of Housing and Urban Development (HUD). For an ADA issue concerning employment, they can contact the Equal Employment Opportunity Commission (EEOC) for additional information. The Department of Justice has a website they that provides literature about the ADA, Fair Housing Act, and several other laws that protect clients' rights. The Advocacy Centers serve as excellent sources of information and good places to refer clients for attorneys and other professional advocates who are up to date on the laws for adults with developmental disabilities.

2. Read the regulations

Whenever Congress passes a law, it assigns the responsibility for administrating that law to a federal agency. The federal agency's responsibilities include promulgating regulations. Regulations are the "rules" that give meaning to the law and its means of enforcement. For the most part, clinicians will find regulations involving laws protecting individuals with developmental disabilities written in relatively plain and understandable English. As an added bonus, many of these regulations are readily available on the Internet, through the Justice Department bulletin board and sometimes in the library. Clinicians need not fear reading the Fair Housing regulations to find out additional information about a client's housing situation or the ADA regulations to look into a client's discrimination situation. Reading the regulations can make the clinician more knowledgeable and facilitate advocacy.

3. Believe your client/patient has a right

Before clinicians take on an issue, they should believe in the right they seek for their clients. Without this belief, clinicians will not make effective advocates.

4. Organize yourself; document your efforts and get everything in writing

Most people associate the phrase "get it in writing" with attorneys. Only written documents provide the key evidence should the situation rise to a

formal complaint or lawsuit. The prohibition against hearsay testimony—
a popular objection on any television courtroom drama—prevents arguing
over who said what in court. On the other hand, written documents hold
the promise of credibility before an administrative investigator, judge, or jury.

Since many of our clients lack adequate skills for expressing themselves in
writing, practitioners can help advocate for clients by helping them write
letters. They may also write their own letters to engage the services of the
protection and advocacy agency that must investigate the situations adverse
to clients.

Advocates will find keeping a diary an invaluable tool for future reference
in advocacy matters. Dates, places, and events, recorded in the diary, fill in
the blanks for the advocate when memory leaves too many gaps down
the road.

5. Start with the source of the problem

Often advocates can solve problems by going to the source to complain.
Ignorance of the law is often the reason behind many problems faced by
adults with developmental disabilities, especially in the discrimination arena.
Often the person at the "front desk" lacks proper training in the rules of
the ADA or Fair Housing Act. Notifying the source and giving that person
or company an opportunity to do "the right thing" can often solve discrimination problems and avoid future incidents

6. Be specific; tell them exactly what you want

When writing a letter or speaking to someone to advocate for a client,
clinicians should very specific about what is required to resolve the matter.
Advocates should spell out specific steps they want taken before taking action.

7. File a complaint

A good advocate need not "make a federal case" out of everything. Most
of the laws discussed in this chapter provide administrative procedures for
remedying the protected wrongs. In passing these laws, Congress charged
various administrative agencies with the responsibility to promulgate regulations to enforce the law. The regulations include an outline of procedures
one may take to resolve a complaint to enforce the law's protection using
investigators employed by the governmental agency. These procedures allow

the individual with a developmental disability to protect his or her rights without going to court.

8. Follow through

Finally, advocates should not give up but must follow up and follow through on their complaints. Investigations under these laws often take a long time. However, frequent phone calls often accelerate investigations and make things happen.

Ethical Considerations in Advocacy

Occupational therapy clinicians acting as advocates will face many ethical dilemmas. Occupational therapy advocates may take positions that risk their jobs or risk funding. Accepting an advocacy role requires balancing interest in one's job with interest in the client's rights. At all cost, however, occupational therapy clinicians must not try to separate the human side from the clinical side. Therapists who find themselves embroiled in hot ethical issues may consult their institution's ethics committee.

CONCLUSION

There remain critical issues facing individuals with developmental disabilities. The uncertainty of health care reform, limited funding, and cuts in disability benefits will ultimately affect their quality of life. Clinicians committed to the provision of quality services should keep abreast of the laws that affect the lives of developmentally disabled persons. Informed clinicians make the best advocates.

REFERENCES

Alliance for the Mentally Ill et al., v. City of Naperville, 8 NDRL ¶28 (N.D. Ill. 1996).
Americans With Disabilities Act, Pub. L. No. 101-336 (July 26, 1990).
Americans With Disabilities Act, Title III Regulations Title III, 28 CFR §36.101 *et seq.*
Association for Retarded Citizens [ARC]. (1992). *Human rights for people with mental retardation.* [Position statement]. Arlington, TX: Author.
Bangertner v. Orem City Corp., 46 F.3d 1491, (10th Cir. 1995).
City of Cleburne, TX v. Cleburne Living Center, 473 U.S. 432 (1985).
City of Edmonds v. Oxford House, Inc., 114 S. Ct. 1776 (1995).
Developmental Disabilities Act, 42 U.S.C. §6000 *et seq.* (Supp. 1989).

Fair Housing Amendments Act of 1988, 42 U.S.C. §2601 *et seq.*

Fair Labor Standards Act of 1938 as amended, 29 U.S.C. §201 *et seq.*

Hasazi, S.B., Collins, M., & Cobb, R.B. (1988). *Implementing transition programs for productive employment.* Baltimore, MD: Paul H. Brookes.

H.R.Rep No. 711, 100th Cong., 2nd Sess., at 18 (1985).

Larson, S.A., & Lakin, C.K. (1989). Deinstitutionalization of persons with mental retardation behavioral outcomes *Journal of the Association for Persons with Severe Handicaps, 14,* 324–332.

Mangan, T., Blake, E.M., Prouty, R.W., & Lakin, K.C. (1993). *Residential services for persons with mental retardation and related conditions. Status and trends through 1991.* University of Minnesota.

Nelson Souder, et al., v. Secretary of Labor, et al., 367 F. Supp. 808 (1993).

Oxford House, Inc., v. Township of Cherry Hill, 799 F. Supp. 450, 462, n. 25 (D. N.J. 1992).

Parry, J. (1990). The Americans with Disabilities Act (ADA). *Mental and Physical Disability Law Reporter, 14,* 292–294.

Potomac Group Homes Corp. v. Montgomery County, 823 F. Supp. 1285 (D. Md. 1983). Rehabilitation Act of 1973, 29 U.S.C. 791 (1973).

Scheffer, A. (1994, Nov.–Dec.). People with disabilities move into their own homes, little opposition reported. *The NIMBY (Not In My Back Yard) Report.*

Shea, A., & Forrest, C.B. (1993). *Patterns of supported living: A resource catalog.* California Department of Developmental Services.

2

Quality of Life

A Guiding Framework for Practice with Adults
Who Have Developmental Disabilities

Rebecca Renwick, PhD, OT(C)

INTRODUCTION

The importance of quality of life has been rapidly growing over the past decade. Most recently, this attention has been reflected in the emphasis on developing outcome measures of quality of life and their use for demonstrating intervention effectiveness and accountability. This chapter summarizes some of the major advantages, as well as the potential disadvantages and risks, of this increasing attention to quality of life, especially within the developmental disabilities field. Further, two interrelated meanings of "quality" and their relevance to the concept of quality of life are discussed. The idea of using quality of life as a guiding framework for occupational therapy practice with adults who have developmental disabilities is examined.

A brief review of the key themes of recent, major conceptual frameworks of quality of life is presented to provide a context for the introduction of the Centre for Health Promotion (CHP) approach to quality of life.

- The background and essential features of the CHP conceptual model are described.
- The importance of having a conceptual framework, particularly one that centers around quality of life, to organize and guide assessment, intervention, and program-planning with this population is discussed.

▌Examples of application of the CHP model to these aspects of occupational therapy practice are presented.

The chapter concludes with a discussion of other potential applications of the model, for example, to research, policy development, and advocacy.

INCREASING EMPHASIS ON QUALITY OF LIFE

Over the last 20 years, but particularly in the last decade, there has been an increasing interest in understanding quality of life and in planning services that enhance quality of life. Several factors have contributed to this growing attention. Fiscal constraints (with the associated trend toward rationing of funding for health and social services) and managed care have exerted pressure to measure and maximize the outcomes of intervention. In essence, the drive toward "getting better results with fewer resources" (Brown, Renwick, & Nagler, 1996, p. 3) has been a powerful influence. However, changes in policy and legislation that emphasize equality, human rights, and independent community living for persons with disabilities have also played a significant role (Brown, Renwick, & Nagler, 1996). This policy and legislation have arisen during a period of strong activism around the issues of empowerment and inclusion in society for persons with disabilities (Renwick & Friefeld, 1996). While this activism has frequently focused on specific issues—new definitions of disability, environmental factors in disability, societal attitudes, and empowerment—one of its ultimate goals can be characterized as fostering and enhancing quality of life. (The forces contributing to this burgeoning interest in quality of life are discussed in detail in Brown, Renwick, & Nagler, 1996, and Renwick & Friefeld, 1996.)

Not surprisingly, many professionals and researchers from a variety of disciplines have begun to develop approaches and programs that will contribute to and support quality of life for persons who have disabilities (Renwick, Brown, & Nagler, 1996). In the current climate of fiscal restraint and with resources available from governments diminishing, ensuring that members of vulnerable populations enjoy a good quality of life is essential. In fact, it is a matter of social justice (see the principles discussed by Jongbloed & Chrichton, 1990, and Townsend, 1993).

The field of developmental disabilities has been at the forefront in attempting to develop these kinds of approaches and programs (Schalock, 1990, 1996, 1997; Goode, 1994). For example, several authors have identified key issues concerning quality of life and articulated the need to employ specific principles of quality of life in planning and evaluating services for persons with developmental disabilities (Dennis, Williams, Giangreco, & Cloninger, 1993; Goode, 1990; Landesman, 1986). Further, a number of new approaches to conceptualizing quality of life has been developed recently (Brown, Brown, & Bayer, 1994; Felce & Perry, 1996; Renwick & Brown, 1996).

Within the developmental disabilities field, several attempts to apply quality of life principles to practice have been reported in the literature (Brown, Brown, & Bayer, 1994; Renwick, Brown, & Raphael, 1994; Schalock, Keith, Hoffman, & Karan, 1989). This area continues to develop. For instance, much work is still needed to make application of theory to assessment and intervention clearer and more explicit. This is particularly important for occupational therapists working with this population, since the profession's literature does not yet provide much guidance concerning either conceptual approaches to quality of life or their application to practice with persons who have developmental disabilities. This chapter is intended to help link a potentially useful theoretical framework to practice with adults in this population.

THE MEANING OF QUALITY OF LIFE

Even though there have been many attempts to understand and measure quality of life (Bowling, 1991, 1995), this concept is often discussed without ever discussing what the term really means (Renwick & Brown, 1996). Quality of life sounds like such a simple idea at first glance, but, once what it really means in the context of people's lives is considered it becomes more complex. Indeed, considerable philosophical and conceptual material can be drawn into a discussion about the meaning of quality of life. However, for the purpose of this chapter, a summary of some important ideas is a more useful approach.

Two Meanings of Quality

Quality has two related meanings. First, it is characteristic of something (Brown & Renwick, 1996). We define objects by their characteristics or qualities. For example, a book is usually rectangular in shape, has a cover, and contains printed paper pages bound together. We understand what a book is because of the characteristics or qualities that are common from one book to another. Human life also has characteristics or qualities. Specifically, people have physical bodies, thoughts, and feelings. People seek shelter and a place to call their own. We need and seek the comfort, companionship, and support that relationships with others can provide. We also seek meaningful and productive activity, leisure activity, and a variety of activities that allow us to learn about ourselves and to grow as individuals. These characteristics or qualities of life are readily understood because they are common to all human beings. Quality of life embodies those characteristics that we consider are shared and expressed in some way by human beings (Brown & Renwick, 1996).

Second, quality means excellence. Thus, when we speak of a high quality of life we also imply an excellent life, a life full of experiences that are thoroughly felt and enjoyed, a life full of meaning. Most people want quality in their lives and strive to attain it. However, a life of great quality is the ideal, and, for most people, life is not ideal. There are some aspects of our lives that we could improve, to varying degrees, and other aspects of our lives that we would like to minimize or eliminate in order to have a "high-quality life" (Brown & Renwick, 1996).

Relationship Between the Two Meanings of Quality

When we use the term *quality of life,* we are referring to both meanings simultaneously—both to those qualities or characteristics of life common to people and to the degree to which life is excellent or approaches this ideal. In other words, quality of life for people means the degree of excellence (quality) of the characteristics (qualities) of human life. So, in asking about a person's quality of life, we are really asking: "Considering the qualities of human life, how good is your life for you?" (Brown & Renwick, 1996). This question is relevant to the quality of life of all people, whether or not they have a developmental disability.

QUALITY OF LIFE AS A FRAMEWORK FOR PRACTICE

Integrating and Organizing Practice

Quality of life can be seen as a organizing framework that can readily guide practice with this population. The material discussed in this chapter and elsewhere (Brown, Renwick, & Nagler, 1996; Renwick & Brown, 1996; Renwick, Brown, & Raphael, 1994; Renwick, Brown, Rootman, & Nagler, 1996) provides a rationale for adopting quality of life as the integrating concept around which all aspects of practice are centered. These aspects of practice include assessment, intervention, program-planning and evaluation, and research, as well as advocacy efforts targeted to securing funding and policy development. Since fostering, enhancing, and maintaining quality of life is often stated as the ultimate goal of occupational therapy, quality of life is a particularly appropriate concept for guiding and integrating practice (Renwick & Friefeld, 1996).

Of course, a clearly articulated and detailed theoretical formulation is required in order to use quality of life as a guiding concept for practice. Several potentially appropriate theoretical frameworks are noted, and one particular approach is discussed in detail in later sections of this chapter.

Advantages

There are advantages associated with using a quality of life framework to guide, integrate, and evaluate practice. It can improve accountability to clients and their families, as well as to the broader community, to specific funders of programs for persons with developmental disabilities, and to the occupational therapy profession. It can also add coherence and provide a solid foundation for practice, that is, provide a theory-based explanation for practice and an integrated set of guidelines for assessment, intervention, and other aspects of practice. Such a theoretical foundation is also consistent with both the ultimate goal and the client-centered nature of occupational therapy practice. Thus, adopting a quality-of-life guiding framework for practice can enhance the credibility of the profession as a whole.

Some Cautions and Potential Limitations

In the last decade, there has been increasing emphasis on outcome measures to evaluate the efficacy and cost-effectiveness of health and social interventions (Canadian Association of Occupational Therapists, 1991). This idea is apparently both beneficial and a matter of common sense. However, other considerations need to be taken into careful account if quality of life is chosen as a practice framework.

For instance, it may not be feasible or desirable to attempt to continuously improve quality of life, either in all areas of life for an individual or for groups of individuals; nor is this necessarily an appropriate and realistic goal of intervention. Maintenance or prevention of deterioration of quality in some areas of life that they already perceive as satisfactory may be an appropriate goal for some clients. In such situations, care must be taken to clearly specify these quality-of-life goals and the rationale for them so that lack of improvement is not interpreted as a "failure" of the intervention, the client, the therapist, or any combination of the three. Sometimes certain interventions, such as moving to a more community-based setting or starting a new program or job are very stressful for clients and disruptive of their daily routines. Therefore, it may be expected that a client's quality of life may decrease in some areas until she or he begins to adapt to the associated changes in daily life. On the other hand, once quality of life has improved in a particular area of life, the individual's expectations about the desired degree of quality in that area is likely to shift upward, too.

The foregoing considerations highlight the need to assess changes in quality of life regularly and carefully over long periods of time. Such repeated assessment is appropriate with a population for whom change is often a slow process. Further, reliable and valid standardized outcome measures are often considered desirable for formal program evaluations. However, care needs to be taken that such instruments have been rigorously validated, found to be psychometrically sound when tested with adults who have developmental disabilities, and are appropriately matched to the goals of the intervention. (Availability of one instrument package that meets these criteria is noted in a later section.) Qualitative information that is consistent with the guiding conceptual framework can also be collected to provide a meaningful context in which to interpret the quantitative outcomes, collected with standardized instruments. If a less-formal approach to evaluation is used, therapists can gather qualitative information through their regular assessment process with clients. However, many of the same cautions noted above concerning appropriate, realistic quality-of-life goals are still applicable.

RECENT CONCEPTUAL APPROACHES TO QUALITY OF LIFE

In recent years, the field of developmental disabilities has been a rich source of conceptual approaches to quality of life (Felce & Perry, 1996; Goode, 1994; Schalock, 1990, 1996). These approaches have suggested some essential themes that taken together, form the foundation of a useful conceptual framework for quality of life.

One major theme is the need to accord the greatest importance to the perceptions of persons with developmental disabilities concerning the quality of life they experience (Goode, 1990; Brown, Bayer, & McFarlane, 1989; Brown, Brown, & Bayer, 1994; Schalock, Keith, Hoffman, & Karan, 1989). This emphasis is often reflected in the concept of satisfaction, as experienced by the individual, usually within each of several areas of life or with life as a whole. A second key theme is embodied in the concept of well-being experienced by the individual and frequently expressed in terms of material and psychological resources and physical health. Other themes include personal growth of and mastery by the individual (Brown, Brown, & Bayer, 1994; Felce & Perry, 1996) as important aspects of quality of life. Finally, the notion of connections between the individual and important others in his or her life is a common theme (Felce & Perry, 1996; Halpern, Nave, Close, & Wilson, 1986). The Centre for Health Promotion (CHP) approach to quality of life encompasses these themes, although it does so by considering broad areas of life essential to all people. The CHP approach also interweaves these themes with other, new concepts to offer a unique conceptualization of quality of life (Renwick & Brown, 1996).

THE CHP QUALITY OF LIFE FRAMEWORK

Development and Assumptions

The CHP approach was developed by the author and a small, multidisciplinary group of researchers at the Quality of Life Research Unit of the Centre for Health Promotion at the University of Toronto. The conceptual framework was developed by means of three concurrent processes that included:

1. a thorough review of the literature
2. consultation with other researchers and experts working in the areas of disability and quality of life
3. most importantly, consultations with individuals and groups with and without disabilities.

These consultations consisted of focus groups and in-depth interviews about what makes life "good" and "not so good" (Renwick & Brown, 1996).

Although the development of the quality-of-life conceptual framework was intended to guide research concerning quality of life experienced by individuals with developmental disabilities, the researchers soon realized that this emerging model had broader relevance, that is, it applied to people with any kind of disability as well to people without disabilities. Thus, during the process of formulating the model, it was tested by means of case studies of the lives of individuals with and without disabilities.

A number of broad assumptions guided the development of the CHP model (Woodill, Renwick, Brown, & Raphael, 1994; Renwick & Brown, 1996). Several of these assumptions are useful to consider here. Specifically, persons are best understood in an holistic way, which is congruent with contemporary, client-centered approaches to occupational therapy practice (Canadian Association of Occupational Therapists, 1991). Quality of life emerges from the dynamic relationship between the person and the environment and thus can change over time. Quality of life also has several dimensions that may change at different rates and in different ways (positively or negatively), and some dimensions may not change at all over the life course. The basic dimensions or aspects of quality of life are the same for individuals with and without disabilities. These dimensions are consistent with broad contemporary perspectives on health (World Health Organization, 1986), including the view that social factors, such as poverty and unemployment, can significantly affect a person's health (Evans & Stoddart, 1990).

Essential Concepts and Features of the Framework

Defining Quality of Life.   The CHP conceptual framework is based on a specific definition of quality of life: It is "the degree to which a person enjoys the important possibilities of his or her life" (Renwick & Brown, 1996, p. 80). Possibilities consist of the balance between opportunities and constraints in the various areas of a person's life (described in the next section). This means that a person encounters many possibilities in life, but it is those possibilities that have particular importance to an individual and his or her way of life that have the greatest implications for quality of life. For instance, exercise is part of many people's lives, but it can take on special significance for individuals attempting to reach or maintain a healthy weight or improve cardiac fitness, for those who walk their dogs several times daily, for people who like to play softball or jog with their friends, for athletes training for the Special Olympics, or for parents of lively, young children.

Possibilities depend upon the dynamic interplay of characteristics of persons and their environments. Some possibilities may be influenced or controlled to varying degrees by individuals through the choices and decisions they make, for example, regarding what they do for fun and with whom, where they work, or how they spend their time and their money. Other possibilities are very difficult to influence or cannot be controlled or changed like the time in history and place of their birth, serious disabilities present at birth, and ethnicity. The enjoyment component of the definition of quality of life refers to the satisfaction people experience from the balance of constraints and opportunities (or possibilities) in their lives.

Dimensions of Quality of Life. Quality of life has a number of dimensions that correspond to broad, fundamental areas of people's lives. The CHP model focuses on the possibilities that arise in three broad, major areas of life: *Being, Belonging,* and *Becoming.* Each of the three areas encompasses three subareas. These nine aspects of quality of life are listed and briefly described in Table 2.1. These dimensions of quality of life are congruent with both the domains of concern to occupational therapists and contemporary occupational therapy principles, particularly the use of an holistic, client-centered approach that is guided by a social justice perspective (Townsend, 1993).

Being includes three dimensions of life concerned with who the individual is as a person. *Physical Being* focuses on the body and physical aspects of health. Included here are exercise and fitness, mobility and agility, and nutrition, as well as grooming, hygiene, and physical appearance. *Psychological Being* refers to the person's thoughts, feelings, and mental health. This dimension encompasses self-esteem, self-concept, self-control, coping with anxiety, and initiating positive, independent activities. *Spiritual Being* centers

TABLE 2.1 Major Areas and Subareas of Quality of Life

Area/Subarea of Life	Brief Description
Being	Who You Are as a Person
Physical Being	Your body and your physical health
Psychological Being	Your thoughts and feelings; your mental health
Spiritual Being	The beliefs, values, and standards by which you live
Belonging	The Fit Between You and Your Environment
Physical Belonging	Where you live and your surroundings
Social Belonging	The people in your life and around you
Community Belonging	Access to and links you have with community resources
Becoming	What You Do to Fulfill Your Goals and Hopes
Practical Becoming	Your practical, daily, or regular activities
Leisure Becoming	Activities you do for enjoyment and/or relaxation
Growth Becoming	Activities you do to learn, change, or develop as a person

around beliefs, values, and standards by which the person lives. Embodied here are an understanding of right and wrong, attaching meaning to life, feeling at peace within oneself, and celebrating special events in life, such as birthdays, Thanksgiving, Christmas, Hanukkah, and other holidays. It also includes helping others, and involvement in such transcendent experiences as music, poetry, nature, and religious activities.

Belonging refers to the degree of congruence between the person and his or her environment. *Physical Belonging* is concerned with the physical aspects of the person's home, work/school/program setting, neighborhood, and community. The major issues here are privacy, security, having personal possessions and a place to display them, and feeling "at home" in one's physical surroundings. *Social Belonging* refers to bonds and connections with significant people in his or her life as well as others with whom he or she regularly interacts. This dimension includes meaningful relationships with a partner or special person, friends, and family members. Relationships with acquaintances, coworkers, and neighbors, as well as members of the person's cultural, faith, or social group are also encompassed here. *Community Belonging* is concerned with linkages the person has with community resources. Having access to events, places, facilities, and services typically available to members of one's community is the major issue here. Some usual community resources are employment, a source of money or income, education, health and social services, shopping facilities, and public events.

Becoming means what a person does to fulfill his or her hopes, goals, and aspirations. *Practical Becoming* subsumes practical activities a person does, or wants or needs to do, on a daily or regular basis. Some examples are involvement in paid work or unpaid work (volunteering, household chores, caring for self, children, or others), school, or other programs. It also includes making and meeting appointments with providers of health, social, and educational services. *Leisure Becoming* centers around what people do for fun, relaxation, or both. Examples of Leisure Becoming include involvement in solitary, group, organized, or spontaneous activities, which may be related to sports, hobbies, games, entertainment, and socializing. This dimension also includes taking brief breaks from routine activities—a weekend away or a night out during the week—and vacations. *Growth Becoming* emphasizes activities associated with learning, change, and personal development. Growth may involve acquisition of new skills or enhancement of existing skills in formal ways, through courses or programs, or the more informal ways of learning from friends, a social group, or "how to" books. The skills learned or further developed may be physical, interpersonal, or related to independent living. This dimension also includes seeking new challenges and adapting to changes in life.

Basic Quality of Life.   Quality of life within each of these nine dimensions of life consists of both the degree of *satisfaction* and the degree of *importance* the person associates with possibilities that arise from the ongoing relationship with his or her environment. These determinants of *basic quality of life* are summarized in Table 2.2.

Personal Control.   Personal control consists of two moderating factors that either can contribute to or detract from the degree of basic quality of life experienced by the individual in each of the nine areas of life. One of these factors consists of the *decisions* and choices a person makes. The other factor consists of the range of *opportunities* available to the person as he or she makes these choices and decisions. Together, these two influencing factors constitute *personal control* (see Table 2.2).

APPLYING THE CHP FRAMEWORK IN PRACTICE

The CHP model has a number of potential applications to occupational therapy practice with adults who have developmental disabilities. Given the focus of this book, the major applications examined here pertain to direct service and include assessment, intervention, program planning, and program evaluation. Other applications will be noted briefly in a subsequent section.

The CHP framework can be applied to identify those aspects of a person's life that are adding to and detracting from quality of life. Its application can also serve to identify the priority areas for goal-setting, program-planning, and intervention. Finally, it can provide a way of determining a baseline

TABLE 2.2   Factors Determining and Influencing Quality of Life

Each of the four factors below is considered for each of the nine areas of life:	
(a) Two Factors Determining Quality of Life	
Importance and Satisfaction ⇨	Basic Quality of Life
(b) Two Factors Influencing Degree of Quality of Life	
Decisions and Opportunities ⇨	Personal Control

against which subsequent changes in a person's quality of life can be compared.

It is essential to note that, wherever possible, the perceptions of the person with developmental disabilities concerning his or her own quality of life should serve as the therapist's major source of information. Further, the client should have as active a role as possible in assessment, program-planning, and intervention. As much as possible, evaluation of program effectiveness for a client or clients should draw most heavily on client experiences. According to the CHP approach, at every stage of occupational therapy involvement, the client should be as active a participant as he or she is able to be (Renwick, Brown, & Raphael, 1994). Others who know the person well, such as family members, people who provide informal supports, and other service providers, can provide additional or supplementary information. This kind of information becomes much more important when clear communication between client and therapist is difficult and the probability of misinterpretation of the client's perceptions is great, for example, when the client has a low level of cognitive functioning or ability to express thoughts and feelings. When this is the case, information should be sought from at least two others who know the client well. Having adequate information from appropriate sources is critical in the assessment process.

Assessment.   Assessment guided by the CHP framework may be quantitative in nature, that is, instruments based on the framework can be used to determine the degree of quality experienced by the individual in each area of life. (Availability of such instruments is noted in a subsequent section.) Assessment can also be done using a more informal, qualitative approach, that is, through the systematic application of the CHP framework to the process of interviewing the client and others, as appropriate (see above). Whatever approach is taken, if assessment is done carefully and thoroughly, the potential for planning a meaningful intervention with the client and achieving a positive outcome is greatly enhanced.

Since a qualitative interview approach is more likely to be used by therapists providing direct service, this application of the framework to client assessment will be examined further. All nine areas of the client's life can be assessed in terms of basic quality of life, specifically, how much importance and enjoyment or satisfaction the client attaches to the items included in each area of life (see Table 2.1 and the *Dimensions of Quality of Life* section above). The items associated with each area can also be assessed with respect to personal control. Specifically, assessment would focus on the extent to which the client perceives that he or she makes choices and decisions, as well as the range of opportunities available to the client from which to make such choices and decisions.

In assessing personal control, it is essential for the therapist to explore how much control the client is comfortable with, feels he or she can deal with, and wants to have in each area of life. For example, a client may be quite comfortable with making more decisions and choices related to Physical Being:

■ when to wash one's hair
■ choosing to have a bath instead of showering
■ choosing what to eat for breakfast
■ deciding to get some exercise by going for a swim.

He or she may wish to have more variety in the available opportunities when making these choices and decisions. On the other hand, he or she may feel comfortable with the amount of personal control he or she has in other areas, such as Leisure Becoming:

■ being able to watch favorite TV programs every week
■ going bowling every Thursday with fellow group-home residents
■ being able to make arrangements to stay at a sister's apartment for the weekend once a month.

However, in other areas of life, the person may feel overwhelmed by the number and kinds of choices and decisions that he or she feels pressured to make. For instance, if Growth Becoming presents this kind of problem, the individual may be finding it difficult to decide what social or independent living skills to improve. He or she may need more structure, assistance, or guidance to facilitate decision-making concerning this aspect of life.

One important aspect of assessment is the exploration of the range of opportunities available to the client in the areas of life in which quality most needs to be enhanced. This process requires thorough consideration of the options, that is, the constraints relative to the opportunities present in each area. In essence, alternative resources—people, groups, settings, programs and activities, and strategies or courses of action—that the person can draw upon to enhance quality in a particular area of life should be balanced against factors that would make improvement difficult or impossible. For instance, some resources may be too costly, may require too much travel time, or may require a lengthy waiting period for the client to obtain access.

Further, some strategies may be inappropriate to the client's current levels or repertoire of skills.

Another crucial aspect of assessment is careful attention to how much the client's environment promotes (or could potentially promote) or detracts from quality in each area of life. The environment in which the client lives, works, goes to school, and engages in leisure activities should be included in the assessment. Consideration should be given to all major aspects of the environment: physical, social, cultural, economic, legal, and political.

Two levels at which the environment can contribute to quality of life should also be explored. First, quality-promoting environments are those that support the individual's basic requirements of human life, such as food, warmth, safety, and social contact. Second, such environments also offer the client a range of choices and opportunities to make decisions that are congruent with his or her capacity and comfort level and have the potential to result in supporting or enhancing enjoyment (satisfaction) in at least several of the nine ares of life. Assessment of the client's environment using the CHP framework can help the therapist identify those areas of life in which the client's environment for living, working, and so forth is likely to promote quality and those areas where it is not likely to do so.

Program Planning and Intervention. The assessment will enable the therapist, with as much participation as possible by the client, to identify which areas of life most require quality enhancement, in particular those areas that are very important but not currently satisfying to the client. These priority areas become the major focus for program-planning (including goal-setting) and intervention. These two interdependent processes should focus on strategies targeted to increasing the client's enjoyment (satisfaction) in the areas he or she finds most important and decrease dissatisfaction with activities he or she does not enjoy doing. It is also essential to increase the amount of personal control in the areas of life in which the client wants to exert more influence. At the same time, the amount of control by the client can be decreased in those areas where the demands to exert more personal control are making him or her feel pressured and very anxious. Increases or decreases in the amount of personal control can be achieved by expanding or narrowing the range of opportunities for choice and decision-making and increasing or decreasing the environmental demands on the client to exercise personal control.

If the environmental assessment indicates that the client's living or work environment does not promote quality or, in fact, undermines it, some environmental modification strategies may need to be planned and built into the intervention. For instance, such modifications could include:

▮ identifying and cultivating opportunities for the client to meet new people
▮ trying new activities
▮ exploring new settings or programs.

Evaluation.   Application of the CHP framework to evaluation of how well the intervention addressed the program goals can be done with individual clients or with groups of clients (those who share common program goals, have similar needs, or live in the same group home). As with the initial assessment and establishment of baselines for the client, evaluation may employ a more formal, quantitative approach using validated instruments or a qualitative approach.

Follow-up assessments (quantitative or qualitative) can be done regularly to determine whether the client's quality of life is improving, deteriorating, or remaining unchanged. The main focus of the evaluation is to determine whether satisfaction has increased in the areas important to the client and dissatisfaction has decreased in areas of less importance. Attention should also be given to determining whether control has increased or decreased to a desired or manageable level for the client. Finally, the therapist should ascertain whether a range of opportunities has been made available to the client of which he or she can potentially take advantage with or without facilitation by the therapist. If the client's goals are not being reached, the results of these reassessments will help the therapist to make adjustments in these goals or the overall program plan and intervention strategies.

Other Potential Applications

The CHP framework is already being used to guide a large-scale longitudinal study (1994–1998) of quality of life for adults with developmental disabilities who live in the Canadian province of Ontario. The provincial government's Ministry of Community and Social Services is implementing policy designed to move these individuals from institutional settings to more community-based settings for living, working, and participating in educational and other programs. The study is being carried out by the author and other researchers from the Quality of Life Research Unit (Centre for Health Promotion, University of Toronto) using a psychometrically sound instrument package.

This instrumentation is based on the elements of the CHP model. The instruments and associated training in their use are expected to be available from the Quality of Life Research Unit by the spring of 1998. Future research could be designed to use these instruments as outcome measures to test the relative efficacy of various interventions with adults in this population.

The framework can also be used to guide the analysis and evaluation of existing policy, without necessarily conducting a specific research study of the kind noted above. It could be employed—in qualitative examination of policy or in summarizing existing statistical reports—to help determine whether current policies adequately address the key aspects of quality of life encompassed by the model for persons in this population. This application could also identify the aspects of quality of life that the policy was not addressing adequately or, perhaps, not at all, and indicate, in general terms, how these gaps might be filled. Further, the framework could be potentially useful in guiding development of new health and social policy designed to target or include this population.

Finally, the CHP approach can help identify priority issues that can constitute the focal point of advocacy for this population. Use of the framework can provide shape and direction for efforts aimed at changing policy, securing funding, and establishing or enhancing programs to support good quality of life for adults with developmental disabilities.

CONCLUSION

This chapter describes the CHP conceptual model and discussed its usefulness as a coherent, systematic guiding framework for occupational practice with adults who have developmental disabilities. Several aspects of this model make it appropriate for application by occupational therapists working with this population. It is consistent with the holistic view of persons and the client-centered approach that are hallmarks of the profession. Further, the CHP framework focuses clearly, and in detail, on the nature of quality of life and how it might be promoted, fostered, and enhanced. This focus is congruent with the frequently-noted overarching goal of occupational therapy: to maintain or improve clients' quality of life. Because it is clearly conceptualized and grounded in the real-life perceptions of people with and without disabilities, the concepts associated with the model can be readily applied to all major aspects of occupational therapy practice: assessment, intervention, and evaluation. Finally, the framework has already been used successfully over time in a large-scale research study of quality of life experienced by adults with developmental disabilities. The research team that designed and is conducting this study includes occupational therapists. In summary, the model offers an opportunity to organize and integrate practice with adults who have developmental disabilities within a conceptual framework that is consistent with the principles central to occupational therapy.

ACKNOWLEDGEMENTS

The CHP framework and associated instrumentation were developed in the context of the Quality of Life Project funded by the Ministry of Community and Social Services (Ontario, Canada). However, the views expressed here do not necessarily represent the views of the Ministry or the Government of Ontario. Since 1993, Dr. Ivan Brown, Project Manager of the Quality of Life Project, and the author, a Principal Investigator on the project, have done a series of presentations and workshops on linking the CHP framework to practice for professionals who provide services to adults with developmental disabilities. This chapter includes several core issues and concepts discussed during those presentations.

REFERENCES

Bowling, A. (1991). *Measuring health.* Milton Keynes, UK: Open University Press.

Bowling, A. (1995). *Measuring disease.* Buckingham, UK: Open University Press.

Brown, I., & Renwick, R. (1996). *Improving quality of life.* Toronto: Quality of Life Research Unit, Centre for Health Promotion, University of Toronto.

Brown, I., Renwick, R., & Nagler, M. (1996). The centrality of quality of life in health promotion and rehabilitation. In R. Renwick, I. Brown, & M. Nagler (Eds.), *Quality of life in health promotion and rehabilitation: Conceptual approaches, issues, and applications* (pp. 3–13). Thousand Oaks, CA: Sage.

Brown, R. I., Bayer, M. B., & McFarlane, C. (Eds.). (1989). *Rehabilitation programmes: Performance and quality of life of adults with developmental handicaps.* Toronto: Lugus.

Brown, R. I., Brown, P. M., & Bayer, M. B. (1994). A quality of life model: New challenges arising from a six year study. *Quality of life for persons with disabilities: International perspectives and issues* (pp. 39–56). Cambridge, MA: Brookline.

Canadian Association of Occupational Therapists. (1991). *Occupational therapy guidelines for client-centered practice.* Toronto: Author.

Dennis, R. E., Williams, W., Giangreco, M. F., & Cloninger, C.J. (1993). Quality of life as a context for planning and evaluation of services for people with disabilities. *Exceptional Children, 59,* 499–512.

Evans, R. G., & Stoddart, G. L. (1990). Producing health, consuming health care. *Social Science and Medicine, 31,* 1347–1363.

Felce, D., & Perry, J. (1996). Exploring current conceptions of quality of life: A model for people with and without disabilities. In R. Renwick, I. Brown, & M. Nagler (Eds.), *Quality of life in health promotion and rehabilitation: Conceptual approaches, issues, and applications* (pp. 51–62). Thousand Oaks, CA: Sage.

Goode, D. A. (1990). Thinking about and discussing quality of life. In R. L. Schalock (Ed.), *Quality of life: Perspectives and issues* (pp. 41–57). Washington, DC: American Association on Mental Retardation.

Goode, D. A. (Ed.). (1994). *Quality of life for persons with disabilities: International perspectives and issues.* Cambridge, MA: Brookline.

Jongbloed, I., & Chrichton, A. (1990). A new definition of disability: Implications for rehabilitation practice and policy. *Canadian Journal of Occupational Therapy, 57*, 32–38.

Halpern, A. S., Nave, G., Close, D. W., & Wilson, D. (1986). An empirical analysis of the dimensions of community adjustment for adults with mental retardation in semi-independent living programs. *Australia and New Zealand Journal of Developmental Disabilities, 12*, 147–157.

Landesman, S. (1986). Quality of life and personal satisfaction: Definition and measurement issues. *Mental Retardation, 24*, 141–143.

Renwick, R., & Brown, I. (1996). The Centre for Health Promotion's approach to quality of life: Being, belonging, and becoming. In R. Renwick, I. Brown, & M. Nagler (Eds.), *Quality of life in health promotion and rehabilitation: Conceptual approaches, issues, and applications* (pp. 75–86). Thousand Oaks, CA: Sage.

Renwick, R., Brown, I., & Nagler, M. (Eds.). (1996). *Quality of life in health promotion and rehabilitation: Conceptual approaches, issues, and applications.* Thousand Oaks, CA: Sage.

Renwick, R., Brown, I., & Raphael, D. (1994). Quality of life: Linking a conceptual approach to service provision. *Journal on Developmental Disabilities, 3*, 32–44.

Renwick, R., Brown, I., Rootman, I., & Nagler, M. (1996). Conceptualization, research, and application: Future directions. In R. Renwick, I. Brown, & M. Nagler (Eds.), *Quality of life in health promotion and rehabilitation: Conceptual approaches, issues, and applications* (pp. 357–367). Thousand Oaks, CA: Sage.

Renwick, R., & Friefeld, S. (1996). Quality of life and rehabilitation. In R. Renwick, I. Brown, & M. Nagler (Eds.), *Quality of life in health promotion and rehabilitation: Conceptual approaches, issues, and applications* (pp. 26–36). Thousand Oaks, CA: Sage.

Schalock, R. L. (1990). *Quality of life: Perspectives and issues.* Washington, DC: American Association on Mental Retardation.

Schalock, R. L. (Ed.). (1996). *Quality of life—Volume I: Conceptualization and measurement.* Washington, DC: American Association on Mental Retardation.

Schalock, R. L. (Ed). (1997). *Quality of life—Volume II: Applications to persons with disabilities.* Washington, DC: American Association on Mental Retardation.

Schalock, R. L., Keith, K., Hoffman, K., & Karan, O. (1989). Quality of life: Its measurement and use. *Mental Retardation, 27*, 25–31.

Townsend, E. (1993). Occupational therapy's social vision. *Canadian Journal of Occupational Therapy, 60*, 174–184.

Woodill, G., Renwick, R., Brown, I., & Raphael, D. (1994). Being, belonging, and becoming: An approach to quality of life of persons with developmental disabilities. In D. A. Goode (Ed.). *Quality of life for persons with disabilities: International perspectives and issues* (pp. 57–74). Cambridge, MA: Brookline.

World Health Organization. (1986). *Ottawa charter for health promotion.* Ottawa: Canadian Public Health Association.

PART 2

A
Profile
of
Needs

3

Adults With Developmental Disabilities and Work

What Can I Do as an Occupational Therapy Practitioner?

David J. Wysocki, MS, OTR/L, ATP
Ann T. Neulicht, PhD, CRC

The American Occupational Therapy Association (AOTA) recognizes *work and productive activities* as one of three areas of human performance along with *activities of daily living* and *play or leisure* (AOTA, 1994, p. 1047). It describes these *performance areas* as including "activities that the occupational therapy practitioner emphasizes when determining functional abilities." AOTA goes on to define *work and productive activities* as "purposeful activities for self-development, social contribution, and livelihood" (AOTA, 1994, p. 1052). This reflects the fact that paid employment bears both pragmatic and psychosocial consequences. It not only offers a means by which a worker can contribute to his or her daily needs; it also sustains a social context for meeting an array of social values and needs (Crist & Stoffel, 1992; Mitchell, 1985). Within the context of self-development, work offers one a sense of mastery over the environment, as well as a sense of accomplishment and competence leading to a heightened self-esteem.

Occupational therapy practitioners serving adults with developmental disabilities often express a sense of isolation. This is complicated by a dearth of current occupational therapy resources in the area of developmental disabilities (DD) and work. For instance, as we prepared for this chapter, our literature search revealed a minimal number of current occupational therapy references. Even taking advantage of the vast high-tech resources of AOTA's online Bibliographic System (*OT BibSys*), the Internet, and the World Wide Web (see below, "Resources for the Occupational Therapy Practitioner"), our efforts produced little. Despite limited resources, occupational therapists acknowledge that the field is rewarding and offers an array of interesting practice experiences ("Adults with Developmental Disabilities," 1995). The field of developmental disabilities and work is not new to occupational therapy (Kirkland & Robertson, 1985; Weeks, 1988) and it is rapidly gaining importance. With the advent of deinstitutionalization in the 1970s and 1980s, the adult consumers with DD traditionally served in institutions moved into the community, leaving many of their occupational therapy services behind. Today, the opportunities for increased community-based involvement (Spencer, 1990), coupled with the comprehensive nature of the population, offer a challenging and rewarding environment for the occupational therapy practitioner as part of an interdisciplinary team.

This chapter offers an overview of *work,* as a practice area, with adults who have DD. It is presented in the belief that work is intrinsic to humankind and that a life without the choice of work is incomplete. The scope of DD, presented in this chapter, includes mental retardation, cerebral palsy, autism, and acquired brain injury. For those new to DD, or readers familiar with work primarily as a practice in industrial rehab and work hardening, the chapter can serve as a comprehensive outline of the field, its history, and prevalent practices. For the more experienced occupational therapist in DD, it can serve as a common framework for a practice underrepresented in current occupational therapy literature. For all readers, the chapter can be a resource of contemporary information within the field, and a report on the progressive changes of vocational perspectives in DD, including some exciting examples of how those changes are being manifested. The chapter includes:

- an overview of DD issues as they apply to work
- a background briefing on work and vocational programs for people with DD
- a description of service and work settings for the adult DD consumer
- a summary of the types and areas of practice for the occupational therapist
- a view on preparing DD consumers for the modern information age of work
- a listing of resources in the field, including a discussion on the information superhighway.

COMMON ISSUES FOR CONSUMERS WITH DEVELOPMENTAL DISABILITIES AND THEIR IMPACT ON WORK

A Range of Issues from Severe to Mild

Developmental disabilities represent a wide range of etiologies, diagnoses, issues, and severity (Reed, 1991). This is important to consider, because the global nature of many developmental disabilities may have a far-reaching affect on functional occupational performance. The issues, their severity and depth, all can have a significant and distinctive impact on the targeted programs, goal expectations, and potential outcomes of any work-based intervention. It is essential, as with any type of occupational therapy, to perform appropriate assessments in developing a treatment plan for the individual consumer. Familiarity with the population, and a sense of the impact a particular disability can have on work performance, will guide the experienced DD therapist in identifying the areas to assess. As a guide to the less acquainted occupational therapist, this section will present common DD and work issues as they relate to mental retardation, autism, cerebral palsy, or acquired brain injury. This section will close with a case vignette of Jerry, to help illustrate the nature of some issues commonly addressed in an individual's work performance. Jerry's case will be revisited at the end of the section on areas and types of occupational-therapy practice in DD and work, and after the section covering modern employment options for people with DD.

Performance Areas

As discussed in the introduction, work is listed as a *performance area* under the *Uniform Terminology for Occupational Therapy* heading of *Work and Productive Activities* (AOTA, 1994). Although the functional outcome focus of this chapter is on the *Vocational Activities* subsection of *Work and Productivity* (see below), an individual's vocational performance can be readily affected by the other *performance areas*. A comprehensive vocational program will consider the needs and strengths of a consumer in all applicable areas, as well as the interactive relationship among the areas. These areas are presented below as listed in the *Uniform Terminology:*

    A. *Activities of Daily Living*
        1. *Grooming*
        2. *Oral Hygiene*
        3. *Bathing/Showering*

      4. *Toilet Hygiene*
      5. *Personal Device Care*
      6. *Dressing*
      7. *Feeding and Eating*
      8. *Medication Routine*
      9. *Health Maintenance*
    10. *Socialization*
    11. *Functional Communication*
    12. *Functional Mobility*
    13. *Community Mobility*
    14. *Emergency Response*
    15. *Sexual Expression*
B. *Work and Productive Activities*
      1. *Home Management*
        a. *Clothing Care*
        b. *Cleaning*
        e. *Money Management*
        g. *Safety Procedures* (also as they apply to the workplace)
      3. *Educational Activities*
      4. *Vocational Activities*
        a. *Vocational Exploration*
        b. *Job Acquisition*
        c. *Work or Job Performance*
        d. *Retirement Planning*
        e. *Volunteer Participation*

Functional Components and Areas

Because of the global and pervasive nature of the developmental disabilities discussed, virtually any functional component can be affected. The severity of the condition also may determine the depth of the disability as experienced by any one consumer. With this in mind, a list of the more common issues experienced within this population is offered when applying occupational therapy services to *work*. This is intended as a guide (not an exhaustive listing) to the areas that may be commonly addressed, as they pertain to the consumer's vocational performance. These functional components and areas include:

■ *Sensory:* Tactile, proprioceptive, vestibular, visual, and auditory reception and sensory processing

■ *Perceptual:* Kinesthesia, pain response, right/left discrimination, and visual perception (e.g., visual discrimination, form constancy, visual memory, figure-ground, spatial relations, visual closure, visual sequential memory, and depth perception)

▮ *Neuromusculoskeletal:* Primitive reflexes, range of motion, muscle tone and spasticity, strength, endurance, postural control, and postural alignment

▮ *Motor:* Gross and fine motor coordination, crossing midline, bilateral integration, motor control, motor learning, motor planning, visual-motor integration, and oral motor control

▮ *Cognitive:* Arousal level, orientation, recognition, attention to task, initiation/termination of activity, memory, sequencing, categorization, concept formation, spatial operations, problem-solving, learning, and generalization

▮ *Psychosocial:* Values and interests, self-concept, social conduct, interpersonal skills, self-expression, coping skills, time management, and self-control

Performance Contexts

In addition to performance areas and functional components, the individual's work environment can have a significant impact on occupational performance. These external or environmental factors are represented in *Uniform Terminology* as *performance contexts* (AOTA, 1994) and defined as "situations or factors that influence an individual's engagement in desired and/or required performance areas." These conditions can have an impact on *anyone* in *any* work situation. Generally, the fields of industrial engineering, architecture, and ergonomics have addressed these issues in the workplace. However, this is seldom done with regard to the disordered effects these contexts can have on the performance of a person with a developmental disability. This becomes an important consideration when elements such as lighting, noise, or social contexts can exacerbate the issues with which an individual with a DD already has to contend. An occupational therapist addressing these issues may recommend treatment and training for the consumer, changing the contexts within the work environment, or a combination of both. The environmental contexts include:

▮ *Physical:* Lighting quality and intensity, noise levels, visual and auditory distractions, visual elements of work surfaces (including video terminals), contact surfaces, vibrations, spatial positioning

▮ *Social:* Physical proximity of other workers, physical and social relationships of significant others in the work environment, supervisory practices, role expectations, social routines

■ *Cultural:* Facility rules (both formal and informal), customs, beliefs, activity patterns, predisposition to disability and disability awareness, support for accommodations

Jerry: A Case to Follow

The following case vignette illustrates, from an occupational therapy perspective, how an individual's multiple issues, associated with DD, can affect the performance area of work:

> Jerry, a man in his early thirties, was recently placed in a community group home from a MR/DD residential institution. He was diagnosed with moderate mental retardation (MR) and mildly spastic quadriplegia. Jerry had worked in the sheltered setting, located at the institution, shredding paper and assembling tool packets for a local electronics company. Jerry's new placement put him in a new job in the community, at a footwear distribution warehouse. His duties included assembling and sorting boxes, by picture, number, and color. The boxes were used for bulk footwear that was sorted and packed before shipping to retail stores. Jerry's employer was not completely happy with Jerry's job performance. Jerry had been working at the distributor for almost 2 months. Although Jerry was always on time and attended his job regularly, boxes were not always being assembled and sorted correctly, and some coworkers had complained of hygiene issues. The incorrectly assembled and sorted boxes caused other problems down the line where the barcodes on the boxes were scanned by other employees prior to packing. Jerry was scheduled to receive a comprehensive occupational therapy evaluation in response to his new community placement. During the occupational therapy evaluation, Jerry demonstrated problems with visual perception, especially with form constancy and spatial relations. In addition, Jerry exhibited a mild nystagmus and difficulty in ocular motor tracking and accommodation. Jerry was eager to perform well during the evaluation, but the heightened stress of the assessment revealed a significant increase in his upper extremity muscle tone which interfered with both gross and fine motor control. The added stress also appeared to increase Jerry's salivation and drooling that lead him to continually wipe his chin and mouth with his hands and shirt sleeves. Jerry's hypertonal spasticity was primarily in his extremities, and he exhibited hypotonicity in his trunk. This affected his endurance, especially while under the stress of performing the assessment tasks. Jerry demonstrated excellent attention to task, good functional problem-

solving skills, and functional memory. However, Jerry also had a history of difficulties when changing jobs or environments, revealing a potential difficulty with immediately generalizing learned skills from one setting to another.

OVERVIEW OF WORK: SERVICES AND SETTINGS FOR ADULTS WITH DEVELOPMENTAL DISABILITIES

Controversy over the care of persons with developmental disabilities and mental retardation has existed for over 130 years (President's Committee on Mental Retardation, 1977). In the 19th century, training schools were erected by enlightened individuals who believed retardation could be "cured" by education and training. By the early 20th century, professionals were convinced that little could be done to help most individuals with developmental delay. Confinement in an institution for life was usually considered the kindest solution for the individual with retardation, for the family, and for the community. By the 1960s, much more was being learned about the abilities of persons with retardation. Some parents sought alternatives to overcrowded and dehumanizing institutions and began community efforts to organize community programs. Staff and planners at institutions began to realize that many residents of institutions could make greater progress living in the community, and the role of the school and sheltered workshop heightened.

Sheltered vs. Supported Employment

The *sheltered workshop* (now commonly called *community rehabilitation facility*) was intended as a long-term but transitional placement for persons with disabilities. Program goals included skill training and work adjustment to prepare individuals for remunerative work in the community. A service continuum of vocational evaluation, preemployment training, work adjustment, job placement, and time-limited employment services was developed to facilitate independent paid employment. Work tasks have traditionally involved labor-intensive benchwork, assembly, packaging, and collating tasks that are routine, repetitive, and unskilled in nature. Remuneration is typically subminimum wage, and there may be much "down time" in a consumer's workweek or other rehabilitative services, such as compensatory education. Although the meaning of *long term* was intended as "for as long as necessary" and consumers were to remain in a workshop only long enough to become ready for competitive employment (Olshansky, 1971), workshops have been severely criticized for maintaining a segregated setting with little hope of long-term success in competitive employment (Parent, Hill, & Wehman, 1989). In fact, results indicate that only 12 percent of sheltered-workshop participants move into competitive employment annually, with only 3 percent maintaining competitive employment status after 2 years (Bellamy, Rhodes, Bourbeau, & Mank, 1986).

Although a *sheltered* setting may be necessary for some individuals with severe disabilities, current trends in the field emphasize inclusion and integration for persons with DD. *Supported employment* has developed as an alternative vocational option to accommodate the individual needs of persons with severe disabilities. Supported employment is defined as:

> paid work in a variety of settings, particularly regular work sites, especially designed for handicapped individuals (i) for whom competitive employment at or above the minimum wage is unlikely; and (ii) who, because of their disability, need intensive, ongoing support to perform in a work setting (*Federal Register*, 1984, p. 17509).

Supported employment was intended to provide services on an ongoing basis, for as long as the individual required assistance, as well as provide flexibility in employment alternatives. The supported employment model does not require that an individual be "job ready" before placement can occur. Often the necessary work and social skills are taught in a work setting, using a train-place-train-follow-up (Lagomarcino, 1986) or a place-train-follow-up (Wehman, 1986) model. Current supported employment approaches include:

- *Individual placement*: individual placement in an integrated, competitive employment setting with one-to-one job coach support. Support is continued, as needed, for as long as the worker is employed. It is also described as a *supported, competitive employment model.*
- *Enclave*: employment of a full-time supervisor and a small group of individuals (not to exceed eight) with severe disabilities at an industry or corporation, where work is performed in an integrated setting. The supervisor and/or supported employees may be employed by the industry itself or by an employment-service program. An enclave may be also described as *work stations in industry.*
- *Mobile work crew*: employment of a full-time supervisor and a group of individuals (no more than eight supported employees) who travel together to multiple work sites in the community, where they engage in contracted work.

▎ *Entrepreneurial business:* a private business operated on a subcontract basis or as a prime manufacturer. The business employs a group of individuals, no more than eight of whom are supported employees. Integration is provided by including individuals without disabilities as coworkers and/or through regular, ongoing contact with the general public.

▎ *Transitional employment:* paid work performed by consumers with integrated business and industry settings that is time limited in nature and typically lasts between 3 and 9 months. Work is typically part-time with continued involvement in other services or support activities.

▎ *Supported jobs model:* individuals are integrated into an employment site, but they are paid subminimum wage based on productivity and receive ongoing training and advocacy from a job coach (Hill, Hill, Wehman, Revell, Dickerson, & Noble, 1987; North Carolina Vocational Alternatives Task Force, 1992).

Support involves activities to assist the employee to acquire, strengthen, and maintain the physical, intellectual, emotional, and social skills needed to perform the specific job tasks, work routine, and personal life activities that are critical to employment success. Support is not time limited and may involve years of service that will ebb and flow with work/life changes. Intervention involves identifying and analyzing jobs in the community, completing functional consumer assessments, writing task analyses, matching job requirements with consumer skills, utilizing behavioral-training strategies, developing environmental/job modifications and negotiating for additional community support when needed. Job carving may be necessary to define a component of a job for a person with a disability who may be unable to perform all essential tasks. The individual responsible for providing employment training is typically called a *job coach.* A job coach actively assists a worker in learning a job and meeting employer expectations, provides advocacy, including the fostering of worker-coworker relationships, natural supports, as well as monitors of the worker's progress and employer satisfaction.

Components critical to the success of a supported employment model include job opportunities in an integrated setting, decent pay for meaningful work, community-based training that reflects labor-market needs, knowledge of vocational alternatives, and vocational choice (Wehman & Moon, 1987). Community-based facilities and school-transition programs that provide supported employment services have undergone an organizational-change process in converting services from a segregated, center-based approach to an integrated community-based service. This has required changes in goal definition, program implementation, funding, staff training, and attitudes.

The beliefs of consumers, parents, staff, and employers that individuals with severe disabilities are not capable of integrated competitive work are being challenged.

Much like contracted work in sheltered settings, supported employment outcomes are typically characterized by labor-intensive benchwork, assembly, distribution, or food, building, and grounds service occupations, often with part-time hours, little or no opportunity for upward mobility or promotion, and few, if any, benefits (Kiernan, McGaughey, & Schalock, 1988). Unfortunately, the implementation of supported employment remains incomplete, as evidenced by low wages, lack of career choices, poor employment retention, and little opportunity for social integration (Dwyre & Trach, 1996; Wehman & Kregel, undated manuscript). Expanding consumer choice and self-determination, as well as promoting meaningful employment outcomes, (not just initial, entry-level jobs) must be considered as we face the challenges of employment for persons with disabilities.

School-to-Work Transition

The school system has a unique set of issues as a service agency offering work programs for people with DD. One of the concerns of the school system is the transition of emerging adults (ages 14 to 21) with DD from school services into the community. During this transition, consumers and their families are forced to negotiate the shift from one federally-mandated system of services to another. This occurs simultaneously with a change in role expectancy for the consumer moving from childhood to young adulthood. Recent studies have shown that this transition into the community and into the role of worker has not been as successful for the disabled population as it has for the nondisabled group. (Barber, McInerny, & Struck, 1993; Ward, 1996). While the national unemployment rate from the late 1980s to the mid-1990s ranged from between five to nine percent, the unemployment rate for youth with disabilities ranged between 44 to 64 percent as a total group. This figure increases dramatically to 85 percent for emerging adults with multiple handicaps. This can be compared to the unemployment rate of 38 percent for emerging adults in the general population. The federal government has responded to the need to incorporate school-to-community transition services into public education. In 1984, school-to-work transition was prioritized nationally by the Office of Special Education and Rehabilitation Services in the U.S. Department of Education, emphasizing that the goal of education and transition was sustained employment (Adelstein, 1992). In 1990, Congress amended the Education for All

Handicapped Children Act to include transition services in the Individualized Education Plan (IEP) for students age 16 and over (and from age 14, when appropriate) (Costello, 1992). This was amended in 1997 with the mandate that transition services begin by age 14 (Public Law 105–17, IDEA).

There is growing recognition in schools of the need for systematic transition planning, starting as early as possible in the student's life. Key factors of a best-practice, comprehensive school-to-community transition program include (Brollier, Shepherd, & Markley, 1994; Carrasco, 1993; Costello, 1992; Mitchell, Rourk, & Schwarz, 1989; Ward, 1996):

- an interdisciplinary/interagency service delivery system, consisting of individual, vocationally-based assessments, program-planning and implementation
- consumer involvement
- parental involvement
- business-community involvement
- prevocational programming, including independent-living and social-skills training, beginning before high school
- vocational training, started by age 16, including job-sampling experience with job analysis, accommodation, and matching services
- successful, paid, supported employment placements before leaving the school system
- postprogram follow-up of former students to evaluate the effectiveness of the transition program.

A number of model programs have been implemented around the country that have successfully included elements of these key factors into their services. They include The Little People's School and The Gaebler Children's Center in Massachusetts, The Career Training Workshop in North Carolina, Project S.T.R.I.V.E. in the Boston Public Schools, and a computer-assisted Salem County Board for Vocational Education training program (Adelstein, 1992; Brollier, Shepherd, & Markley, 1994; Carrasco, 1993; Costello, 1992; Mitchell, Rourk, & Schwarz, 1989). These programs offer examples of how a more intensive and systematic response to transition issues can make a difference in the life of consumers and their communities.

Residential-Institutional Settings

Despite deinstitutionalization and the movement to more integrated and normalized employment opportunities, large residential MR/DD centers still exist in most states across the country (Prouty & Lakin, 1996). The populations in these centers tend to be more severely and multiply-disabled, some with significant medical or behavioral issues. The centers are faced with increased difficulty in transitioning their consumers into the community. In many states, a lack of openings in group homes and community-based programs, due to funding and an incapacity to cope with the severe population, has lead to a significant reduction in community placements. Out of the 342 large state MR/DD facilities operating in the U.S. between 1960 and 1995, the total closed during that period was 119, with peak closure occurring between 1988 and 1995. The average closures during this period were ten facilities per year. However, the total planned closures of large facilities by the year 2000 is 22, at an average of 4.4 per year (Sandlin, Prouty, & Lakin, 1996). This brings the closure trend back to nearly predeinstitutionalization levels.

Although community transition is still an active goal in DD services, some residential centers have reoriented their strategies for service. In North Carolina, the centers are recognizing their role as both a care facility (for those most medically involved) and a center for community-based outreach services. The community-based outreach offers a core of interdisciplinary expertise for continuing education, evaluations, recommendations, assistive-technology services, and other consulting services. This has developed into more outcome-based collaborative relationships within the community, including schools, work programs, day programs, and group homes, as well as with individual consumers and families. Progressive vocational programs offered by institutions today still provide sheltered work settings, while integrating some of their consumers into more supported employment opportunities. The centers are also using their interagency relationships to increase work and training opportunities for the DD population as a whole, both in and out of institutions.

AREAS AND TYPES OF PRACTICE FOR OCCUPATIONAL THERAPY IN DEVELOPMENTAL DISABILITIES AND WORK

Each setting (community-based facility, school system, or residential institution) will have its unique service protocol and its expectations for occupational therapy involvement. This will depend, in part, on governmental and payer mandates, the facility's culture and philosophy, their history with occupational therapy services, and the level of occupational therapy marketing and education that is performed locally and statewide. The level and types of services expected of the occupational therapist can also be affected by the occupational therapist's employment status. A therapist may be employed as a direct employee, indirectly as a contract therapist, or as a self-employed, private-practice occupational therapist. In general, an occupational therapist can be expected to provide evaluations and treatments directly to consumers, perform as a member of an interdisciplinary team, and offer consultative services for intervention to be provided to the consumer by other disciplines. These services may be directly involved with the consumer's work program as *work-based* interventions (for example, performing a job analysis or developing simulated work), or be *supplemental* to the work program (for example, seating/positioning or activities-of-daily-living assessment). The literature reviewed offered a wide variety of ways that an occupational therapy practitioner can serve people with DD in the field of work. It reflects the broad-based profession of occupational therapy and the fact that each practicing occupational therapist brings with him or her a unique background and set of competencies. If a therapist has proficiency in an appropriate occupational therapy service, which is meaningful to the consumer, that service should be considered within the consumer's interdisciplinary service matrix.

Settings and Occupational Therapy

Settings that are federally-funded are mandated to offer interdisciplinary team services that include occupational therapy. For adults in both community-based and large residential-based services, the consumer's program will be team developed, monitored, and maintained as their Individual Program Plan (IPP) or Individual Habilitation Plan (IHP). The IPP/IHP will include long- and short-term goals, as well as assessments and recommendations for health care, educational, and vocational needs. Occupational therapy services may fit into any of these program areas. The community-based IPP will tend to have a greater orientation to independent-living skills and vocational programming, whereas the residential IPP may have more emphasis on the healthcare plan. The schools' team-based consumer program plan is called the Individual Education Plan (IEP). The IEP's purpose is to meet the consumer's needs for a free and appropriate education. Since 1990, it has been federally mandated to include a school-to-community transition plan, called Individual Transition Plan (ITP), in the IEP which must address the student's vocational preparedness. Although occupational therapists have been historically oriented toward earlier intervention in the schools, they could fill an important role in school transition vocational services as well (Brollier, Shepherd, & Markley, 1994; Ward, 1996).

Vocational Teams

A treatment *team* is integral to providing an effective vocational intervention plan. The team will vary among settings and may include from only a few or many service providers. In addition to occupational therapists, the team can include vocational professionals (for instance, rehabilitation counselor, job analyst, vocational evaluator, job developer, job coach), educators, community-oriented professionals (social worker or case manager), psychologists, rehabilitation engineers, physical therapists (as needed, primarily for functional mobility, seating, or orthopedic conditions), and other healthcare providers. The occupational therapist's role will vary among facilities. It will be up to the occupational therapist to identify where best to complement the team, based on the consumer's needs, team composition, and the occupational therapist's knowledge.

Types of Practice: Work-Based

A variety of interventions can be performed by an occupational therapist for consumers with DD specific to work-based practice. These include:

- prevocational assessment and training
- vocational assessment and intervention
- functional capacity evaluation
- job analysis
- environmental assessment and modifications
- assistive technology/work jigs.

Many work-based interventions require a degree of specific experience or training and are often done in partnership with vocational professionals. The occupational therapist's contribution to the team-based assessment can lead to direct occupational therapy treatment or to consultations with other team members to establish goals and provide the services, so that the consumer can attain those goals.

Prevocational Assessment and Training

Prevocational intervention is often used for, but should not be limited to, consumers not yet in the work force. It can be especially effective as part of a school, community, or job transition plan and should be implemented as early as possible before the expected transition. As part of a comprehensive vocational plan, prevocational services look at the consumer's *vocational readiness.* Vocational readiness is defined as "the process of assessing and treating deficits in performance components that interfere with the individual's ability to participate in productive occupations throughout the life span" (Kirkland & Robertson, 1985, p. 2). Prevocational intervention addresses job and career preferences, job-getting and job-keeping skills, social living, community living, personal care, and leisure activities (Brollier, Shepherd, & Markley, 1994; Reynolds-Lynch, 1985; Ward, 1996). These performance areas are dynamically integrated and should be considered together with the effective performance components and contexts as found in occupational therapy's *Uniform Terminology* (that is, sensorimotor, cognitive and psychosocial components, and temporal and environmental contexts).

Vocational Assessment and Intervention

Vocational intervention also addresses vocational readiness but usually as it applies to consumers already in or about to enter the workforce. A vocational evaluation should be as inclusive as the prevocational assessment, but oriented to the consumer's immediate, functional relationship with his or her respective job situation. If prevocational intervention has occurred, there should be less emphasis on work objectives and preferences and more focus on work performance. For the consumer preparing to enter the workforce, this may also include simulated work, work sampling, supervised job experiences, internships, or monitored volunteer work. For the consumer about to enter the workforce or who has already begun working, the vocational assessment can be geared to issues more specific to their prospective work situation. Vocational intervention should include a *functional capacity evaluation* (FCE—also called a physical or work capacity evaluation). In industrial rehab the FCE is geared more to physical issues, including functional strength and endurance (sitting, standing, lifting, carrying, pushing, bending, repetitive use, grasping). This is important to the consumer with DD as well, but the design of the FCE should integrate the physical and cognitive issues relevant to the consumer's DD status and prospective work. It is important to consider both the consumer's present functional ability and the therapist's perceived potential for improvement. The occupational therapist's contribution to the vocational assessment (ADL and work performance areas; sensorimotor, cognitive and psychosocial components; and temporal and environmental contexts) should be integrated into recommendations for remedial and compensatory consumer treatment, leading to an improved ability for the consumer to work (Kornblau, 1996).

A *job analysis* is part of a comprehensive vocational plan and is critical to matching prospective work with the prospective worker. The objectives of a job analysis include:

■ identification of the elements of a job, including the essential and nonessential functions, tasks, and duties

■ determination of the skills required to perform the variety of job tasks

■ exploration of the potential compatibility of the job with the consumer, as well as the adaptability of the job to the consumer.

The job analysis is an assessment of the job's physical and cognitive demands, aptitudes, educational/training requirements, stress factors, objectives or outcomes, required tasks, equipment used, environmental conditions, and safety issues (Blackwell, Conrad, & Weed, 1992; Havranek, 1992; Jacobs & Wyrick, 1989; U.S. Department of Labor, 1991a).

The *environmental assessment* is an integral part of a comprehensive job analysis. Environmental factors can have a significant effect on the success of a person with disabilities entering the work force (Kielhofner, 1992; Velozo, 1992). The sense of mastery of one's environment, elicited through the physical, cognitive, and psychosocial accessibility of the workplace, can greatly affect the potential for a meaningful and fulfilling work experience (Kielhofner, 1992). An environmental assessment should consider the total facility and not be limited to the immediate task surroundings. For example, the physical, cognitive, and psychosocial accessibility of the coworkers, supervisors, personnel representatives, front door, restrooms, lunch and break rooms, snack machines, emergency exits, safety equipment, reference materials, etc., takes on significant importance for an individual with DD. The assessment should consider all the environmental contexts of the setting, including the physical, social, and cultural contexts (as described under *Performance Contexts* earlier in this chapter).

The occupational therapist can facilitate a change in the worker's environment to improve conditions that may adversely affect their performance. These *environmental modifications* can occur within any of the environmental contexts. Environmental modifications are a compensatory intervention and may be considered concurrently with remedial consumer treatment. A physical modification could include increasing accessibility to the bathroom, changing the quality of lighting in the work area, adjusting the position of a computer monitor to reduce glare, or using other assistive technology to increase access to the work station. A social modification could include changing the proximity of a significant other to the consumer, educating coworkers on disability awareness, or facilitating natural supports. An example of a cultural modification could include education of management on Americans with Disabilities Act (ADA) mandates, leading to an employer-directed change in the environment. This could include a physical change, as well as nonphysical change, such as an adjustment in the worker's schedule.

Assistive Technology Services

In *Assistive Technologies: Principles and Practice,* assistive technology (AT) is defined as "a broad range of devices, services, strategies, and practices that are conceived and applied to ameliorate the problems faced by individuals who have disabilities" (Cook & Hussey, 1995, p. 5). AT devices can range from low to high tech; can be custom, off-the-shelf, or modified, and can include products designed specifically for the disability population or standard consumer products used in an assistive manner. An AT device can be general and applied to a variety of environments or be a specific modification of the workplace or job. A type of AT frequently referred to in work environments for people with DD is a *jig.* A jig is a device that is often custom-made. It is designed to increase a worker's cognitive or physical ability to perform a particular task. Examples of jigs include paper folders, templates used in assembling multiple pieces, or work holders. An example of a modern work jig (though not referred to as such) could be a computer key guard, expanded keyboard, or a switch-adapted track ball.

Assistive technology service includes team-based assessment, identification, recommendation, procurement, delivery, training and follow-up. An AT team should consist of the consumer, caretaker or family member, direct service providers, case manager or leader, therapists, and the appropriate technology practitioners. If off-the-shelf AT is being considered, the team may also include an AT supplier. A rehabilitation engineer is an additional team member who can provide an array of technical support for vocational intervention (Gordon & Kozole, 1984). For vocational AT services the team should also include the vocational service providers and may include the employer.

Assistive technology is a broad, dynamic, and increasingly interdisciplinary field. The Rehabilitation Engineering and Assistive Technology Society of North America (RESNA) has responded to the many features of the field by developing ethics and standards for AT practice as well as a credentialing program for both AT practitioners and AT suppliers (ATP and ATS, respectively) (Minkel, 1995, 1996). The RESNA AT certification is a value-added supplement for an already practicing rehabilitation professional, including occupational therapists. Because of the extensive and dynamic nature of the field, most AT specialists concentrate in only one or two practice areas (e.g., computer access, seating and positioning, environmental controls, work modifications). With the possible exception of a rehabilitation engineer, the AT practitioner will often play a combined role as both a regular member of the vocational intervention team (for example, occupational therapist, educator, vocational professional) and as an AT practitioner. If the consumer has multiple AT needs, the team may have more than one AT consultant with different backgrounds. For example, the team could have an occupational therapist specializing in work place modifications and another occupational therapist with a seating and positioning background. In addition to occupational therapists with specific AT backgrounds, occupational therapists with a general awareness of AT can contribute greatly to the team (Angelo & Gross, 1994). For example, an occupational therapist who has extensive experience in DD assessment and intervention can team up with an occupational therapist specializing in general computer access, offering a more complete and effective service to the consumer.

Occupational Therapy Practice: Supplemental to Work

In addition to work-specific intervention, occupational therapy can contribute globally to the vocational success of an individual with DD. As a team contributor to the consumer program plan, an occupational therapist can perform a comprehensive occupational therapy evaluation. The information garnered from an occupational therapy assessment can be applied to specific program goals, including vocational planning and treatment. An occupational therapist can help the team to identify areas that may interfere with the consumer's success at work and make recommendations for strategies and services to respond to those issues. For example, an occupational therapist can analyze performance issues in activities of daily living, such as grooming, hygiene, and mobility; then the occupational therapist can evaluate the consumer for factors contributing to these issues. These factors may include cognitive, sensory, perceptual, and motor performance components. With the information attained by the occupational therapist, the team can better address the consumer's needs as they relate to both current and potential skills and abilities. An occupational therapist can be a key team member in helping to identify *any* potential inhibitor to work performance and help guide the team to the best ways to address those issues.

Other Elements Affecting Vocational Services for Adults With Developmental Disabilities

Other programs exist that can have both direct and indirect influences on vocational programs for people with DD and the provision of occupational therapy services. They include Technology-Related Assistance grants, State Vocational Rehabilitation (VR) Services, and the Americans with Disability Act (Crist & Stoffel, 1992; Metzler, 1995; Shelly, Sample & Spencer, 1992). The Technology-Related Assistance for Individuals with Disabilities Act of 1988 (Public Law 100-407) is commonly referred to as the Tech Act. Its purpose is to increase access to and awareness of assistive technology. Most states have received federal funds, matched by state monies, and established projects to promote systems change and increase interagency coordination in the provision of AT services. Occupational therapists with AT interests can contribute to the development and the applications of state Tech Act programs, which may include services for people with DD and work issues. State Vocational Rehabilitation (VR) services are generally funded through the Rehabilitation Act of 1973 (Public Law 93-112 and its amendments). Through state VR services, people with disabilities including those with severe DD can receive community-based vocational services to enhance employability and independent living. Services include:

- performing a vocational evaluation
- developing a vocational rehabilitation plan
- utilizing rehabilitation facilities and support services (including occupational therapy, physical therapy, rehabilitation engineering, and assistive-technology services)
- providing education and training assistance
- providing school-to-work transition planning, work adjustment, supported employment, job placement assistance, and follow-up as necessary (see Rubin & Roessler, 1995, for more information)

Another avenue for consumer job opportunities is the Americans with Disabilities Act of 1990 (Public Law 101-336). The ADA is a far-reaching civil rights law promoting *full* participation in community-based life, including work, for people with disabilities. It includes comprehensive legislation regarding public access, employment, transportation, and telecommunications. Under the ADA, employers with more than 15 employees must not discriminate against qualified persons with disabilities in hiring, firing, advancement, compensation, training, and other employment-related areas. The ADA mandates *reasonable accommodations* that may allow qualified individuals with disabilities to work. Reasonable accommodations may include on-site modifications to the job tasks, environments, or work schedules. Occupational therapists may be useful in the process of identifying the essential job functions, the environmental or job modifications, and any appropriate assistive technology to enable the consumer to work (AOTA, 1992).

Jerry: A Case Revisited

As a result of Jerry's occupational therapy evaluation (see "Jerry: A Case to Follow"), the team agreed to several additional interventions to help improve Jerry's work performance at the footwear distributor:

■ Jerry was referred to a vision-therapy clinic, with an occupational therapist on staff, for more extensive vision assessments and recommendations for vision therapy.

■ Jerry's group home staff was consulted by his occupational therapist to help Jerry learn socially acceptable and improved ways to manage his drooling.

■ A team comprising his occupational therapist, rehabilitation counselor, and a job coach performed a job analysis, including an environmental assessment, at Jerry's work site. They also performed an adapted functional capacity evaluation (FCE) with Jerry.

The vision assessments showed that Jerry had potentially treatable problems with visual perception. They identified vision exercises that Jerry could do to improve his visual accommodation and help remedy his visual perception issues. Jerry's nystagmus was very mild and consistent with his increased spasticity under stress. The environmental assessment and job analysis revealed a number of key areas for further intervention. Jerry had broken new ground as the first employee there with a developmental disability, and Jerry's employer cared about him and wanted to employ more people with DD. However, a general lack of disability awareness existed at the site. The assembly and sorting problems with Jerry's work included missorted boxes, primarily by number, and assembled boxes with the barcode partially covered. The identifying numbers for sorting were the last two digits. They followed a set of four numbers and a dash, but the two distinguishing numbers were often present in the first set of four, as well. Jerry had no work station. He had to stand over the palettes of unassembled boxes, using them as a makeshift work table on which to perform the assembly operation. The palettes were located in the back stacks of the warehouse, near a drafty freight door where the palettes were delivered regularly and where lighting was poor. Jerry's FCE revealed a problem with endurance, especially while standing and bending constantly for a period of time.

Additional recommendations were made, based on the updated information. They included:

■ A disability awareness program for company employees, directed by Jerry's employer, was created based on standardized information modules (educational packets using printed materials and videos) supplied by the team.

■ A pathway was opened allowing the box palettes to be transported to an area with better lighting and climate control, and in better view of the other employees.

■ A work station was set up with a height-adjustable work table and an adjustable height chair with a back providing lateral support. The work station needed adequate visual access for Jerry, where easy-to-follow patterns for assembling the boxes could be placed.

■ Clearly marked sorting bins on wheels were made and positioned for Jerry's easiest access, helping him place assembled boxes. The wheeled bins allowed for easier transport to the packing area by the other employees.

■ A work jig was developed for Jerry to use with assembled boxes that shields the nonidentifying numbers, allowing him to sort more easily and accurately.

■ Another jig was designed to help Jerry with the folding and holding tasks on smaller boxes.

■ Jerry was assigned a job coach during his transition period for supported learning of the new job skills and to develop natural supports with the other employees.

■ A schedule change allowed Jerry to balance the more physically demanding periods with less demanding times.

PREPARING CONSUMERS WITH DEVELOPMENTAL DISABILITIES FOR THE INFORMATION AGE OF WORK: WHAT *MORE* CAN I DO AS AN OCCUPATIONAL-THERAPY PRACTITIONER?

A columnist recently wrote that the only things in the world that are not affected by technology are truth, beauty, love, and the hiccups . . . however, even love has been altered by the Internet, and it is likely that truth, beauty and the hiccups are not far behind. The increased use of technology has changed the way societal transactions are conducted by creating a constant demand for fast access to and analysis of information. This directly affects the knowledge, skills, and abilities required of both producers and users of goods and services.

A Case for Modernizing Work Options for People With Developmental Disabilities

By the year 2000, labor-intensive work will represent only 15 percent of the workplace, and the unskilled person will be structurally unemployable in the United States (Daggett, 1995). Although some routine, labor-intensive jobs will always exist, they will require the ability to interface with technology. The work world will be characterized by increased automation and robotization, flexible production schedules requiring frequent resetting of assembly lines, and a greater use of information technologies, computer interfaces, and computer-mediated processes. Workers will be required to perform multiple skills, utilize a multidimensional knowledge of products, processes and procedures, and use higher-order skills to interact with symbols on a computer. The work force will shift from production, assembly, and task oriented work, to knowledge, service, and outcome work (Ryan, 1995).

In the new-information age, the challenge will include the ability to:

- interface with multiple platforms (Windows®, Macintosh®, etc.) in a constantly changing environment
- adapt to job demands that are assignment-specific, rather than task-specific
- periodically relearn and retool
- interpret symbolic, verbal, oral, and visual representations
- independently execute tasks that require problem-solving and decision-making
- fund and train personnel to provide multiple interventions and long-term follow-up.

While computers and technology present challenges, they also create opportunities. Technology offers:

- a method for performing complex and multidexterous tasks using standard user-to-computer interfaces or access

▎ accommodations for physical, sensory, perceptual, cognitive, and performance limitations

▎ reduction of multiple-step commands to single buttons, symbols or icons

▎ activities that are consistent in format and content

▎ analogous operating concepts for similar tasks across different platforms.

Historically, employment outcomes for persons with developmental disabilities demonstrate that many are placed in the very jobs that are expected to stagnate or decline in the future (Kiernan, McGaughey & Schalock, 1988; U.S. Department of Labor, 1995). Further, education and skills training has been task-specific with little or no integration of learning for a functional purpose. Persons with disabilities are often unable to develop a career path or meet the needs of new environments because they are not given the opportunity to develop employability and transferable skills. They are placeable in specific jobs but not employable in a changing environment.

To increase employability for information and automated work environments, training strategies that integrate critical thinking, decision-making, and problem-solving with social and job-related skills are essential. Computer technology offers a window of opportunity. In recent years, teachers, therapists, and researchers have discovered the power of computer technology as a tool for circumventing learning difficulties associated with disabilities. Computers are a motivating medium, one that enables individuals with disabilities to fully experience the information world. By their very nature, computers expose an individual to language and enhance their ability to read, understand, and communicate. Computers can provide useful reading and writing opportunities, as well as options for the understanding and execution of instructions, the development of decision-making and problem-solving skills, and the internalization of cause and effect. Independence in cognitive skills (learning, decision-making, and problem-solving) is inherent in the successful execution of computer tasks. When combined with an integrated program that addresses other critical vocational behaviors such as job-seeking skills, and social, community, and personal living competencies (Krantz, 1971), options for employment and employability are enhanced.

The computer has become a prevalent work tool of modern business, including rehabilitation settings (Burkhead & Sampson, 1985; Sampson, McMahon & Burkhead, 1985; Schmitt & Growick, 1985). Today's office, communication, clerical, and administrative support tasks are largely being done with the help of computers. Computers have created entrepreneurial opportunities as well as options for job sharing and home offices (Murray & Kenny, 1990). Use of computers and assistive technology has expanded access to new work environments by persons who have been traditionally excluded from work because of severe physical or cognitive disabilities. Computers are also evident in many "nontechnology" positions. Even in low-skill, highly labor-intensive positions, the ability to interface with a keypad or keyboard is necessary to clock time, enter employee or job numbers, and access benefits. Leisure, daily living activities, and access to routine services, such as banking, customer service, and libraries, often require the ability to type information to obtain services.

Pioneering Efforts to Expand Available Work Options

Results of computer-skills training programs with individuals who are developmentally disabled indicate that the training provides a number of benefits, including increases in communication skills, concentration, memory, perceptual skills, reading skills, dexterity, cognition, independent functioning, vocational development and exploration, self-esteem, and socialization (Armstrong, & Rennie, 1986; Fiedorowicz, 1986; Links & Frydenberg, 1988; Wood, 1986). Successful computer-training efforts with individuals who are developmentally disabled include

- Careers in Automation for Persons with Severe Physical Disabilities (Lash & Licenziato, 1995)
- Project COMPETE (Mann & Svorai, 1994)
- Goodwill Industries, Hartford, Connecticut (Ross, 1991)
- Hawaii State Planning Council on Developmental Disabilities Computer Training Project (Peet, Saka, & Nakasone, 1985).

Several successful programs in North Carolina have provided computer and technology training and jobs to individuals with physical and cognitive limitations. Through Adaptive Technology Centers, Inc., over 280 individuals with severe disabilities have been served since 1988. Over 78 percent of those trained have had a positive employment outcome in positions, such as office clerk, data entry clerk, mail clerk, and shipping/handling/order processing (S. Primlani, personal communication, January 8, 1997). COPYMATIC is a company started in 1989 by United Cerebral Palsy of North Carolina, using the entrepreneurial business model. It offers copying, computer graphics, database, and mailing services and employs and integrates severely- to moderately-disabled adults with nondisabled employees. The company employs over 50 workers with disabilities in all aspects of the business in five North Carolina cities (Ranii, 1994; S. Collura, Director, COPYMATIC, personal communication, February 14, 1997).

COMPuter Utilization Training for Employment (Project COMPUTE) was a 2-year project in North Carolina designed to encourage changes in the delivery of services and vocational outcomes for persons with developmental disabilities through the development of a computer-skills training model (Neulicht, Primlani, & Chewning, 1995). Grant activities also included a study tour of existing training programs, labor market analysis, multidisciplinary assessment, a program guide and videotape. COMPUTE involved 12 consumers, aged 21 to 42, most with multiple impairments, including mild mental retardation, autism, cerebral palsy, severe visual impairment, and psychosis. The only criteria for inclusion into the training model was a desire to learn to use a computer to improve vocational options. Three of the consumers were not literate, and the rest of the group read and wrote minimally. Ten consumers worked in a traditional workshop, performing assembly and production tasks prior to computer training. Average training time to develop both general and job specific skills was 350 hours. The program provided 16 hours of training per week, over a 12-month period (two groups of six consumers). Staff-to-consumer ratio was predominantly 1:6 but varied by consumer and activity. One-to-one instruction was utilized for clerical skills and literacy instruction. Consumers who trained through Project COMPUTE demonstrated a marked increase in their abilities to access and utilize computers. They also demonstrated significantly increased self-esteem, self-confidence, and work-appropriate behaviors.

Project TechWork, as a progression of COMPUTE, is a grant-funded project designed to provide the methods and means for persons with severe developmental disabilities to obtain gainful technology-based employment through the use of assistive technology. The consumers range in mental retardation from severe to moderate, with other severe to mild physical and mental disabilities. The project is a multiagency collaborative effort led by Murdoch Center, a state residential MR/DD facility. It involves consumers from Murdoch Center, INCO, a community rehabilitation facility and supported-employment contractor, and the Granville County Schools Transition Program. Other state agencies have collaborated in support of the project including Vocational Rehabilitation services, the regional community college, the North Carolina Assistive Technology Project, and the University of North Carolina at Chapel Hill. To date, a three-part screening tool for adults with developmental disabilities has been developed and used to assess, identify, and prioritize candidates for vocational-technology services. Over 120 referrals have been screened and training has begun for the Murdoch Center residents. A 12-section computer-based access evaluation has been developed and is used to identify job-access issues, assistive-technology recommendations, and consumer-training needs. Two TechWork jobs have been contracted that involve updating customer mailing lists and printing labels (a value-added service to the already existing job of folding mailers) for bulk mailing services. Software has been developed that adapts existing business-based data management systems to the literacy, cognitive, and physical needs of the consumers. The software is used to augment consumer computer-skills training and to enable consumers to perform in the mailing jobs. Additional marketing to develop jobs that involve barcoding and document imaging has been initiated and includes partnering with a leading international document imaging systems company. Several graduating high school students have been successfully placed into job sampling sites, and one student applied for and attained a permanent competitive-wage, computer-based inventory restocking system job. Ongoing vocational technology assessment and training services for north-central North Carolina have been integrated into North Carolina's state DD Services 10-Year Plan.

Modern Job Market Areas for People with Developmental Disabilities

The job analyses and industry interviews conducted through Project COMPUTE and TechWork confirmed how much the work world has become information-based. To be used effectively, information has to be generated, updated, stored, and distributed, and the computer is the most prevalent tool.

Work involving computer-based technologies involves both the operation of equipment and the management of data. The data can range from simple to complex and continuous text and graphics. Operating procedures can range from simple to complex, multistep instructions. Computer tasks can be categorized as: command and control, discrete data entry, document processing, graphics, and systems integration including programming. The focus in Project COMPUTE's and TechWork's labor-market research was on jobs involving production, maintenance, and distribution of information.

Of most promise for persons with severe disabilities are command and control tasks. These tasks include those where the operator makes routine selections from datasets or a computer interface operating the equipment. Examples include touch-screen interfaces to operate high-volume copiers, mail-handling equipment, and communication equipment, such as phone/modem/fax machines. Automated copiers perform a range of collating, binding, and stapling tasks, producing bound and loose-leaf documents. Discrete data entry tasks—such as entering or updating a database, order-processing, payment/remittance processing, or inventory clerking—offer other viable employment options. Potential document-processing tasks include imaging, paging and formatting, cutting and pasting, archiving, assembly of boilerplate, as well as the printing of form letters. An interesting position was developed at a newspaper office, where individuals paged copy to meet the publisher's requirements. Another potential market is on-line transcription of messages for a telephone paging company. Even though it is production work, such messages can be abbreviated, lending themselves to standardized message formats and reducing the number of keystrokes required.

We found that office automation itself can be considered an accommodation with positive vocational outcomes for individuals with severe disabilities. For example, the industry trend is to reduce decision-making to limited parameters and standardized operating procedures, using barcodes for data input, icons/symbols to graphically represent tasks, and scanning to reduce keystrokes. Further, automated conveyor belts, hydraulic lifts, spring-loaded carts and trays reduce material handling and physically demanding lifting and carrying tasks. The manufacturing sector also proffers many machines that are operated by computerized touch pads.

Additional examples of "mainstream accommodation" include hand-held microcomputers with keypads and barcode scanners. These tools help manage inventory both in stores and in distribution centers. The input devices have been designed to accommodate all types of users, including a hands-free device. The warehouse clerk, micrographics technician, or order processor must understand only the codes for location and item prior to entering the number of units requested. Manual tasks are often reduced to shelving/removing of items and literacy demands are low.

Program Planning in a New Work Age: Staff, Equipment, Support, Consumer Assessment, Job Marketing, Training, and Job Procurement

Prior to starting a computer-skills training program, one must consider staff and equipment resources. Instructors, including job coaches, and job-development specialists must themselves be computer-literate in order to train and effectively market services to the business community. Equipment must be in working order and able to support all desired applications. As with any new service, attitudes and the acceptance by staff, family, and employers may be guarded at first. Active community involvement through a Business Advisory Council or Employment Advisory Board is necessary to develop volunteer/internship experiences and jobs. Funding through private, community, state, and federal grants, should be solicited to begin this effort and a fee for service agreement, through the Division of Vocational Rehabilitation, should be utilized to maintain and expand training and placement.

A profile of the consumers' issues and strengths is important for modern job matching. Some issues that are common to people with DD become especially important to consider when preparing consumers for the information age. For example, literacy remediation is likely to be an issue for DD consumers and must be considered as part of an integrated program, not an "add on" service. In addition, visual and visual processing issues, such as ocular motor control, visual tracking, visual-motor integration, field deficits, visual acuity, visual accommodation, and visual perception become critical when planning for visual access to modern equipment such as computers (Cook & Hussey, 1995). Cook and Hussey cited a 1979 study by R. Duckman of 25 children with cerebral palsy that revealed substantial and extensive vision issues within the study group. Ninety-two percent of the participants had ocular motor dysfunction, 40 percent had significant refractive errors, 56 percent exhibited strabismus, 100 percent demonstrated accommodation deficiencies, and 78 percent had issues with visual perception. Often, these issues remain hidden unless the consumer is evaluated for these components, or until the more demanding functional requirements of computer access come into play. Other critical sensory areas to consider are hearing (as used for auditory computer feedback), and tactile and proprioceptive issues (for computer input). The latter become especially important when adapted computer input is used, and visual and auditory cues are not immediately available.

A consumer-centered, comprehensive vocational plan is essential to placing persons with DD in the modern workplace. The inclusive vocational plan, coupled with an awareness of the particular issues related to modern jobs, can greatly increase the consumer's chances for success. Programs must make a commitment to analyze the job market, develop the profile of consumer skills, and create a job match that goes beyond traditional food service and janitorial positions, so that individuals with developmental disabilities can be employable in the new information age.

Consumer Case Examples

The following case examples illustrate individual personal and professional progress as a result of computer skills training.

Jake

Jake, a 22 year old gentleman with Down's Syndrome, earned a high school certificate through participation in a self-contained Educable Mentally Handicapped (EMH) program. Jake functioned in the moderate range of mental retardation and was not literate. A baseline evaluation revealed that Jake was unfamiliar with basic punctuation marks and rules for capitalization. Verbal skills were limited to simple phrases. Prior to training, computer experience was limited to games on an Apple IIG with nonrhythmic random keyboarding. During training, Jake required both verbal instruction and demonstration, as he had difficulty with written instructions. Jake also demonstrated social immaturity with mildly inappropriate social behaviors and hygiene issues. A word-prediction program was used to enhance generative writing and improve language ability. Jake's training plan goals included a focus on reading and following instructions, maintaining and following a schedule, and increasing social and vocational maturity by teaching job expectations and behaviors.

At the conclusion of approximately 500 hours of training over a 4-year period (200 hours in a 2-year school-based model), Jake was independent in his use of the keyboard and mouse. He demonstrated functional use of MS Windows®, drop menus, and other keyboard commands. His keyboard speed using the complete keyboard was 12 wpm, keypad at 15 wpm, and data entry at 1600–1800 keystrokes per hour (kph). He learned to recognize and interpret standard icons and symbols, use basic commands to independently operate WordPerfect 5.1 for DOS and Windows, transcribe text, copy simple letters and memos, generate simple sentences, as well as perform database update tasks such as data entry, searching, and correcting from source material, including alphanumeric and coded information. He also learned to sort alphabetically and numerically using a sorter and became independent with most clerical and bulk-mailing tasks.

Jake has been competitively employed full-time for 7 months as an office clerk. He now independently rides public transportation to work. His duties include using a computer to enter weekly time sheets for all employees at a temporary agency, sorting incoming mail, metering and preparing outgoing mail, and operating a copier and document shredder. He is independent in his tasks and follows a general routine with occasional variation. Jake is now aware of his personal appearance and behaviors. He has decided to change his eating habits so as to avoid burping in public, and, as a special note, for Valentine's Day, he bought candy for his coworkers. He has transitioned from a self-contained EMH class—with job expectations in food service/janitorial work—to competitive employment in an office setting, using technology, computers, and natural supports.

Michelle

Michelle is a 24-year-old woman with cerebral palsy and moderate mental retardation who uses a wheelchair for mobility. Activities using fine-finger dexterity, grip, and grasp were impaired. She exhibited motor control and planning issues, as well as problems with visual tracking and accommodation. Difficulty sequencing, categorizing, and comprehending multistep verbal instructions were noted. Michelle was a nonreader, with limited sight word vocabulary and decoding strategies. Michelle's strengths included excellent interpersonal skills, good verbal communication and conversational skills, and she was highly motivated to learn and perform new tasks well.

Michelle had no exposure to a computer or keyboard prior to training. During the initial evaluation, she entered text without spacing or knowledge of punctuation and capitalization. She needed frequent repetition of verbal and modeled instructions and needed affirmation for each keystroke. Michelle's training plan goals included increasing sight word (work) vocabulary, executing single-word, stepped, written instruction, maintaining a schedule, and increasing self-confidence.

At the conclusion of 320 hours of training over a 6-month period, Michelle was keyboarding using a nonrhythmic 10-finger method at 8 wpm, keypad at 8 wpm, and data entry at 980 kph. She was functional with simple list menus and learned keyboard commands. She could enter text with spaces between words and some punctuation as well as simple alphanumeric data into a single screen. Her decision-making confidence dramatically improved, and she was able to tell professionals at a national conference to give people like her a chance "because we can do it."

Michelle is now employed full time, with natural supports, in a competitive position as a greeter. She maintains a flexible schedule and has received compliments from her employer regarding her learning ability. Michelle has transitioned from performing below competitive standards in a workshop setting to competitive employment with natural supports. She has since married and has moved into her own apartment.

Jerry: What the Future Could Hold

Let's look back in on Jerry, after his successful transition to community-based work, and peer into what the future could bring:

> Jerry improved significantly on his job at the footwear distributor after his team-based vocational intervention. He was able to improve on his visual and perceptual skills well enough that, together with the compensatory environmental and job modifications, his job performance improved to nearly competitive standards. He also received a pay raise reflecting his improved performance. Moving Jerry into proximity with other warehouse workers and designing job modifications that helped everybody and increased coworker interaction significantly opened favorable relations among Jerry and the other employees. Jerry's subsequent improvement in social awareness and hygiene skills added to an increased awareness and involvement of his coworkers, creating a positive working environment.
>
> Based on his favorable experience and desire to do more vocationally, Jerry had expressed an interest in gaining some new job skills. The rehabilitation counselor worked with Jerry to identify some interest areas. It was then that his employer and VR services were contacted regarding Jerry's aspirations. One of Jerry's interests was to work in distribution and with the computer. (During the period Jerry had been employed at the footwear distributor, the shipping department had become more automated with a computer-based system.) Jerry's employer was interested in keeping him as an employee and Jerry expressed that he, too, enjoyed where he worked. A computer-access evaluation was performed by an occupational therapy Assistive Technology Practitioner (ATP) with a computer applications background, a vocational counselor, and an evaluator. The evaluation revealed that Jerry could benefit from basic computer-use training and literacy training. It was recommended that his computer access could be improved by using two devices: a switch-adapted track-ball in place of the standard mouse, and a key guard to reduce errant keystrokes caused by his spasticity and motor-control issues. The distribution station would also require some minor access modifications and an adjustable work table. Because the automated distribution system uses barcodes for inventory identification and shipping lists, it was recommended that Jerry begin by

spending part of his day performing some of these tasks. His employer agreed and initiated the natural supports to begin training Jerry on the new tasks. Based on a commitment from Jerry's employer, VR services implemented a training program that included an adapted computer class and literacy training. After some discussion between VR services and Jerry's employer regarding financial responsibility for the implementation of recommended job accommodations, an agreement was reached. Jerry would be loaned his assistive technology by the State Tech Act Project during his training classes. After successful training, Jerry's employer would take advantage of the tax adjustments offered through the ADA and implement all necessary job modifications at the company's cost. With support and the appropriate intervention, it appears that Jerry is on his way to modern-based employment in his community.

RESOURCES FOR THE OCCUPATIONAL THERAPY PRACTITIONER IN WORK AND DEVELOPMENTAL DISABILITIES

The Internet, a Rapidly Expanding Source of Information: *Hitch a Ride, Hire a Cab or Take a Bus, . . . But, by All Means, Get Moving on the Information Superhighway!*

The Internet is here and, from a 1998 perspective, it arrived almost overnight! Although the Internet may seem intimidating to many, very recent developments are making the Internet, the World Wide Web, and the various on-line services continuously easier to access and use (Crumlish, 1996). Computer, software, and information-based technology companies are committing tremendous amounts of their resources to this global information system (Hof, 1997). Hof underscores this when he quotes Microsoft Corporation Chairman Bill Gates: "The Internet is the most important thing going on for us. It's driving everything at Microsoft." According to Hof, in addition to allocating enormous amounts of its $2.1 billion research and development budget for Net products, Microsoft has recently spent $750 million investing in 20 Internet-related companies. Such a market emphasis, coupled with dramatically increased accessibility, is making the Net a pervasive entity of modern life. It will not pay to ignore the information superhighway. It probably will not go away, and it will likely affect almost everyone's life.

The Internet is important to both professionals and consumers of disability services and products. New Websites are being posted at a rate of thousands per week. Some of these sites are rehabilitation- and disability-related, including professional, service-agency, and disability-related company Websites. AOTA, state occupational therapy associations, RESNA, ARC (Association for Retarded Citizens), United Cerebral Palsy, Job Accommodations Network, among many others, have sites. A recent look at an occupational therapy-related Website (InternOT) revealed a listing of over 30 other occupational therapy sites available at that time. Disability consumers and professionals now have access to a world of services, product information, software, bibliographic databases, sociability and even work opportunities, all via computer and modem. Communication with colleagues internationally is easily supported through e-mail, while groups of individuals can communicate with others of like interests through e-mail listservers. An example of this is the AOTA Technology Special Interest Section listserver, where members may pose questions to the group and participate in discussions regarding assistive-technology applications. Collaborative efforts such as writing and research can occur remarkably well through Internet communications. This chapter, for example, was cowritten by authors in two locations with all literature searches, resource searches, document transfers, and revisions among the two authors occurring over the Net. Efforts to promote access to and use of the Internet's resources are offered to consumers and professionals alike. For example, in addition to the work-related computer training projects in North Carolina cited earlier, another grant-funded project, Partnerships in Assistive Technology (PAT), is fostering consumer access to the Net and assistive technology. It includes a consumer-drive Website with numerous professional and consumer resources, including assistance in acquiring hardware and Internet access, as well as training.

The information superhighway is not without its disadvantages. For instance, increasing reliance the Internet poses access issues, and it becomes essential to ensure that people with disabilities may freely use the information superhighway. The Trace Research and Development Center at the University of Wisconsin-Madison is one of the pioneers in addressing these concerns, and its Website offers a significant number of papers and reports on these efforts. Trace Center's Webpage also lists four other programs contributing to the effort of "curb cuts" on the information superhighway.

Probably one of the most important questions that arises regarding the Internet today is: "How do I access it?" Fortunately, just as occupational therapy-related Websites abound, so do opportunities to learn to gain access to them. Introductory sessions offered at conferences or local continuing-education programs can be extremely helpful. This can be combined with one of many publications on the subject, along with taking advantage of the competitive offers made by the on-line service companies. It all comes down to taking the leap and trying it out. Because of the nearly *warp-speed* growth of the Net, it is important to use the most updated resources available when you do take that plunge.

Organizational Resources for Practitioners and Consumers

Because of the community-based nature of most DD work intervention, the available resources come from a combination of professional and consumer-related organizations. Many of these organizations have state or local chapters. Some key organizational resources include:

American Occupational Therapy Association
Developmental Disabilities Special Interest Section (SIS)
Technology SIS
Work Programs SIS
PO Box 31220
Bethesda, MD 20824-1220
Phone: (301) 652-2682; TDD: (800) 377-8555; Members: (800) SAY-AOTA
Internet/Website: http://www.aota.org/

Americans with Disabilities Act Document Center
Internet/Website: http://janweb.icdi.wvu.edu/kinder/#home

The Arc (Association for Retarded Citizens)
National Headquarters
PO Box 1047
Arlington, TX 76004
Phone: (817) 261-6003; TDD: (817) 277-0553
Internet/Website: http://thearc.org/welcome.html

Association for Persons in Supported Employment
1627 Monument Avenue
Richmond, VA 23220
Phone: (804) 278-9187 Fax: (804) 278-9377
Internet/Website: http://www.apse.org
E-mail: apse@apse.org

Brain Injury Association Inc. (formerly: National Head Injury Foundation)
1776 Massachusetts Avenue, NW, Suite 100

Washington, DC 20036-1904
Phone: (202) 296-6443; Fax: (202) 296-8850
The toll free information and resource number is: 800-444-6443
Internet/Website: http://www.biausa.org

Closing The Gap, Inc.
PO Box 68
526 Main Street
Henderson, MN 56044
Phone: (507) 248-3294; Fax: (507) 248-3810
E-mail: info@closingthegap.com
Internet/Website: http://www.closingthegap.com

The Down Syndrome Research Foundation and Resource Center
3580 Slocan Street
Vancouver, BC V5M3E8
Phone: (604) 431-9694; Fax: (604) 431-9248
E-mail: dsrf@sfu.ca
Internet/Website: http://fas.sfu.ca/kin/ds/

Job Accommodation Network (JAN)
West Virginia University
PO Box 6080
Morgantown, WV 26506-6080
Phone: (800) 526-7234
Internet/Website: http://janweb.icdi.wvu.edu/

National Down Syndrome Society
666 Broadway, 8th Floor
New York, NY 10012-2317
Phone: (212) 460-9330; (800) 221-4602
Internet/Website: http://www.ndss.org/

National Association for Down Syndrome
PO Box 4542
Oak Brook, IL 60522-4542
Internet/Website: http://www.nads.org/

National Down Syndrome Congress
1605 Chantilly Drive, Suite 250
Atlanta, GA 30324-3269
Phone: (800) 232-6372
Internet/Website: http://www.carol.net/~ndsc/

National Rehabilitation Association
633 South Washington Street
Alexandria, VA 22314-4293
Phone: (703) 836-0850

National Rehabilitation Counseling Association (NRCA)
8807 Sudley Road, #102
Manassas, VA 22110-4719
Phone: (703) 361-2077; Fax: (703) 361-2489
E-mail: nrcaoffice@aol.com
Internet/Website: http://www.nationalrehab.org

National Rehabilitation Information Center (NARIC)
8455 Colesville Road, Suite 935
Silver Spring, MD 20910-3319
Phone: (301) 588-9284; (800) 346-2742
Internet/Website: http://www.naric.com/naric/

President's Committee on Employment of People with Disabilities
1331 F Street, NW, Suite 300
Washington, DC 20004
Phone: (202) 376-6200; FAX: (202) 376-6219; TDD: (202) 376-6205
Internet/Website: http://www.pcepd.gov/

RESNA (Rehabilitation Engineering and Assistive Technology Society of North America)
1700 North Moore Street, Suite 1540
Arlington, VA 22209-1903
Phone: 703-524-6686; Fax: 703-524-6630; TTY: 703-524-6639
Internet/Website: http://www.resna.org/reshome.htm

Trace Research and Development Center
S-151 Waismen Center
University of Wisconsin-Madison
Madison, WI 53705-2280
Phone: (608) 262-6966; TDD: (608) 263-5408
Internet/Website: http://trace.wisc.edu/

United Cerebral Palsy Associations, Inc.
1660 L Street, NW
Washington, DC 20036-5602
1-800-USA-5UCP

Phone/TDD: (202) 776-0406; Fax: (202) 776-0414
Internet/Website: http://www.ucpa.org/
E-mail: ucpanatl@ucpa.org

Vocational Evaluation and Work Adjustment Association (VEWAA)
200 East Cheyenne Mountain Boulevard, Suite N
Colorado Springs, CO 80906
Phone/TDD: (719) 527-1800; Fax: (719) 576-1818
Internet/Website: http://www.impactonline.org/vewaa
E-mail: 76101.3626@compuserve.com

Virginia Commonwealth University
Rehabilitation Research and Training Center on Supported Employment
1314 West Main Street
PO Box 842011
Richmond, VA 23284-2011
Phone: (804) 828-1851; TDD: (804) 828-249
Internet/Website: http://www.vcu.edu/rrtcweb

SUMMARY

Work is essential to our development, social contribution, and livelihood. It is a means by which we contribute to our daily needs, and it sustains a shared context for meeting social values and needs. Work offers us a sense of mastery over our environment, as well as a sense of accomplishment and competence, leading to a heightened sense of self-esteem. All too often, opportunities to experience these same qualities of life are thwarted for persons with developmental disabilities. However, with appropriate and comprehensive vocational-related services, people with DD have been able to contribute more to the quality of their lives and to their community. Occupational therapy practitioners can play a pivotal role in providing the team-based services that can impact on work and community outcomes for this population.

Vocational services for adults with DD have gone through significant changes since the beginning of this century. Since the 1970s, shifts in services have opened new opportunities for more meaningful community-based living, bringing about an array of increased challenges for consumers with DD and their service providers. Because of the range of associated issues and their impact on work, these opportunities and challenges vary among individuals and their service-delivery environments. An awareness of these issues is critical to providing appropriate and effective vocational services to the consumer.

With the shift to more community-based services, there is an increasing need for effective occupational therapy services in community settings. Occupational therapists can contribute to the vocational intervention team with specific work-based practices or with more general occupational therapy services. As part of the team, an occupational therapist's role is to help identify potential and actual inhibitors to a consumer's work performance. The occupational therapist can make the recommendations necessary to help remediate and compensate for the identified issues, leading to the consumer's improved occupational performance.

Assistive technology is becoming an increasingly applicable tool to facilitate successful work outcomes for people with disabilities. This is an added component that may be an expected part of occupational therapy service provision. Occupational therapists can now provide AT services as a RESNA Certified Assistive Technology Practitioner or Supplier or use their general awareness of AT to refer the consumer and team to an AT service provider.

The workplace has become less labor-intensive and more computer-based, and consumers with DD need to be prepared for employment opportunities associated with the technological demand. Knowledge of both contemporary job market trends and the specific consumer's issues and strengths is important for job matching. Issues such as literacy, vision and visual processing, physical, cognitive and cultural access to work and equipment, and cognitive performance (for example, attention to task, distractibility, left-to-right sequencing, and learning) are common to people with DD and must be considered when preparing consumers for the information age of work. A consumer-centered, comprehensive vocational plan is essential to placing persons with DD in the modern workplace. Further, an awareness of the particular issues related to modern jobs will greatly increase our consumers' chances for success as members of our communities today. In conclusion, as Radabaugh (1988) so eloquently said, "Technology makes things easier for most people. For individuals with disabilities, technology makes things possible." There are limitless opportunities for those who take the challenge.

ACKNOWLEDGEMENTS

The authors gratefully acknowledge the assistance of Martin Rice, Ph.D., OTR/L, Medical College of Ohio, for his review and comments on a draft of this chapter; Bob Robertson, OTR/L, Murdoch Center, for his review and comments on sections of the draft; and Denise Plachcinski, MEd, Murdoch Center, for her contributions to the chapter's knowledge-base through her work and leadership on Project TechWork.

REFERENCES

Abbott, M., Franciscus, M., & Weeks, Z. R. (1988). An overview of occupational therapy. *Occupational therapy careers* (pp. 1–11). Lincolnwood, IL: VGM Career Horizons, National Textbook Company.

Adelstein, L. A. (1992). Work-related treatment for youth. *Work, 2*(2), 7–10.

Adults with developmental disabilities. (1995, Fall). *OT Week for Today's Student*, 16.

Angelo, J., & Gross, K. (Eds.). (1994). Special issue on relationships with colleagues and clients [Special issue.] *Technology Special Interest Section Newsletter, 4* (2).

American Occupational Therapy Association. (1992). White paper: Occupational therapy and the Americans with Disabilities Act. *American Journal of Occupational Therapy, 46*, 470–471.

American Occupational Therapy Association. (1994). Uniform terminology for occupational therapy—third edition. *American Journal of Occupational Therapy, 48*, 1047–1059.

Armstrong, J., & Rennie, J. (1986). We can use computers too: The setting up of a project for mentally handicapped residents. *British Journal of Occupational Therapy, 49*(9), 297–300.

Barber, M., McInerny, C. A., & Struck, M. (1993). Training for independence: Transition from school to work. AOTA, *Work Programs Special Interest Section Newsletter, 7*(2), 1–2.

Bellamy, G. T., Rhodes, L. E., Bourbeau, P. E., & Mank, D. M. (1986) Mental retardation services in sheltered workshops and day activity programs: Consumer benefits and policy alternatives. In F. R. Rusch (Ed.). *Competitive employment issues and strategies*. Baltimore, MD: Paul H. Brookes.

Blackwell, T. L., Conrad, A. D., & Weed, R. O. (1992). *Job analysis and the ADA: A step by step guide*. Athens, GA: Elliott & Fitzpatrick.

Brollier, C., Shepherd, J., & Markley, K. F. (1994). Transition from school to community living. *American Journal of Occupational Therapy, 48*, 346–353.

Burkhead, E. J., & Sampson, Jr., J. P. (1985). Computer-assisted assessment in support of the rehabilitation process. *Rehabilitation Counseling Bulletin, 28* (4), 262–273.

Carrasco, R. C. (1993). Work-related programs for children and adolescents: Part I. AOTA, *Work Programs Special Interest Section Newsletter, 7*(1), 1–4.

Cook, A. M., & Hussey, S. M. (1995). *Assistive Technologies: Principles and practice*. St. Louis, MO: Mosby-Year Book.

Costello, C. (1992). School-based supported work/supported employment. *Work 2*(2), 11–14.

Crimando, W., & Goodley, S. H. (1985) The computer's potential in enhancing employment opportunities of persons with disabilities. *Rehabilitation Counseling Bulletin, 28*(4), 275–282.

Crist, P. A., & Stoffel, V. C. (1992). The Americans with Disabilities Act of 1990 and employees with mental impairments: Personal efficacy and the environment. *American Journal of Occupational Therapy, 46,* 434–443.

Crumlish, C. (1996). *The Internet for busy people.* Berkeley, CA: Osborne/Mc-Graw-Hill.

Daggett, W. R. (1995). Technology: What is it? Keynote address. Schenectady, NY: International Center for Leadership in Education, Inc.

Dwyre, A. E., & Trach, J. S. (1996). Consumer choice for people with cognitive disabilities: Who makes the choices in the job search process? *Journal of Applied Rehabilitation Counseling, 27*(3) 42–47.

Federal Register. (1984). *Employment of handicapped clients in sheltered workshops.* Chapter V, Part 525, 17509.

Fiedorowicz, C. A. M. (1986). Training of component reading skills. *Annals of Dyslexia, 36,* 318–334.

Gordon, R. E., & Kozole, K. P. (1984). Occupational therapy and rehabilitation engineering: A team approach to helping persons with severe physical disability to upgrade functional independence. *Occupational Therapy in Health Care, 1* (4), 117–129.

Havranek, J. E. (1992). Methods and uses of job analysis: Implications for implementation of the Americans with Disabilities Act of 1990. *NARPPS Journal & News, 7*(3): 113–117.

Hill, M., Hill, J. W., Wehman, P., Revell, G., Dickerson, A., & Noble, J. H. (1987). Supported employment: An interagency funding model for persons with severe disabilities. *Journal of Rehabilitation, 53*(3): 13–21.

Hof, R. D. (1997, February 10). Netspeed at Netscape [cover story]. *Business Week* [on-line].

Jacobs, K., & Wyrick, J. (1989). Use of Department of Labor references and job analysis. In S. Hertfelder & C. Gwen (Eds.), *Work in Progress* (23–65). Bethesda, MD: American Occupational Therapy Association.

Kielhofner, G. (1992). Functional assessment: Toward a dialectical view of person-environment relations. *American Journal of Occupational Therapy, 43,* 248–251.

Kiernan, W. E., McGaughey, M. J., & Schalock, R. L. (1988). Employment environments and outcome for adults with developmental disabilities. *Mental Retardation, 26*(5), 279–288.

Kirkland, M., & Robertson, S. C. (Eds.). (1985). *Planning and implementing vocational readiness in occupational therapy.* Bethesda, MD: American Occupational Therapy Association.

Kornblau, B. L. (1996). The occupational therapist and vocational evaluation. AOTA, *Work Programs Special Interest Section Newsletter, 10*(1), 1–4.

Krantz, G. (1971). Critical vocational behaviors. *Journal of Rehabilitation, 36,* 14–16.

Lagomarcino, T. (1986). Community services. In F. Rusch (Ed.), *Competitive employment issues and strategies* (pp. 65–75). Baltimore, MD: Paul H. Brookes.

Links, C. & Frydenberg, H. (1988). Microcomputer skills training program for the physically disabled in long term rehabilitation. *Physical and Occupational Therapy in Geriatrics, 6*(3–4), 133–140.

Lash, L., & Licenziato, V. (1995). Career transitions for persons with severe physical disabilities: Integrating technological and psychosocial skills and accommodations. *Work, 5,* 85–98.

Mann, W. C., & Svorai, S. B. (1994). COMPETE: A model for vocational evaluation, training, employment, and community for integration for persons with cognitive impairments. *American Journal of Occupational Therapy, 48,* 446–451.

Metzler, C. A. (1995). Federal legislation and services for persons with developmental disabilities. AOTA, *Developmental Disabilities Special Interest Section Newsletter. 18*(2): 1–3.

Minkel, J. L. (1995). Assistive technology credentialing: What is RESNA's program and plan? AOTA, *Technology Special Interest Section Newsletter, 5*(3), 1–2.

Minkel, J. L. (1996). Credentialing in assistive technology: Myths and realities. *RESNA News, 8*(5), 1, 6–7.

Mitchell, M. M. (1985). Values. In M. Kirkland & S. C. Robertson (Eds.). *Planning and implementing vocational readiness in occupational therapy* (pp. 45–47). Bethesda, MD: American Occupational Therapy Association.

Mitchell, M. M., Rourk, J. D., & Schwarz, J. (1989). A team approach to prevocational services. *American Journal of Occupational Therapy, 43,* 378–383.

Murray, B., & Kenny, S. (1990). Telework as an employment option for people with disabilities. *International Journal of Rehabilitation Research, 12*(3), 205–214.

Neulicht, A., Primlani, S., & Chewning, L. (1995). *Computer utilization training for employment: A program guide.* North Carolina: Council on Developmental Disabilities.

North Carolina Vocational Alternatives Task Force (1992). *Supported employment in North Carolina.* Raleigh, NC: Author.

Olshansky, S. (1971). Breaking workshop exit barriers. *Rehabilitation Record, 12*(6), 27–30.

Parent, W. S., Hill, M. L., & Wehman, P. (1989). From sheltered to supported employment outcomes: Challenges for rehabilitation facilities. *Journal of Rehabilitation, 55*(4), 51–57.

Peet, W., Saka, T., & Nakasone, D. (1985). *Teaching work processing to young handicapable adults: A manual for the trainer.* Hawaii State Planning Council on Developmental Disabilities Computer Training Project.

President's Committee on Mental Retardation. (1977). *Mental retardation past and present.* Author: Washington, DC.

Prouty, R., & Lakin, K. C. (Eds.). (1996). *Residential services for persons with developmental disabilities: Status and trends through 1995* (Report #48). Minneapolis: The College of Education and Human Development, University of Minnesota.

Radabaugh, P. (1988). *Quality indicators applicable to service delivery programs.* Atlanta, GA: The Smart Exchange.

Ranii, D. (1994, October 29) Thriving on unusual strategy. *Raleigh News and Observer,* pp. 1D, 6D.

Reed, K. L. (1991). Part I—Developmental disorders. *Quick reference to occupational therapy* (pp. 1–86). Gaithersburg, MD: Aspen.

Reynolds-Lynch, K. (1985). In M. Kirkland & S. C. Robertson (Eds.), *Planning and implementing vocational readiness in occupational therapy* (pp. 175–178). Bethesda, MD: American Occupational Therapy Association.

Ross, M. (1991). Using computers for vocational training. *OT Week, 5*(10), 6–7.

Rubin, S. E., and Roessler, R. T. (1995). *Foundations of the vocational rehabilitation process* (4th ed.). Austin, TX: Pro-ed.

Rusch, F. R., & Hughes, C. (1989). Overview of supported employment. *Journal of Applied Behavior Analysis, 22*(4), 351–363.

Ryan, C. P. (1995). Work isn't what it used to be: Implications, recommendations, and strategies for vocational rehabilitation. *Journal of Rehabilitation, 61*(4), 8–15.

Sampson, Jr, J. P., McMahon, B. T., & Burkhead, E. J. (1985). Using computers for career exploration and decision making in vocational rehabilitation. *Rehabilitation Counseling Bulletin, 28*(4), 242–261.

Sandlin, J., Prouty, R., & Lakin, K. C. (1996). Large state MR/DD facility closures, 1960–2000. In R. Prouty & K. C. Lakin (Eds.) *Residential services for persons with developmental disabilities: Status and trends through 1995* (Report #48) (pp. 30–41). Minneapolis: The College of Education and Human Development, University of Minnesota.

Schmitt, P., & Growick, B. (1985). Computer technology in rehabilitation counseling. *Rehabilitation Counseling Bulletin, 28*(4), 233–240.

Shelly, C., Sample, P., & Spencer, K. (1992). The Americans with Disabilities Act of 1990 expands employment opportunities for persons with developmental disabilities. *American Journal of Occupational Therapy, 46*, 457–465.

Spence, J., Woods, J. N., & Young, P. L. (1984). The computer: Expanded uses in a sheltered workshop. *Journal of Rehabilitation, 50*(3), 64–65, 67.

Spencer, K. C. (1990). Supported employment: The role of occupational therapy at the job site. *Occupational Therapy Practice, 1*(2), 74–82.

U.S. Department of Labor. (1991a). *The revised handbook for analyzing jobs.* Washington, DC: U.S. Government Printing Office.

U.S. Department of Labor. (1991b). *The dictionary of occupational titles.* Washington, DC: U.S. Government Printing Office.

U.S. Department of Labor. (1995). *Occupational outlook handbook.* Washington, DC: U.S. Government Printing Office.

Velozo, C. A. (1992). Work evaluations: Critique of the state of the art of functional assessment of work. *American Journal of Occupational Therapy, 43*, 203–209.

Ward, K. M. (1996). School-based vocational training. In Kurtz, L. A., Dowrick, P. M., Levy, S. E., and Batshaw, M. L. (Eds.), *Handbook of developmental disabilities: resources for interdisciplinary care* (pp. 237–248). Gaithersburg, MD: Aspen Publishers.

Wehman, P. (1986). Competitive employment in Virginia. In F. Rusch (Ed.). *Competitive employment issues and strategies* (pp. 23–33). Baltimore: Paul H. Brookes.

Wehman, P., Hill, J. W., Wood, W., & Parent, W. (1987). A report of competitive employment histories of persons labeled severely mentally retarded. *Journal of the Association for Persons with Severe Handicaps, 12*(1), 11–17.

Wehman, P., & Kregel, J. (undated manuscript). At the crossroads: Supported employment ten years later. Richmond, VA: Virginia Commonwealth University Rehabilitation Research and Training Center on Supported Employment.

Wehman, P. H., & Moon, M. (1987). Critical values in employment programs for persons with developmental disabilities: A position paper. *Journal of Applied Rehabilitation Counseling, 18*(1), 12–16.

Wood, R. L. (1986). Rehabilitation of patients with disorders of attention. *Journal of Head Trauma Rehabilitation, 1*(3), 43–53.

4

An OTR's Description of the Legacy, Current Environment, and Clinical Issues Characterizing Adults with Profound Disabilities

Hollis A. Kellogg, OTR/L

Paula is a 23-year-old who spends her day in a wheelchair. She keeps her hands and arms in a flexed position. She does not use her hands to reach, grasp, or hold any objects, including food. She is nonverbal and does not utilize any gestural or pictographic communication. When upset, she yells. She is thought to be cortically blind. She is totally dependent in all aspects of self-care, and records indicate she has been so since birth. Such an individual, and others not nearly so dependent, are the subjects of this chapter.

Individuals who have mental retardation make up 2.5–3 percent of the population. Of this 3 percent, 13 percent have IQs under 50, and have serious limitations that require institutionalization or special care (ARC, 1982). Within this 13 percent, there is a still smaller percentage of individuals such as Paula. When compared to the entire mentally retarded/developmentally disabled (MR/DD) population, this is a small number of people. Many programs do not adequately serve their needs, and clinicians are not routinely taught about this very small population in baccalaureate-level programs. As states began to downsize large, overpopulated, and substandard institutions in the 1970s, the most dependent residents were often the last to be relocated. These people were described as a small but very difficult to serve population averaging 1,000 per state. Techniques for training them to leave the facilities had not been adequately developed (Stark, Baker, McGee, & Menousek, 1982), so the highest functioning residents were deinstitutionalized first.

In New York, this trend was seen in the state institutions. In 1977, 46 percent of the institutionalized residents were considered profoundly handicapped, 86 percent were toilet-trained, and 25 percent had behavioral disorders. By 1987, 62 percent were seen as profoundly impaired, and those with behavioral disorders and toilet dependency increased by 20 percent (Lakin, Hill, and Hadyn, 1989). This was due primarily to the placement of the higher functioning residents into small group homes and day programs. In order to complete the closing down of the state facilities, some day programs had higher functioning consumers discharged from their facilities to make room for the most dependent consumers still awaiting placement. At present, New York has mostly completed this first phase, and some day programs have at present a large census of those considered the most dependent. The next trend might be the phasing out of day programs, causing elimination of or changes in clinical services to the participants.

As these cost-cutting trends swing in various directions, clinicians working with those who present the greatest challenges will need frames of reference, methods, and information resources.

It is difficult to take people with developmental disabilities as a whole and then to clearly separate those with the most-challenging deficits from the rest. Generally, these are people who are defined as profoundly retarded, with an IQ of 20 or less as determined by standard psychological tests such as the Vineland or Stanford Binet scales. Terms such as *profound, severe, moderate,* and *mild* are still used to describe degrees of retardation, just as the old terms *cretin, idiot, moron,* and *imbecile* were used until they became anathematized. Another classification system contains the terms *educable, trainable,* and *subtrainable.* The terms *educable* and *trainable* were adapted by the White House Conference on Children and Youth in 1930. The term *trainable* was a catch-all for the most dependent, and what then may have been known as *subtrainable* individuals were included. Programs for this group were almost nonexistent then (Dussault, 1989).

The American Association on Mental Retardation also no longer wishes to use the *mild* to *profound* labels, instead emphasizing strengths and weaknesses across four dimensions:

▮ intellectual/adaptive skills
▮ psychological/emotional considerations
▮ physical/health/etiological considerations
▮ environmental considerations.

These areas are assessed after administering a formal intelligence test. Then, levels of support are assigned four levels of intensity:

▮ intermittent
▮ limited
▮ extensive
▮ pervasive (The Arc, 1996).

The subjects of this chapter could be described as those who generally require extensive to pervasive support across all four dimensions.

Etiology

The group of individuals marked by extreme dependency have etiologies similar to the general MR/DD population, such as Down's syndrome, Fragile X, fetal alcohol syndrome, and low birth weight. However, these and other etiologies do not indicate accurately the degree of handicap an individual will demonstrate in later life. For example, a study showed that only 20 percent of very low birth-weight babies had significant handicaps, with the rest described as intellectually competitive (Stahlman, Grogaard, et al., 1988). Children with retardation may be developmentally delayed at birth by genetic abnormalities or prenatal damage from alcohol or drugs. A child who is normal at birth may suffer postnatal neurological insult from ingesting toxins such as lead paint, or suffer from head trauma, hydrocephalus, and various diseases that destroy or damage parts of the brain. Those born normally who experience significant central nervous system damage before the age of 21 may be classified as retarded. Those who suffer such damage after 21 are considered brain injured and generally will not be placed into the MR/DD system.

Other factors weigh significantly in degree of dependency. Some have dual diagnoses: developmental delay plus mental illness. Affective disorders are reported to occur in 3–6 percent of the general MR/DD population, but rates are much higher for adults than for children under the age of 10 (Reiss, 1996). Adults with dual diagnoses who test in the severe or moderate range can exhibit behaviors that inhibit independent functioning, and this may subsequently place them in a profound level of function. Cerebral palsy, in its most severe quadriplegic forms, and other diseases that significantly affect motor function may seriously decrease the functional capacity of individuals and place them in the most dependent status. Since adults with mental retardation have been living longer, the incidence of age-related dementias and Alzheimer's disease has become more prevalent in this population. For example, virtually 100 percent of those with Down's syndrome over the age of 40 have significant Alzheimer's neuropathology (Haxby & Shapiro, 1992). Another secondary diagnosis is familial or environmental deprivation. When a child with retardation is raised in a dysfunctional family or in a barren environment within an institution, the initial handicaps that result may be amplified or compounded by adulthood.

Characteristics and Capabilities

In this population, deficits may be seen in all or nearly all areas but are *very* varied. Sensory functions may be intact, absent, or impaired, or may indicate sensory integration problems. Motor function may or may not be impaired. Some may be fully ambulatory and even show good fine-motor skills. Others may ambulate with a stable if primitive gait, while others require assistance or a wheelchair. Fine-motor skills can range from being able to tie shoelaces, to gross grasping, to not using one's hands in any functional manner, even for feeding. Self-stimulatory and/or self-abusive behavior may be seen. Self-stimulation often is in the form of

- rocking, twirling, or head rolling (vestibular)
- string fixation or finger weaving (visual/tactile)
- sexual self-stimulation
- auditory self-stimulation in the form of vocalizations.

Self-abuse may be seen in the form of hitting the head with hands or on surfaces, grinding teeth (bruxism), picking skin, and biting hands or other body parts.

The individual may exhibit obsessive, sometimes sensory related problems, such as disrobing, fecal smearing, tearing clothes, licking floor and objects, flinging objects, eating paper, dirt, or other nonedibles (pica), and many other, even more bizarre behaviors that are difficult to analyze.

Communication is limited, with expressive capacity usually lagging far behind receptive ability. Some may be minimally verbal, use a few signs, or point to pictures or objects they want, while others will only show preference when food or stimuli are offered to them, and they accept or they refuse in the form of pushing away or becoming agitated.

History: The Effect of Long-Term Institutionalization

At the present time, many adults with severe developmental disabilities attend day programs and live in state-run or proprietary residences. Some of these adults still live with their families. Many day program attendees may have a long-term state institutional background.

Large-scale, long-term institutionalization of persons with retardation has a troubled past. Through the first half of the 20th century, it was a common belief that the retarded were hereditary aberrants and the defective results of "bad stock." In the manner of criminals, it was felt appropriate that they should be separated from society. This belief was particularly easy to maintain with the most dependent, such as someone who could not engage in basic self-care or effectively communicate, as opposed to an adult considered "feeble minded" (that is, someone who could perhaps help out in the grocery store on the corner). At that time, institutionalization was heavily utilized by poor families who had no resources to support their disabled child at home. In many states, large numbers of these individuals, born during the 1930s up to the beginning of the 1970s, were placed in state facilities that eventually housed several thousand. Some spent their childhood and much of their adulthood in such settings.

In New York, these settings deteriorated severely due to the withdrawal of funds during the 1960s, and it took a class-action lawsuit to begin reform. Willowbrook (the Staten Island Developmental Center, New York) was so bad that some residents who were relocated from it were placed under a "Willowbrook decree" and assigned public advocates. At one time in this facility, many residents huddled unclean, half-clothed or naked in bare, filthy rooms and got the barest minimum of custodial care, with one staff member to 30 or 40 residents (Kihss, 1977). The Faribault state institution in Minnesota in the late 1960s was equally horrible. Other states had similar situations, and at one time an estimated 92,000 adults with retardation were living in comparable substandard conditions in the United States (Thompson, 1971).

The legacy of this kind of long-term neglect is that day programs at present have hundreds, perhaps thousands, of residents who were formerly in state institutions. Even though the number of survivors diminishes with each day, these people will continue to be a presence through the year 2000. Of this population, those residents with severe and profound handicaps appear to have suffered the most. With impaired mobility or confinement to a wheelchair, with sensory impairments, with little or no capacity or opportunity to make needs and wants known, and with little more than a shoelace or scrap of paper to play with for year after year in a bleak ward, these individuals show the effects of neglect. I have observed that individuals with profound disabilities who lived for many years in underfunded institutions tend to show more deficits than similar individuals raised in home environments.

In 1954, a child named Eric was 2½ years old. He was born with Down's syndrome and showed profound developmental delay, and on the advice of a doctor his family placed him in a large state institution at that time. No early intervention services were easily available, whether through state, federal, or private sources. For 32 years, he lived in a limited, highly-segregated environment in which funds for adequate supplies and staffing were gradually withdrawn. In 1986, the state instituted reforms, and he was moved to a small group home. In 1988, he was enrolled in a day program, and I met him for the first time. I found a 44-year-old man, ambulatory but with a minimal interest in his environment. His only interest was string, which he would dangle in front of his face and make "suckling" motions while he fondled it. Was this type of limited, repetitive, self-stimulatory behavior caused by a sensory-deprived childhood? What would have happened to Eric if, in his infancy, he was placed in a well-run, early intervention program? Answers to these questions are subject to discussion, but I suspect that Eric and others like him were affected in a very negative way by institutionalization and with better care would have matured with a significantly higher skill level.

Justification of Service and the Professional's Challenge

Why serve those who show a minimal level of independent purposeful function? I once met a professional who felt that individuals who function at the very lowest levels should simply be euthanized. For the slightly higher functioning, he felt most therapy was a waste of time. A therapist, however, is a practitioner of health who is concerned with maximizing and maintaining function. Regardless of whom a therapist is asked to treat, the therapist should have a commitment to maximizing each consumer's potential: assessing, finding a problem, and redressing the problem.

The problems related to deficits in self-care, work, and leisure areas are so numerous that a beginning therapist may be overwhelmed and not know where to begin. These problems are further magnified by public underfunding and apathy. The adult with developmental delay who cannot work even in a sheltered workshop, and who needs a great deal of support and supervision, is seen by the general public as a burden on society like other chronically-disabled people. Most facilities for adults with retardation are remnants of old, underfunded state-run programs or Medicaid-supported county not-for-profit institutions, or proprietary programs run on shoestring budgets. There are exceptions, in the form of well-financed private programs, but these are usually inaccessible to those of low income and are few in number. The therapist choosing to work with this population will more often than not find an underfunded program with underdiagnosed and underserved consumers, just as one would expect to find in agencies serving the chronically mentally ill and impoverished. These facts alone justify intervention with this population, in which well-trained and dedicated professionals probably always will be in very short supply.

In the facility where I work, I am required to cover the needs of over 200 adults in three different day programs. This type of case load forces ethical decisions on the therapist. An adult who is able to speak in simple sentences, work independently on simple tasks, and make simple decisions is a far better candidate for a variety of therapy interventions than a nonverbal adult who shows poor adaptive skills and limited receptivity to verbal and physical prompts. In making such a choice, a therapist has to weigh different factors and develop a priority system. The main questions will be: What resources do I have and, given these resources, with whom can I accomplish the most?

Resource Questions

1. *Equipment:* Do I have what I need? If I want vestibular stimulation, do I have a swing, rocking chair, or similar device?

2. *Environment:* Is the consumer's present environment conducive to my therapy goals? Do I need space, quiet, and accessibility?

3. *Time:* Can I accomplish my goals in a reasonable amount of time? Will a specialized sensory program, designed to change a consumer's behavior, produce results that will be worth the time invested?

4. *Assistance:* If I am an OTR, do I have a COTA or therapy aide capable of understanding and carrying out my therapeutic ideas? If I am a COTA, does my supervising OTR support my ideas and give me a case load I can realistically handle? Do other clinicians (PT, ST, RN, psychologist) support or agree with my therapy ideas?

5. *Carry over of therapy by nonprofessionals:* How much of what I hope to accomplish is dependent on nonclinical staff?

The last question is of particular concern. An OTR's interventions with this population often depend on staff showing understanding and following recommendations. Most adult day programs have a job description for direct-care staff, and one of the basic job duties is to "follow clinical staff's recommendations." As many clinicians who have worked in this field will report, compliance can be far below average. Many direct-care staff I have encountered have no college or specialized education related to MR/DD and leave the field in a year or less. Some agencies experience a turnover rate of 50–100 percent within a year (Gardner & Chapman, 1985). Some direct-care staff have attitudes detrimental to any kind of therapeutic relationship: "he doesn't need therapy; he is just lazy"; "clinicians make big bucks; we don't need them"; or "clinical recommendations are unimportant and a nuisance; we won't bother to follow them." I have encountered direct-care staff and even some program administrators with these kinds of attitudes, and getting therapy carried over with such people in charge is nearly impossible. However, most agencies may have as many or more people who are supportive of the clinician's ideas and therapy programs. The therapist must not give up hope.

In summary, the therapist serving the needs of those with profound disabilities will need to:

- obtain a physician's referral
- establish the consumer's functional needs
- prioritize who will be treated
- identify resources available such as equipment, professional assistance, environment, staff support, and time.

Functional Category Guidelines for Treatment Intervention

In order to assist the therapist in developing appropriate programs and expectations, some classification of those with profound disabilities is useful. Some have argued against this, stating that "advocates for persons with profound retardation are often caught in the classic bind of simultaneously articulating the deficits or differences that characterize this particular group of individuals. ... [T]he standards, expectations, and criteria that have emerged in the field for persons who are 'moderately' and 'severely' handicapped apply perhaps equally to those who are the most profoundly disabled" (Evans & Scotti, 1989). This reasoning is laudable on the point of preventing overly-negative expectations, but if different criteria are used for different categories in a careful and methodical manner with full consideration that one may move from one category to another, then this "labeling" will be helpful rather than harmful.

Knowledgeable and informed professionals will be aware of "normalization" needs and will not segregate or neglect people just because they fall into a category. The following is a simple protocol that will help to organize the deficits and develop appropriate methods of intervention.

CATEGORIZATION GUIDELINES FOR THE MOST DEPENDENT

Category I

1. The consumer is nonverbal, does not use signs or point to picture symbols.
2. All movements of the body are limited. The individual usually is severely physically handicapped but, if not, will only show limited movement.
3. Little or no interest in or interaction with the surrounding environment is shown. The individual will not reach, grasp, hold, or manipulate most objects. He or she may insert their hand in their mouth, chew on clothing, or make other repetitive or stereotypic movements but generally will not respond to external stimuli. If responses are made, they are "short chain" in nature, such as a startle reflex or withdrawal response and do not lead to learning or adaptive patterns.
4. The individual may show little or no visual regarding. Looking at faces or objects may be very transitory if seen at all. Those that do show some ocular motor function or sustained gaze will not use this function to obtain objects.
5. The individual usually will not feed him or herself.
6. The individual usually will be incontinent of bowel and bladder.

These individuals usually have significant differences from the profoundly handicapped population as a whole, but they are often grouped with others without regard for their special status. Some of the words used to describe states of awareness after a head injury form an interesting description with which Category I individuals correlate. For example, *stupor* indicates spontaneous movement and groaning in response to various stimuli. This term is not used with the MR/DD population but may depict the functional level often seen in Category I. Category I individuals make up a very small number of those with developmental disabilities. In a day program setting where I have worked, five people qualified out of a census of 80. In another setting I counted approximately 10 out of a population of 130. Different states and different institutions will vary in the number of these individuals placed in one setting.

Category II

The individual in Category II shows some awareness of and interaction with the environment. They may look at faces or objects, and reach for them. They may hold objects and manipulate them. They may have some primitive but consistent means of communication. They will show some connection with the world around them, unlike the consumer in Category I, who appears to be only interested in his own body. Even if their interactions with the environment are primitive and repetitive, there are observable connections that are not seen with the Category I consumer. These consumers may have their cognitive deficit compounded by problems in one or more of the following areas: mobility, perception, and behavior. Because of their great diversity, the consumer in Category II is hard to separate from others of higher function. Some may have splinter skills, such as self-feeding and toileting, but may be extremely dependent in nearly all other areas. Two elements stand out to distinguish them from others less dependent:

■ an apparent lack or utilization of long-term memory
■ initiation of purposeful activities.

The majority of those who attend day programs often present the characteristics of Category II.

In point of reference, Category I individuals correspond to the lowest segment of the profoundly retarded with IQs of 10 or much less. Those in Category II may also be classified as profound (with IQs of 20 or less) but may also test within the severe range (20–35). Those who test in the upper severe and moderate ranges (approximately 30 to 36 IQ) and who are functioning within average expectations for this range are not seen as qualifying as subjects of this chapter.

Category III

Category III persons have mobility and communication impairments that are so severe that they are totally dependent in nearly all domains. However, they have cognitive capacities that are significantly higher than their physical capacities. If they did not have these physical restrictions, they might conceivably be working in a sheltered workshop, and showing independence in activities of daily living (ADL) routines.

An example is Ronald, a 43-year-old man who tests in the severe IQ range and might score in the moderate range, if his motor abilities were not so impaired. He has spastic quadriplegic cerebral palsy and is confined to a wheelchair he cannot self-propel. His only intact functional movement is in his head, face, and left hand. He is able to feed himself with a universal cuff and other adaptations. He is nonverbal but can draw attention by yelling and is able to point to a wide variety of pictures with good accuracy. His memory for people and day-to-day events is good. His attention span is also good in comparison to his peers, and he is cooperative and friendly. Such a person is a good candidate for occupational therapy but also can present great challenges. In my experience, this type of day program attendee is rare. In 8 years, I have encountered only 3 or 4 people who fit this description.

In some facilities, such people may be grouped together so a teacher or therapist can maximize their potentials with assistive technology, such as computers and environmental control devices. Unfortunately, many day programs or group homes do not have the budgets to provide such expensive items or to hire clinicians skilled in their use. There also may be little incentive to spend a lot of scarce funds on just one or two individuals. Some individuals are given expensive and sophisticated communication and mobility equipment in their school-age years, which may not be used later on when they enter a day program. If the equipment needs repair, modification, or replacement, funding that was available when they were of school age may be unavailable now that they are adults. Often this equipment requires assistance and encouragement from others for the consumer to use. Some direct-care staff may be unfamiliar with the function or importance of the device and will not use it, causing it to be virtually abandoned. Assistive technology does not always guarantee a consumer significantly more function. Without these devices, extra staff support, and specially-adapted activities, a Category III individual may be grouped with the most dependent, just because he or she cannot physically work on the tasks that others in higher functioning groups can.

A person can drift between Category I and Category II status, and conceivably a Category III person may decline in function and qualify as being in Category II or I. If a person considered Category I shows a Category II action, then that action should be encouraged and promoted. The purpose of the categories is simple: to have a frame of reference from which to build interventions. Not everyone who is classified as being in one of the above categories will necessarily stay there for the duration of his life, but the characteristics of one category will often predominate.

Assessment and Choosing Areas of Intervention

Assessment of adults with severe and profound handicapping conditions is difficult. Traditional means of evaluation are often inappropriate. The primary focus when working with people with profound disabilities is: *What does the individual initiate?* Those in Category I may only initiate a limited repertoire of movements. Those in Category II may initiate little more than feeding and stereotypic behaviors. This means that the therapist must have excellent observational skills and an open mind with which to interpret what seems to be meaningless and aimless behaviors. Some common characteristics to watch for are:

▮ a receptive capacity or an ability to follow simple directions that is far greater than expressive capacity

▮ odd behaviors that may be related to sensory-processing abnormalities

▮ significant challenges associated with the initiation of purposeful or adaptive actions.

In behavioral terms, the last would indicate a lack of operant behavior in the environment.

Each individual, even someone who is extremely dependent, tends to show some kind of distinctive pattern of response and arousal to stimuli. These patterns should be considered when making assessments of ability to perform a purposeful action. Although it seems the functional capacity of these individuals can be determined relatively quickly, the therapist must be wary of making judgments based on two few observations made in only one or two environments. The consumer may not exhibit specific abilities to some examiners or will show certain actions or behaviors only in certain environments. I recall a case of an adult care worker who tried unsuccessfully for several years to get one of the adults in her care to write his name. He would make a few letters only poorly. Then one day, when he did not know she was looking, he wrote his full name legibly. Another man presented himself to me as nonverbal and would not utter a sound in all of our interactions. However, with others, he would speak in sentences. These types of circumstances may often be seen with the autistic individual, who may demonstrate a splinter skill in an unpredictable manner. Another typical situation often encountered is when the parent or house caregiver states, after hearing about how the individual behaves in a day program: "Bobby never shows that behavior with us." In view of this, the therapist must interview different staff and observe the individual in as many different environments as possible in order to get the most accurate information.

Establishing Priorities in Providing Therapeutic Interventions in a Day Program

The following is an example of a typical day program classroom.

The classroom is a 25′ × 12′ room with one entrance, a wall with some windows, and a few old battered metal cabinets, tables, and chairs. Two training specialists are assigned to a group of six consumers. The two staff have little with which to work. Their cabinets are mostly filled with bibs, diapers, and economy foodstuffs. They have an odd mixture of program materials: children's toys, a "Mr. Potato Head," preschool puzzles with missing pieces, pegboards, and many homemade items. There is a dirty cardboard box with empty bent-up soda cans, parts of broken toys brought in from home, shoe boxes of clothespins, straws, beads and popsicle sticks, old clothing, stuffed toys, plastic Easter eggs, and piles of ragged women's magazines. The training specialists are young with little knowledge of developmental or physical disabilities. They also have limited knowledge of the needs or past histories of their consumers. They are given a brief introduction to the people to whom they are assigned and then are expected to supervise and provide a goal-based program for nearly 4 or 5 hours, 5 days a week. In classrooms for the most dependent, a great deal of time is spent toileting. Because toileting and changing some individuals may take over 20 minutes, often six or more consumers are supervised by only one training specialist. Because the program budget will not allow the hiring of enough direct-care staff and because of high staff turnover and absentee rates, clinicians and program administrators frequently need to spend time in the classroom to provide coverage.

This particular classroom contains six individuals, all conforming to Category I–III criteria. The characteristics of all these individuals are closely based on real persons with whom I have worked.

> *Ray* is a 42-year-old man with tubular sclerosis, is hyperactive. He runs about the room, grabbing any object he sees, and quickly flinging

it when it no longer interests him. The staff have resorted to hiding most all materials to prevent them from being flung or broken or accidentally striking another consumer.

Nate is a 38-year-old man who has severe spastic quadriplegia. He is positioned in a wheelchair he does not self-propel, is nonverbal, and has severe visual impairments. When taken out of his chair, he assumes a fetal position. He has contractures in various joints and does not use his arms to reach for any nonedible objects placed within his reach. He is often constipated and may "dig" himself, necessitating a major clean-up operation.

Mildred is 56 years old and blind. She will not work on any tabletop activities, but sits rocking, singing to herself, and chewing on her shirt. Occasionally, after she is tired of sitting, she will stand and fling over her chair.

Richard is a 42-year-old man with right hemiparesis. He is fully ambulatory and has good use of his left arm and hand. He has lived at home all of his life, and has been fed, dressed, and toileted by his mother. He will not eat in the day program and will not use the toilet, having adjusted himself to only doing those things at home. He does not engage in any purposeful task in the day program, preferring to wander, to sit in a rocking chair, and occasionally to have a tantrum when he is bothered by certain noises or redirected.

Margret is a 34-year-old with a severe self-abusive problem. On a daily basis, she will strike her head with her hands or bang it on hard surfaces sometimes causing bleeding. It may take two or more staff to stop her from self-abusing. At other times she will be calm and may fall asleep.

Joseph is a 41-year-old man with spastic quadriplegia and is positioned in a wheelchair he cannot self-propel, like Nate. Unlike Nate, he shows good awareness of people and objects. He is nonverbal but can gesture and point to some picture symbols with accuracy. He is very mobility impaired and feeds himself with difficulty, using adapted devices. He is friendly and recognizes favorite staff, greeting them with a yell.

The six disparate people making up this classroom present a therapist with multiple problems.

▮ Which of the six should be treated with a formal therapy program?

▮ Who should be treated first?

▮ What types of therapeutic interventions should be used?

The occupational therapist with a background in holistic thinking should have many questions with which to deal.

To begin, I gathered all the known information I could on each individual: the past history, past therapies if any, diagnoses, and, as available, descriptions of the family or institutional environments in which he or she had lived since birth. My clinical decisions were as follows.

Ray

Ray was treated first. His grabbing and flinging behavior was disrupting the entire classroom, making it very difficult for staff to use materials or give any attention to others in the room. First, I observed Ray in the day program environment. I considered him a Category II. He would not sit for much more than a few seconds, despite concerted efforts to train him. He would run about the room, grabbing all manner of objects, observe them, shake them briefly, and then fling them. Often he would return to the flung object and pick it up, only to quickly fling it again. He would be extremely restless and forage about obsessively, damaging property, and sometimes knocking people over to get something. I provided the classroom with a large, brightly-colored box in which I put a number of interesting objects and worked one-on-one with Ray for several weeks. He was allowed to choose whatever he wanted out of the box, but if he flung it, he had to pick it up and put it back in the box. This was partially successful. Then, I observed that some objects seemed to interest him longer than others. A large rubber spider was particularly interesting to him, giving him visual stimulation to which he did not quickly habituate. Eventually I made him a spider-like object: a sturdy plastic ring with short lengths of rope attached. This became his object and held his attention through most of a program day. His foraging and destructive behavior greatly decreased. I also felt it was important for a hyperactive and restless person like Ray to get outside his room; so I took him outside and around the building for walks. This provided him with significant amounts of proprioceptive, visual, auditory, and other stimulation, and he did not need his object when on the walks. The fact that he did not need this "stimulator" on these walks indicated that the classroom space provided inadequate movement and stimulation. The walking activity also provided me with opportunities to work with him on simple ADL routines, like putting on and taking off his coat.

Nate

Nate was not as high a priority as Ray. He did, however, require some intervention. He was seen as possibly falling into a Category I status, largely because of his severe limits in mobility. His marginal self-feeding needed some monitoring of his adaptive equipment, which consisted of a high side dish and a spoon in a universal cuff. He needed sensory stimulation because he could not explore or reach for objects. A range-of-motion maintenance program was developed by the occupational and physical therapy departments. His staff was instructed in techniques for a) guided movement (described later), b) maintaining his self-feeding, and c) providing adequate sensory stimulation. His digging problem—not uncommon with those who are constipated and incontinent of bowel and bladder—was monitored by staff and addressed by providing movement and keeping a regular changing schedule.

Mildred

Mildred required intervention to address her chair-flinging behavior, which had a high potential for injuring others. A chair with a heavy base fixed to the legs was fabricated by a COTA and use of this prevented her from tossing it. By why did she do this? Perhaps she needed to walk. Perhaps she felt unable to walk by herself because of blindness. She did not show the requisite skills to learn cane use or blind mobility techniques like trailing. In her attempts to walk she would often get up and bump into something before staff members could get to her. Staff members were often unable to leave the room to walk with her, because they had to supervise the others. Intervention in a case like this might involve putting her into a sensory environment designed so she could not hurt herself but in which she could explore freely. If this were not possible, arrangements could be made to give her walks and multi-sensory experiences suited to her needs.

Richard

Richard was seen as having a number of problems, including sensory integration deficits. He showed hypersensitivity to noise. He was dependent in basic self-care skills. He was self-abusive and aggressive towards others at times. He was nonproductive, even though he showed some potential to follow simple instructions. A program to get him to feed and toilet himself was very difficult, because his mother was unable to relinquish her role as a mother of a dependent son, whom she continued to spoon feed. In her 80s and partially deaf, she was difficult to counsel on Richard's need to be more independent. She also would not cooperate in administering behavior medication to him, and he would not easily take medication from anyone except her. It naturally fell to the OT department to intervene. In this case, an intuitive COTA who had known and worked with him for years was the impetus for positive changes. She went to a conference given by Patricia Wilbarger on sensory defensive behavior and how it can be treated with a tactile stimulation program. This program involved vigorous brushing with a soft plastic brush over arms, legs, and back. Richard tolerated this program well and appeared to show some improvement in behavior. This treatment alone was not sufficient; he needed to be trained in purposeful activities. It was known that he immensely enjoyed walking despite a hemiparetic leg. In the past, staff would let him wander about the building. This was structured into something more purposeful. He would stay in a classroom part of the day, and the COTA would come to get him and set him up with some simple tasks like carrying bags of clothes to other classrooms and helping to push wheelchair-bound consumers around the day program. Gradually, his self-abusive and aggressive behavior decreased.

Margret

Margret showed a severe self-abusive problem. In her case, it appeared that the primary reason for her behavior was a craving for specific stimuli. After consulting with a therapist who had worked with her in the past, it was found she craved vestibular stimulation in the form of spinning. A large, pediatric floor saucer was found, and fortunately this woman was small and could fit into it. All self-abusive behavior ceased immediately when she experienced gentle spinning, and the effect would sometimes last for hours after a session.

Joseph

Joseph fit into Category III. He had certain capacities but was so physically impaired that he could do very little. His mother and brother felt that he could "do nothing" for himself. After evaluation, it was found that he was able to do certain things with adaptive devices. He could feed himself with adaptive equipment. He could press switches to turn on a radio, fan, or battery-operated toy. He remembered people and objects, could follow simple instructions, and point to pictures. With these capacities, the therapist could facilitate some independence.

The individuals described above illustrate the three categories of those with profound challenges and suggest certain methods of intervention. Also, the need to prioritize problems is demonstrated. These individuals were co-existing together in a confining space, and the actions of one individual could affect all the others. For example, treating Ray first was important, because his behavior would have undermined interventions that the therapist would attempt to do with others.

Key Treatment Considerations

Positioning

Positioning problems are most frequently seen with Category I and Category III consumers. Kyphosis and scoliosis of the spine may keep them in a poor posture. Hemiplegia may cause lateral leaning and other problems. Those who sit for long periods and who are unable to shift weight are at risk for decubitus ulcers. When intervening with such problems, the therapist should know as much as possible about the individual's specific orthopedic pathology. Often the individual has already been placed in some kind of customized wheelchair or seating arrangement. Over time, this seating system may need modification. The therapist needs to get a full workup of the diagnosis and any past interventions that have already been done or attempted. Then the therapist must examine the individual in his or her environment. Is the positioning problem affecting eating, working on tasks, or mobility? For example, one very dependent consumer who needed to be spoon fed had a tendency to extend his head while eating. This head position created a higher risk for aspiration, so a head rest was installed. Another consumer was partially ambulatory and used a regular armchair to sit in, but he tended to lean significantly to one side. A small, firm, rectangular cushion was custom-made to support him in a more upright posture on that side.

A very common problem is table height and dangling feet. Many consumers are of short stature (some under 5′ tall), and standard tables and chairs are not appropriate. Firm cushions can raise consumers up in their seat. Getting their elbows to rest on the table in 90 degrees of flexion is ideal but may be unrealistic, and another position that increases function is often acceptable. Feet should be supported. A foot box can be made to the correct height so feet can rest comfortably. Some may wish to attach the footrest to the chair so its use will be guaranteed, but if the consumer transfers independently, he or she must be able to do so without tripping on the rest.

Some consumers (mostly Category I status) may have what is known as a "tilt-in-space" wheelchair. This is a large, complex chair that enables the entire seating component of the chair to tilt back within the frame; it differs from a reclining back wheelchair, where only the back of the chair tilts. The tilt-in-space chair is used for severely mobility-impaired persons who need to be in an upright posture but also need pressure taken off of the coccyx and ischial areas. Pressure relief is gained by placing them in at least 45 degrees of tilt for part of the day.

Positioning those with severe orthopedic problems is a science in itself. Unless a therapist is particularly knowledgeable, he or she could do more harm than good when attempting significant interventions. It is best to consult with experts. If a whole new seating system is being planned, the therapist needs to work with the physical therapist, orthopedist, wheelchair vendor, and other significant professionals. In this team approach, the OTR may need to speak up on certain issues related to occupational therapy practice. For example, a physical therapist may recommend that a consumer be placed in a fully reclining position due to hip contractures. The OTR, in turn, might indicate the significant perceptual problems such an individual might experience when placed in that position.

Positioning adults who have been accustomed to abnormal postures most of their lives is difficult. They may have developed habits of walking, sitting, or lying that are comfortable or acceptable to them, and interventions at this stage may be uncomfortable or unacceptable because they are simply different. One man with whom I worked had a leg-length discrepancy and hip and back deformities. He could work on simple tabletop tasks, but he preferred to stand and lean on a table to work. I experimented with cushions that put him in a very functional seated position. Since he was verbal, I asked him if he was comfortable, and he said he was. However, he removed all of the cushions after I left and went back to his old pattern of standing and leaning. The therapist must be aware of the pitfalls of intervening in such positioning problems and proceed carefully before spending lots of money or time.

To summarize, the therapist working with positioning must:

1. Have a good knowledge of the consumer's positioning history, diagnosis, and any pertinent pathologies
2. Assess needs as related to respiration, eating, swallowing, task function, stress on joints, functional vision, and safety
3. Consult as needed with others
4. Experiment before ordering or making expensive alterations

5. Be sensitive of how the positioning device will fit into the consumer's lifestyle and be accepted or tolerated by him or her.

SUGGESTED TREATMENT INTERVENTIONS TO TEACH TO STAFF AND USE AS FORMAL THERAPY

Guided Movement

Guided movement as described here is not a special technique and may resemble other methods with the same or with more complex names. It is simply a means to give movement to the consumer who initiates minimal movement. Most importantly, it is meant as a technique that the therapist can teach to direct-care staff. The Category I consumer is most frequently suited to this type of intervention, but some Category II consumers may benefit also. The consumer would usually be in a wheelchair. He or she would tend to keep the limbs in one position often making some limited, repetitive, self-stimulatory movements. He or she may or may not have contractures. To guide movement, the staff members would first let the person know that they are going to move their arms or legs. This is especially important if the person startles easily and should be done regardless of whether the consumer understands what is being said. The staff may say: "I am going to move your arm up so your hand can touch your head." Staff then gently guides the person's arm in that direction. If the person begins to pull away, the staff member goes with the consumer's movement. The staff should not try to move the limbs in directions in which the consumer resists moving, or cannot move, due to range-of-motion limits. Instead, the staff should attempt to guide the limbs to move in ways they might move if the consumer showed more cortical control and motivation to do so. Some Category I consumers will favor a fetal-like position with flexed arms. Gradually, they may develop contractures and lose range, first in shoulder flexion, and then elbow and wrist extension. While it may slow this loss, guided movement is not passive range of motion (PROM). If passive range of motion is recommended by the occupational or physical therapist, the therapist treats the consumer. Guiding or encouraging movement, however, is not the specific stretching of soft tissues with outside forces. It can be done by nonclinical staff. Some therapists may feel it is risky to train nonprofessionals to do this. However, direct-care staff make the consumers go through such movements anyway (when they dress, toilet, and transfer them). Some staff also need this training to feel less inhibited about touching the people to whom they are assigned. Furthermore, one therapist cannot go about a program with 100 consumers and do all the therapeutic handling that is required.

The basic tenets of guided movements are:

1. They are not performed to passively stretch joints in order to maintain ROM but to give proprioceptive and tactile stimulation, as well as to maintain a consumer's sense of his or her own body.
2. They can be taught to direct-care staff. The therapist makes the judgment as to the capability of the staff members to learn the technique with a specific consumer and then trains them with the consumer.
3. The staff goes with the self-initiated movements of the consumer and gently guides the movements and expands on them. For example, a consumer fixates on twirling the hair on the left side of her head. The staff encourages and guides the consumer's hand to her ear or other body parts.
4. All movements are slow and gentle. If the consumer pulls in a direction opposite to the staff, the staff goes in that direction. The staff stops the procedure if the consumer becomes agitated or too resistive.
5. Guided movement should be a part of the Category I consumer's daily multisensory experiences.
6. Staff performing this procedure are regularly monitored by a clinician.
7. They are often used with Category I consumers and sometimes with Category II consumers who show limited volitional movement.

Assisted Function

Unlike Category I consumers, many Category II consumers are reaching, grasping, and moving their limbs in purposeful ways. However, many have difficulty completing most actions successfully. For example, they may grasp a spoon but are unable to use it to feed themselves. When someone uses a hand to guide/prompt a consumer's movement during eating or other functional tasks, the desired movement is being *assisted*. This method can be used for all activities involving reaching, grasping, holding, and placing. If the consumer shows some improvement in completing an action by themselves, then the hand-over-hand assistance can be faded out. This should proceed from distal to proximal, first hand then to wrist, and finally forearm. This basic method has been used a long time with children and adults and has been detailed by Whitman (Whitman, Scibak, & Reid, 1983) and others, but it is amazing how few staff who work with this population apply it.

Category II consumers are usually able to understand some verbal instruction. Verbal prompts alone should be used first before immediately providing assisted function, to check if the consumer needs the physical help. In order to encourage independence, it is good practice for all staff at home as well as at day programs to use assisted function techniques on a regular basis. Assisted function should not be confused with "facilitated communication." The latter was a controversial technique used to assist nonverbal people in communication by providing support to the dominant hand/wrist/arm so that letters could be typed in sequence and, in turn, words could be spelled.

Assisted Function Is Not Used if the Consumer Consistently Does Not Maintain Grasp on Varied Objects

For example: A consumer uses his hands to grasp string to self-stimulate and uses hands to scratch self or suck on fingers. He will consistently not grasp any object, even if it is placed in his hands. However, staff members attempt to hold his hand around a pencil or paintbrush so as to artificially make lines or patterns that he is exerting no effort himself to make. In addition, he shows no awareness of the action or inaction of his limbs in this or other tasks. After evaluation and careful review of the consumer's history, a determination can be made that it serves no purpose to use assisted function. Such an individual is in a Category I status and should receive guided movement as opposed to assisted function.

Basic Tenets of Assisted Function Techniques

1. They are used with consumers who will consistently grasp and hold a variety of objects and who show some awareness of and appropriate response to the external environment.
2. Hand-over-hand assistance should be faded out proximal to distal.
3. They can be used at times with Category I consumers as an experiment, but therapists should counsel staff if they feel guided movement is more appropriate.
4. Verbal prompts should be used first. If there is no or inadequate response, the same verbal prompts should be used with the assisted function.

Other Activities

ADL

Dressing, grooming, toileting, eating, and other activities of daily living seem to be the first areas to address in this population. The therapist, however, should expect to see little significant progress in the development of new skills. Often the consumer has had a lot of self-care training in childhood, and, if not, there may be important behavioral/cognitive reasons.

Nonetheless, an assessment of the consumer's present skills and a concerted effort to preserve these skills should be made. For example, direct-care staff often need frequent reminders not to give full assistance. A 45-year-old man may not be able to signal his need to go to the bathroom and may wear an adult protective garment. With prompts, he will undress and assist in changing himself. A 32-year-old woman will bring a spoonful of food to her mouth but does not scoop the food herself. In both cases, the therapist should make sure the staff is letting the consumer do as much as possible of the task. Sometimes an assistive device will help. Assistive devices for eating, such as high-sided dishes, covered, spouted cups, and built-up handle utensils are often helpful in reducing spillage. Assistive dressing devices, such as long-handled shoehorns, sock aides, and dressing sticks are much more difficult to use with this population. Simpler dressing adaptations that require little or no training are more appropriate. A roller brush that will brush one's hair no matter how the handle is held is much better than a comb or a one-sided brush. Velcro®-tie shoes or elastic shoelaces that transform a tie shoe into a slip-on shoe are preferable as long as they provide support. I have seen many consumers who would have been independent in donning shoes, if staff had used a substitute for laces.

The Use of Toys and Switches

Toys

The use of toys with this population is controversial because of the need to provide age-appropriate activities. While a therapist would be unlikely to give an item to a consumer that is obviously a child's toy, such items often find their way into day programs. Some consumers also may be oriented to certain items that would be considered toys. Often the item may not function as a true toy to a consumer but rather as something that provides sensory stimulation. For example, a consumer may hold a doll and pick at the hair or buttons on it, getting tactile stimulation or visual stimulation while shaking it. The direct-care staff is not always aware of the relationship a consumer has with an object. Since the consumers appear child-like to them, it may seem natural to give them children's toys. The staff may be unaware that the consumer does not have representational thought: an ability to engage in make-believe that is usually seen emerging in normal children at about 4 years. The sensory value of an object should be considered. A ball and a stuffed animal both provide sensory stimulation, but the ball will move more freely when pushed. Different objects need to be introduced to someone so they have a choice. Some adults may seek out a doll or stuffed toy over a more age-appropriate item but should not then only be given those items. Battery-operated toys such as cars or animal figures could be used, but only if the consumer shows some sustained eye contact or response. Ideally, such toys should be hooked up to a switch, so that the consumer can operate them independently. It is often a judgment call as to whether a toy is appropriate for an adult. Obvious infant items such as rattles and teething rings should be avoided.

Some items can be adapted. In the aforementioned case of Ray, a ring with strings attached was a less child-like object than a toy spider. Another caveat is to prevent toys from becoming a fixation like a security blanket from which a person cannot separate. Also, there is a choking risk with small items when used with consumers who mouth items, as well as hygienic concerns.

Switches

Therapists and staff often get excited over the possibilities of switches but may be unaware of their limitations. It is easy to buy or make battery interrupter switches that will activate things when touched. The first problem that arises is: Will the consumer use it? The Category I consumer probably will not. He or she does not show a sense of cause and effect and usually is unaware of how their actions change the environment. A motion switch, however, may be useful to break stereotypic behavior in a Category I consumer. For example, a man always inserts his hand in his mouth. A motion switch is attached to his wrist, and when he lifts his hand to his mouth, it activates a diversionary stimulus such as a vibrator. This may not always work, because the person can habituate quickly to the diversionary stimulus. Switches may be useful with the Category II consumer, but results also will vary considerably. The variance of the stimulus may be important. Such people may "outwit" the purpose of the switch. One Category II consumer simply laid an object on a switch so it would continue to activate a music-producing computer while he walked away from it. This is good problem-solving training, but the therapist will need to make such a system more sophisticated and adaptable if he or she want further purposeful interaction. With Category III consumers, switches are often the most useful. These people are aware of their actions on the environment and desperately need some method to gain whatever independent control can be given to them. The therapist will need to find the right activity, then adapt and position it, so it can be independently used.

What can a switch activate? Some suggestions and problems:

1. A battery-operated toy can easily be hooked up to a switch. The result is usually only a limited amount of repetitive visual and auditory stimulation. These items are often fragile and break easily.
2. Radios and tape players make a good choice if the consumer responds to music and voices, and it can be varied. The consumer will probably need to tolerate headphones, if they are in a classroom, so that others will not be disturbed.
3. Lights are a limited stimulus but may be set up in such a way so it can be varied.
4. Fans, again, are a limited stimulus and somewhat difficult to find in a battery-operated form that is safe, but this has possibilities for some individuals.
5. Computers can also be operated by simple switches and may be a valuable communication device. They are expensive, and the therapist needs access to and knowledge of software and keyboard adaptations.

SELF-ABUSE AND SELF-STIMULATION: TREATMENT CONSIDERATIONS

It is hypothesized that adults with severe and profound retardation who engage in self-injurious behavior (SIB) and stereotypic self-stimulation do so because they lack stimulation from their environment. If the appropriate amount of stimulation is provided, including positive social interaction, then the SIB is expected to decrease or stop. In more sensory-integrative-based theories, the person's internal thresholds for experiencing stimuli may be abnormally high or low. Then, the problem is seen as more neurological, but the result may be the same: the individual engages in SIB or self-stimulation to compensate. Both of these perspectives must be put into the context of the specific individual and not vice versa. There is no simple formula for dealing with such behavior. For intervention, each person will need a custom-tailored program.

This subject covers a large area and is presented here in an introductory manner. The reader is urged to research the literature and consult with psychologists and behavioral specialists. Nonetheless, it is important to note the distinctions between self-injurious behavior and self-stimulatory or stereotyped behavior.

Self-Injurious Behavior (SIB)

SIB is an action that is self-inflicted and causes physical harm. It may be done as a form of temper tantrum, a response to redirection, or frustration. It also may be done in response to internal pain or in response to an outside stimulus such as noise. SIB also may be done as a means to provide neurological stimulation (Belfore & Dattilio, 1990). SIB causes some kind of lasting damage such as a bruise, laceration, or other more serious injury. A common form is head banging: the person strikes his head against a hard surface or slaps or strikes it with hands or fists. People with chronic problems like this are often seen wearing helmets and receiving contingency/reinforcement programs set up by a psychologist. Hand or arm biting may also be seen. Sometimes the skin is broken and blood is drawn; sometimes only calluses are produced. Skin picking, usually on arms, hands, or face may be seen. This can produce a small, mildly-callused or reddened area, or a large area of scar tissue. Hair or fingernails may be pulled out. Finding a specific etiology for SIB is difficult. Although aspects of this behavior demonstrate that it is very likely the result of learning processes, biological causes are implicated as well (Cataldo, 1988). In regard to psychiatric causes, a study of SIB in 251 severely and profoundly retarded individuals found no specific psychiatric disease associated with the behaviors (King, 1995).

Self-Stimulatory Behavior

Self-stimulatory or stereotypic behavior differs from SIB in that it does not usually cause damage to the person. One of the most common examples is rocking while seated or standing. Persons may also engage in twirling or spinning around. They may make repetitive arm or hand movements, such as shaking or flapping a hand in front of their face. They may make repetitive vocalizations or noises. Objects may be used. One favorite object used in self-stimulation is a string; persons fondle or dangle a string, shoelace, or similar object in front of their face.

There may be a blending of self-abusive and stereotypic behaviors. Sometimes a stereotypic behavior such as finger-sucking can produce damage by breaking down the skin. Excessive rubbing of one area of skin can also produce damage. Bruxism (teeth grinding) can damage teeth. Some repetitive behaviors can cause injury by accident. For example, someone who frequently swings his head around may inadvertently strike it on an object. In such cases, the therapist might intervene to provide some environmental adaption to protect the person. In the case of self-stimulatory yelling, something should be done to protect others in the same room from auditory abuse. The therapist or another staff should be able to take the loud consumer out of the room to give the other consumers and staff a respite. Repetitive self-stimulatory behavior that does not injure the consumer or bother others is usually not seen as needing intervention, although such behaviors may upset parents and caregivers who are attempting to get the consumer to behave as normally as possible. The therapist should offer the team members suggestions for activities or methods but should remind them that some behaviors may arise from sensory needs and may be a chronic and "necessary" action for the consumer.

Chronic SIB, especially in its more serious forms, attracts attention. If manifested in childhood, there usually has been some attempt to treat it. The therapist makes note of this, and it is significant if the behavior is of more recent origin. More commonly, the person is profoundly disabled, noncommunicative, and has a history of SIB, usually of a specific nature. In an attempt to analyze a person's SIB, one must look first to an internal pain, such as a toothache, headache, or ear problem (for example, otis media). If pain is ruled out, then one must look to environmental causes. Is the person bothered by stimuli in the environment? Does the person engage in SIB only when certain stimuli are present? For example, one nonverbal man would bite his hand only when objects dropped on the floor or when someone turned on a faucet. SIB also is often a form of tantrum exhibited only when the person is redirected or frustrated.

SIB is sometimes the individual's only means of communication. Some have learned to use SIB as a means of communicating that they want attention or to gain something. One woman learned that by pulling off hangnails and causing bleeding, she could get to go the nurse's office and get a Band-Aid, on which she fixated. These reasons for SIB are usually easy to identify when consistently seen and may be remediated with behavioral approaches, environmental changes, and/or sensory methods.

Interventions for SIB

Sensory Substitution

One simple method to deal with sensory behaviors is sensory substitution. Sensory substitution is finding an alternative way to provide a stimulus the person seems to crave. The substitute stimulation is safe, whereas the original stimulation causes harm. For example, a woman picks the skin on her arms and produces numerous small lesions. She is given a soft plastic brush to rub briskly on her arms, producing a similar sensation without causing harm. In another case, a man strikes his chin, impacting his inner lip on his teeth and causing a lesion. He is offered a vibrator and encouraged to try it on his chin. In both examples a substitute stimulus is used to replace the original, harmful one.

Alternative Activity

When using alternative activities, one is basically using the old behavioral methods of differential reinforcement of incompatible behavior (DRI) or differential reinforcement of other behavior (DRO). In one example, a woman picks at her hand until it bleeds. She is given a computer game to play that occupies both hands. In all cases, the individual is not forced in any way to comply but is shown the activities and encouraged to engage in them. As with all such interventions, the activities are offered *noncontingently*—that is, they are not offered only when the person self-abuses. If they receive the activity or are given attention only when SIB is shown, the risk is present that the SIB will be reinforced.

Somatosensory and Sensory-Integrative Approaches

Somatosensory refers to bodily sensations as distinguished from visceral or cortical influences. Noncontingent sensory stimulation has been suggested as a method to reduce SIB based on the presumption that certain levels of somatosensory stimulation are necessary or desirable for human beings. If such stimulation procedures are successful, direct-care staff could use them to reduce SIB in the severely and profoundly retarded nonambulatory population (Hiramu, 1989). Hiramu completed a study in which SIB was reduced in eight teenage subjects by the use of noncontingent tactile stimulation. The stimulation was in the form of stroking, squeezing, and pressing specific areas of the body.

Sensory defensiveness, most commonly seen in the form of tactile defensiveness, can produce symptoms of SIB or antisocial behavior. Here the person's nervous system is overreacting to familiar stimuli and negative behaviors may result. One somatosensory approach to address this problem in children aged 2–12 was to brush specific areas of the body vigorously with a soft plastic surgical brush. A treatment session was believed to produce effects that would last about 2 hours (Wilbarger & Wilbarger, 1991).

Both of the above techniques emphasize the use of *deep* pressure as opposed to light touch, which has a different neural pathway and affects different behavioral outcomes.

Vestibular stimulation has been frequently used with developmentally-delayed children and is a valuable technique with some adults as well. In the above mentioned case of Margret, vestibular stimulation in the form of gentle swinging in a swing or large floor saucer would immediately calm her down, and she often would remain calm for hours afterward.

To organize one's thinking about sensory-related behavior, the following steps and questions should be kept in mind:

1. Is there any evidence that an acute pain is the cause of behavior? For example, a consumer striking her face is found to have a bad tooth.
2. Does the behavior warrant intervention? Is it harmful to the consumer or to others?
3. Is the behavior best remediated with a behavioral/contingency program? If so, the psychologist/behavioral specialist should intervene.
4. If the behavior is sensory in origin, does it seem to be manifested primarily because of outside stimuli, internal processing problems, or lack of stimuli?
5. Should the approach be in the form of a sensory substitute, environmental adaption, alternative activity, or sensory-stimulation program?
6. Can direct-care staff safely and effectively administer the program?

If treatment is decided upon, the following should be done:

1. Consult with the team regarding the why, the how, and the where of therapy.
2. Secure a physician's order. A specific form should be used with a description of the SIB behavior, prior diagnosis, current medications, and description of treatments to be used. The form should indicate that certain reasons for the SIB have been ruled out, such as a medical condition or means to communicate anger, frustration, or to seek attention. That is important to justify the intervention of an OTR rather than a nurse or psychologist.
3. Make an accurate method of documenting the incidence of the target behavior prior to, during, and after treatment.

Environments: Safe, Suitable, and Sensory-Enriched

Typical day programs and home residences for adults with profound disabilities may often be structured and furnished in ways that are unsuitable for the needs of the consumers. Often a day program may be in an older building designed for a completely different purpose. The building may have been formerly an old factory, department store, or religious seminary. Sometimes the building is fairly new but, due to severe budget restraints, may be greatly lacking in important features. Residential homes can also vary widely in suitability. They may be new modern structures designed to serve mobile independent people, but where in time the beds were given to people with more severe disabilities. They may be large estates "converted" into group homes. Sometimes they are dilapidated structures that pose a variety of hazards and limitations to the residents. The following are important elements for which a clinician should advocate:

1. Handicapped Accessibility and Safety

It seems incredible that people with wheelchairs and physical handicaps can be placed in homes and day programs lacking basic wheelchair accessibility, but this may happen all too frequently. Ramps built to the code of one foot of ramp to one inch of elevation should be in place where needed. Sinks and tables should not have obstructions that prevent consumers in wheelchairs from utilizing them. Consumers of very short stature should have the choice of using small chairs that allow them to sit and have both feet resting on the floor, if they will not or cannot use a foot box. Double railings and grab bars should be provided where required; sharp edges of furniture and other potential hazards should be padded or modified as needed.

2. Adequate Space

Category I consumers have limited or no mobility and may not need a large space. The Category II consumer is more mobile and needs to have the opportunity to explore the environment. Sometimes these mobile consumers are confined to absurdly small spaces and drab "classrooms." Sensory materials and supplies can be brought into these spaces, but the space itself often needs to be changed to deliver the most effective interventions. If mobile consumers have behaviors such as food stealing, tendencies to wander, or are at risk of falling, there is often an attempt to keep them in an enclosed classroom that may be very small and confining. Those are unacceptable reasons to limit their freedom. A large recreational space should be available, where they can move about freely and safely for at least part of every day. An outside area, fenced in and with an area protected from the sun, is essential.

3. Bathrooms and Sinks

Every room should have a sink or be in close proximity to one. Hands and supplies frequently need to be washed for hygienic reasons. As many consumers have toileting accidents, the room they are in should have a bathroom within or in close proximity, equipped with changing tables, lifters, and all needed supplies. This is important not only for consumer-training purposes but also to expedite the whole routine. Otherwise, some consumers end up spending a large part of the day in a toilet routine.

4. Sensory Room

The so-called classroom equipped with tables and chairs is often unsuitable for consumers who are the subjects of this chapter. They need a place to sit, but they are not usually people who work at tables. The rooms in which they are placed should offer them sensory interest. It may be suitable to have mats on the floor and large balls and bolsters about the room. There should be boards with different textures for tactile experiences. Objects such as mobiles and balloons should be suspended from the ceiling to provide visual stimulation. If possible, a special room may be set aside for such an environment where consumers may be brought for part of a day. At the Young Adult Institute in Tarrytown, New York, for example, a sensory "obstacle course" was built in one room. This 20′ × 19′ structure was the product of a multidisciplined core team, composed of an occupational therapist, physical therapist, and a special education teacher. It was carpeted and designed to encourage a consumer to engage in a variety of experiences that stimulate gross motor and sensory functions. This structure contains mats, tunnels, and hanging bolsters, as well as textured walkways, mirrors, lights, music, and a "smell station." Several features of this environment were activated by the consumer via switches. If such an environment as this could be made in units that could be adapted and modified as needed, it would truly be an asset to any house or day program seeking to provide a sensory-enriched environment.

The Therapist as Educator

The treatment team may consist of direct care staff (training specialists), clinicians (occupational, physical, speech, nursing, psychology), a physician, supervisors at the day program, house managers, social workers, parents, consumer advocates, and/or significant others. Each plays a role as part of a team that ideally works together for the consumer's benefit. The occupational therapist communicates with all needed team members. In my experience, I have found that the OT perspective is very important with this population, and OT staff often needs to bring specific issues to the attention of the team. Providing in-services to training specialists and others is also very important.

Sometimes staff, even clinicians, harbor certain attitudes that one may find necessary to address. Staff may need to have neurological and sensory impairments explained to them, as well as why it is wrong to always assume that the consumer is being lazy or engaging in a manipulative behavior when he or she does not meet expectations. Sometimes, a consumer will have a disease, physical/sensory impairment, or drug-induced syndrome, and, additionally, exhibit behaviors that confuse staff. One consumer I worked with developed a Parkinsonian movement disorder and had a long history of being given neuroleptic drugs. At times he would be able to move very fast, and at other times he would become very stiff with "cogwheel rigidity" and would tend to fall. Because of these inconsistencies of movement and because he would smile or show a flat affect to pain and falls, many staff felt he was only exhibiting attention-seeking behaviors. Due to this attitude, these staff members did not respect his disabilities. The therapist needs to intervene in such cases, sharing his or her professional judgment and providing education.

CONCLUSION

Working with this population delivers job satisfaction for those who have patience, persistence, and motivation to meet therapeutic challenges. Key elements needed to achieve meaningful outcomes include:

- making effective, appropriate assessments
- prioritizing treatment issues and empowering direct-care staff for nonskilled issues
- being willing to take calculated risks and try varied approaches
- utilizing resources effectively
- reviewing progress regularly and monitoring for necessary changes.

It is quite possible that with advances in genetics, biomechanics, and early intervention access, the members of this population may decrease in number in the future. They may also be served in programs and with methods that are simpler, more streamlined, and more effective than ones that now exist across the country. The drive to cut costs will continue to harm progress in this area. The essential element to improving quality of care, however, will be a better understanding on the part of the public of the nature of people with these disabilities and of their needs.

REFERENCES

Association for Retarded Citizens (ARC). (1982). Internet resource. *Introduction to mental retardation: How many people are affected by mental retardation? Questions and answers.* http://thearc.org. Posted 9/97.

Association for Retarded Citizens (ARC). (1996). Internet resource. *Introduction to mental retardation: How is mental retardation diagnosed? Questions and answers.* http:// thearc.org. Posted 9/97.

Belfore, P. J., Danttilo, F. (1990). The behavior of self-injury: A brief review and analysis. *Journal of Behavioral Disorders,* Vol. 16, 1, XXX.

Brown, F., & Lehr. D. H. (1989). *Persons with profound disabilities: Issues and practices.* Baltimore, MD: Brookes.

Burkhart, L. (1982). *Homemade battery powered toys and educational devices for severely handicapped children* (2nd ed.) Baltimore, MD: Burkhardt.

Cataldo, M. (1988). Analysis and modification of disruptive behavior. In J. Kavanagh, (Ed.), *Understanding mental retardation: Research accomplishments and new frontiers* (p. 272). Baltimore, MD: Brookes.

Durand, M., & Kishi, G. (1987). Reducing severe behavior problems among persons with dual sensory impairments: An evaluation of a technical assistance model. *The Association for Persons with Severe Handicaps, 12*(1), 2–10.

Dussault, W. (1989). Is policy of exclusion based upon severity of disability legally defensible? In Brown, et al. (Eds.), *Persons with profound disabilities* (p. 45). Baltimore, MD: Brookes.

Evans, I., & Scotti, J. (1989). Defining meaningful outcomes for persons with profound disabilities. In Brown, et al. (Eds.), *Persons with profound disabilities* (p. 84). Baltimore, MD: Brookes.

Gardner, J. F., & Chapman, M. S. (1985). *Staff development in mental retardation services.* Baltimore MD: Brookes.

Haxby, J. V., & Shapiro, M. B. (1992). Longitudinal study of neuropsychological function in older adults with Down's syndrome. In Natel & Epstein (Eds.), *Down's syndrome and Alzheimer's disease* (pp. 35–50). New York: Wiley-Liss.

Heller, L., & Lockwood, J. (1991). *Designing a sensory motor environment.* Presentation at NYS/ADTP Statewide meeting. Young Adult Institute, Tarrytown Day Treatment Program, NY.

Hiramu, H. (1989). *Self abusive behavior: A somatosensory approach.* Bethesda MD: Chess Publishing.

Iwasaki, K., & Holm. M. B. (1990). Sensory treatment for the reduction of stereotype behaviors in persons with severe multiple disabilities. *Occupational Therapy Journal of Research, 9,* 170–183.

Janicki, M. P., Heller, T., Seltzer, G., & Hogg, J. (1995). *Practice guidelines for the clinical assessment and care management of Alzheimer and other dementias among adults with mental retardation.* Washington DC: American Association on Mental Retardation.

Kihss, P. (1977). Court ordered winds of change touch Willowbrook. *The New York Times, 2/26,* pp. 21, 41.

King, B. (1995). *Self-injurious Behavior (SIB) in individuals with mental retardation.* Internet resource. http:WWW.MRRC.NPI.UCLA.EDU/mrrc95/research/clinres/bking.htm.

Lakin, K. C., Hill, B., & Haydn, M. (1989). *Directory of residential centers for adults with developmental disabilities.* Phoenix: Oryx Press.

Luiselli, J. K., (1995). Reinforcement methods and variations in the clinical treatment of challenging behaviors. *The Habilitative Mental Healthcare Newsletter, 14, 2.*

Lynch, K., Kiernan, W., & Stark, J. (1982). *Prevocational education for special needs youth.* Baltimore, MD: Brookes.

Parrete, H., Strother, P. O., & Hourcade, J. J. (1986). Microswitches and adaptive equipment for severely impaired students. *Teaching Exceptional Children,* Fall, 1986.

Peck, C., & Hong, C. (1989). *Living skills for mentally handicapped people.* London: Croon & Helm.

Reisman, J., & Hanschu, B. (1990). *Sensory integration inventory for adults with developmental disabilities: User's guide,* Minneapolis, MN: PDP Press.

Reiss, S. (1996). *Mental illness in people with mental retardation.* Internet resource. Http://thearc.org. Posted 8/96.

Stahlman, M. T., Grogaard, J., et al. (1988). Neonatal intensive care and developmental outcome. In Kavanagh (Ed.), *Understanding mental retardation.* Baltimore, MD: Brookes.

Stark, J., Baker, D., Menousek, P., & McGee, J. (1982). Behavioral programming for severely mentally retarded/behaviorally impaired youth. In Lynch, et al. (Eds.), *Prevocational and vocational education for special needs youth: A blueprint for the 1980s* (p. 215). Baltimore, MD: Brookes.

Thompson, T. (1971). Preface to the first edition. In T. Thompson & J. Grabowski (Eds.), *Behavior modification of the mentally retarded* (2nd ed.). New York: Oxford University Press.

Whitman, T., Scibak, J., & Reid, D. (1983). *Behavior modification with the severely and profoundly retarded.* New York: Academic Press.

Wilbarger, P., & Wilbarger, J. (1991). *Sensory defensiveness in children aged 2–12: An intervention guide for parents and other caretakers.* Santa Barbara, CA: Avanti Educational Programs.

5

Low Vision Intervention for Individuals with Developmental Disabilities

T. Ann Williams, OTR/L

INTRODUCTION

The following chapter addresses visual dysfunction and the adult who is developmentally disabled, but it focuses primarily on the evaluation and treatment of visual dysfunction. It is intended to provide basic knowledge regarding the causes of vision loss, vision evaluation, and treatment of the functional problems that result. All daily living tasks can be affected by visual dysfunction, including self-care tasks, meal preparation, vocational tasks, and leisure activities. No matter what other disabilities the individual has, evaluation and treatment principles of vision loss are the same. As with any intervention used with the population that is developmentally disabled, appropriate modifications should be made for individual cognitive and physical abilities.

BACKGROUND

Persons with developmental disabilities encounter a myriad of obstacles in their attempts to adapt to their environment. These obstacles include a variety of chronic conditions manifested in childhood that include physical, psychological and cognitive impairments. Impairments of the visual system occur with high frequency in this population. It has been reported that the rate of incidence ranges from 48 percent to 75 percent (Manacker, 1993). The most common disorders that affect these individuals include refractive errors, strabismus, amblyopia, and motility problems. The etiology of these disturbances can be categorized as genetic, infectious, traumatic, and congenital.

The *congenital* causes often include abnormal embryologic development that can affect the eye or visual pathways. The ophthalmic problems resulting from these types of disturbances include strabismus, nystagmus, optic nerve hypoplasia, and cortical visual impairment. These conditions are long-lasting and often irreversible.

Ophthalmic findings that result from genetic causes of visual impairment vary in their characteristics. Disability can range from total vision loss to mild impairment. For example, retinitis pigmentosa is a progressive disorder with no known intervention that can cause total loss of vision. On the other end of the spectrum, persons with Down's syndrome often experience nonprogressive visual disturbances, such as high refractive errors, strabismus, and cataracts, which are highly treatable conditions.

Examples of *infectious* processes that can occur at birth or in childhood include toxoplasmosis, cytomegalovirus, and herpes simplex. Retinal scarring resulting from these diseases is common. This scarring is permanent and sometimes progressive, causing significant visual impairment, especially when the macula (the area of best vision on the retina) or fovea (the most acute vision in the macula) is involved.

Traumatic injury is a leading cause of visual impairment and developmental disability in children. Direct injury to ocular or cortical structures, and hypoxia are examples which induce damage. Individuals with developmental disabilities may suffer traumatic visual impairment that is caused by themselves (eye poking, head banging), their care-givers, or peers. Hypoxia is the primary cause of cortical visual impairment in children.

Visual impairments with congenital onset in the developmentally disabled individual should be evaluated and treated as early as possible to ensure the visual system's best chance to mature in a normal fashion. It is estimated that the human visual system matures between the ages of 6 and 7 (Manacker, 1993). Prior to this age, if there is visual deprivation or a disparity in the visual images that the two eyes receive, amblyopia can occur. *Amblyopia* is defined as subnormal visual acuity without a visible organic cause. It can be caused by visual acuity deficits due to asymmetrical refractive errors or by disparate images caused by strabismus. Treatment of the underlying causes, and the occlusion of the better eye, have proven to be successful in normalizing the acuity of amblyopic eyes in young children. After the visual system matures, amblyopia can not be caused or cured. Since a high percentage of persons with developmental disabilities experience the types of vision problems that can cause amblyopia, it is imperative that ophthalmological intervention begin early in life.

The occupational therapist working with the adult developmentally disabled person may be able to provide effective intervention for visual impairment even if it has been present since childhood. Adaptation of the person's environment using the principles presented below could prove beneficial, as could the use of adaptive equipment that would maximize the use of the client's remaining vision. In addition, as the person with a developmental disability ages, new vision impairment may occur that affects his or her ability to function at work or at home. Vision loss in the adult can occur as the result of many conditions. This loss may be due to:

▮ infectious diseases
▮ vascular abnormalities
▮ tumors
▮ traumatic injury
▮ ocular diseases such as macular degeneration and glaucoma.

Functional implications depend upon whether the vision loss is central or peripheral.

The visual system gathers information through central and peripheral fields. This information is processed by the central nervous system simultaneously. Focal vision, which uses the central visual field, is defined as the ability to perceive detailed information about an object. The macula and fovea are the ocular structures that constitute the central visual field. The fovea is the area of most acute vision in the eye. The macula is the 20° of visual field surrounding the fovea. Any area of decreased retinal function or blind spot that is within this 20° field is called a *scotoma* (Schuchard, 1995). Scotomas can be classified by their position on the retina (central or paracentral) and by their sensitivity to light (dense or threshold). Central scotomas are those that involve the fovea. The presence of a central scotoma forces the person to use an eccentric viewing position to view objects (Schuchard, 1995). Since the fovea is the area of best acuity, the person unable to use this area will require magnification to view small objects when using the chosen eccentric viewing position. A paracentral scotoma is one that is in the macula but does not involve the fovea. The person with a paracentral scotoma will continue to use the fovea as the primary viewing position but may miss visual information if it falls within the scotoma or blind spot. Dense scotomas are areas of the retina that do not respond to light at any intensity. Threshold scotomas are areas of decreased sensitivity that respond to light at high intensity but behave as blind spots in low lighting situations (Fletcher, Schuchard, Livingstone, Crane, & Hu, 1994). It is estimated that 83 percent of persons experiencing low vision have dense macular scotomas (Fletcher, Schuchard, Livingstone, Crane, & Hu, 1994). These scotomas can cause the person to miss salient features when trying to identify objects; they can also cause distortion of the visual image that the person perceives.

The peripheral fields are used to gather information about the environment and the person's relationship to it. They work in conjunction with the vestibular and proprioceptive systems to provide balance and are important in maintaining orientation.

The therapist working with individuals who have experienced a decrease in visual function should know which type of vision (central or peripheral) is affected by each diagnosis and should be aware of typical problems that occur with each type of loss. Listed below are brief descriptions of some common causes of vision loss in the adult.

COMMON CAUSES OF VISION LOSS IN ADULTS

Infectious Diseases

Histoplasmosis. This disease is caused by a fungus transmitted by spores found in the dried excrements of animals. It commonly affects vision and can be life threatening if not treated. Histoplasmosis causes scattered lesions on the retina in both the macular and peripheral areas. When the macula is affected, a decrease in visual acuity is present and color vision is often deficient. As with other conditions that cause macular scotomas, contrast sensitivity scores may also be reduced.

Toxoplasmosis. Toxoplasmosis is an intraocular infection caused by *toxoplasma gondii*. It is transmitted through contact with infected animals or ingestion of raw meat. This disease causes retinal lesions, especially in the macular area. The disease is nonprogressive, although new lesions may develop over time. As in all other conditions that affect the macula, a loss in visual acuity, decreased contrast sensitivity scores, and deficient color vision may be present.

Acquired Immune Deficiency Syndrome.   AIDS is caused by the human immunodeficiency virus (HIV) and predisposes the infected person to a host of other diseases that affect vision. Persons with HIV have an increased risk of retinopathy, especially from the cytomegalovirus. Both the macula and peripheral fields are affected. This disease can (and often does) cause complete vision loss in the AIDS patient.

Tumors and Traumatic Injury

Tumors and traumatic injury can cause visual impairment through a variety of means. Damage may be inflicted by direct or indirect injury to ocular or cortical structures. For example, the optic nerve can be directly injured through stretching by sudden deceleration during a traumatic head injury or by a direct penetrating injury to the nerve such as occurs with stab or gunshot wounds. Indirect injury to this same structure can occur by compression from edema, hematoma, or tumor.

The ocular structures and all parts of the central nervous system, including the brainstem, cerebellum, and cortex are vital to the processing of vision. The vision loss resulting from a traumatic injury or tumor depends upon which structures are involved and the extent of the damage caused by such insults. Common problems include visual field loss, ocular motility problems, decreases in acuity, and paralytic strabismus.

Ocular Diseases

Macular Degeneration.   Macular degeneration is any kind of ocular degeneration affecting the macula. The most common type is age-related macular degeneration (ARMD). This is a disease that primarily affects those persons 50 years of age and older. It causes retinal deterioration in the central visual field, thus resulting in decreased acuity, contrast sensitivity, and color discrimination. Peripheral vision is spared in this type of disease process.

There are two types of ARMD: exudative and dry. The exudative type is characterized by neovascular structures that bleed or leak fluid into the space between the retina and underlying structures, thus causing macular swelling and death to the cells of the retina. The person with exudative ARMD can experience a gradual or sudden loss of vision, depending upon the severity of the bleed. Laser treatments are used to seal off these neovascular structures, thus attempting to slow the progression of the disease. However, research has demonstrated that these treatments postpone the onset of severe vision loss only by approximately 18 months. This is because of the high rate of recurrent growth of new vessels. The dry type of ARMD is characterized by gradual onset and has no known treatment. The pigment epithelium is a layer of tissue just beneath the retina and provides nourishment to it. In the dry type of ARMD, the part of this layer that nourishes the macula dies, thus causing these retinal cells to degenerate or to die. The causes of macular degeneration are not known at this time.

Glaucoma.   Adult onset of glaucoma can be of the primary or secondary type. *Glaucoma* is a generic term much like "cancer." It refers to a group of disease processes in which the intraocular pressure is so high that it damages the tissues of the eye, resulting in vision loss. The most common type of glaucoma is primary, open-angle glaucoma. As with all other glaucomas, it is caused by insufficient outflow of the aqueous humor from the eye. The etiology of this condition is unknown. It causes peripheral visual field loss first. Thus the person who has it may not be aware of a visual impairment until late in its progression when visual acuity may be affected. Persons with glaucoma often experience a decrease in contrast sensitivity function and a "washing out" phenomenon when exposed to too much light. This phenomenon is one in which the image at which they are looking fades out when the illumination level is high.

Diabetic Retinopathy

Diabetic retinopathy is the leading cause of blindness in the United States (Gardner & Schoch, 1987). It occurs in those persons who have diabetes mellitus, which is a systemic condition resulting from the lack of insulin in the bloodstream. There are two types of diabetes mellitus. Juvenile diabetes (onset prior to age 20) is the most severe and most difficult to treat. Onset of the disease after age 40 is considered mature diabetes and is generally controlled by oral medication and diet control. The complications from diabetes mellitus depends upon the severity of the disease process and its onset. The ocular problems associated with this disease stem generally from changes in the blood vessels of the eye. However, some early signs of diabetes are the general loss of the ability to accommodate and a fluctuating refractive measurement.

There are two types of diabetic retinopathy: nonproliferative and proliferative. In nonproliferative retinopathy, the changes in the eye are confined to the retina. These changes include dilation of veins, hemorrhages, and edema or exudates in the retina. Proliferative retinopathy involves both the retina and the vitreous and has the worst prognosis. The most damaging feature of proliferative retinopathy is the growth of new blood vessels on the surface of the retina that sometimes extend into the vitreous. These new blood vessels can cause retinal detachment, as well as new hemorrhaging in the eye. Visual impairment depends upon which area of the retina is affected and can vary from one hemorrhagic episode to the next. Fluctuating visual function is a common characteristic of diabetic retinopathy.

EVALUATION

As an occupational therapist working with developmentally disabled adults, one must be able to recognize signs that may point to visual dysfunction. Some common visual symptoms are:

- ocular pain
- blurred vision
- diplopia
- distortion of vision
- photophobia
- flashing lights
- halos around lights
- abnormal color vision
- visual hallucinations
- night blindness
- inability to see details (Gardner & Schoch, 1987).

Many persons with developmental disabilities are unable to accurately describe the symptoms they are experiencing. Therefore, observation by the occupational therapist is critical for early detection of visual problems experienced by this population. If a therapist believes that a client is experiencing visual problems, more formal testing will be necessary to determine the severity of the deficit.

Four areas of visual function that are commonly affected by disease and trauma include contrast sensitivity function, acuity, visual field, and oculomotor dysfunction (Rubin, 1989; Giatnutsos, Ramsey, & Perlin, 1988; Schlageter, Gray, Hall, Shaw, & Sammet, 1993). All daily living tasks can be affected by deficits in these areas including:

- self-care (applying toothpaste, eating neatly, selecting clothing)
- meal preparation (measuring ingredients, cutting or chopping items, identifying foods)
- housekeeping
- work tasks
- shopping (making change)
- community activities (accessing transportation, recognizing acquaintances, negotiating curbs/steps)
- reading and leisure activities (card games, bingo).

Acuity

Conditions that affect the macula, such as macular degeneration, glaucoma, and many infectious diseases can cause decreased acuity, as can trauma to the eye or central nervous system. The function of acuity is to ensure that a sharp image is focused on the retina. It depends upon the transparency of all of the structures between the outside of the eye and the retina, on the length of the eyeball, the closeness of the object, and the integrity of the retina.

Measurement of acuity is simply the evaluation of the threshold for recognition of high-contrast materials at different distances (Lampert & Lapolice, 1995). It is most commonly written in a Snellen fraction (20/40), which in this case means that the examinee was able to see at 20 feet what a person with average normal visual acuity can see at 40 feet. This far distance acuity could affect the person in some mobility tasks and community interaction tasks but may not have any functional implications in the home or work place. Since most activities of daily living are performed at near or intermediate distances (16 inches to 3 feet), it is important to measure the persons's acuity at these distances (Colenbrander & Fletcher, 1992). Due to accommodation, the presence of myopia/hyperopia, and a myriad of other factors, the measurements gained at near and intermediate distances may very well be different from those obtained at a far distance.

Clinical observations that may indicate visual acuity problems include being unable to recognize faces and difficulty in seeing small objects or the salient features of larger objects. A more detailed list of clinical observations can be found at the end of this chapter (Appendix C).

Formal evaluation of acuity can be performed with a variety of commercially-available products. In adults, visual acuity is normally measured with eye charts using letters or numbers, such as the Pelli-Robson and Snellen charts. These tests require the person being tested to have the ability to recognize and name the characters presented. Some developmentally disabled persons have the ability to name letters and numbers, but many do not. Because of this fact, a test designed for acuity measurement in children may be more appropriate for use with this population. The Lea Symbols acuity chart is designed for individuals who are developmentally 18 months of age and above. It utilizes four symbols and a variety of testing tools to allow evaluation of nonverbal and multihandicapped individuals. The test is easy to administer and gives acuity values for the viewing distance at which each chart is most commonly used (10 feet, 16 inches). For persons who are developmentally below 18 months of age, acuity can be measured using grating acuity tests. Because of the skill required to accurately give this test, it is recommended that these persons be evaluated by an ophthalmologist or optometrist familiar with grating acuity measurements. In this type of test, the person detects the presence of parallel lines of decreasing width. The gratings are defined by the numbers of pairs of black and white lines within one degree of visual angle. The examiner presents two targets to the individual. One has the parallel lines on its surface, and the other has a solid gray surface. The person being tested is more likely to look at the patterned surface if they can detect the lines, since there is more visual stimulation than on the gray surface. Acuity is calculated by noting the smallest distance between lines that the person appeared to be able to see.

Contrast Sensitivity

Decreased contrast sensitivity can cause significant functional problems in many daily living tasks, including facial recognition and mobility activities. *Contrast sensitivity function* is defined as the ability to differentiate objects of similar luminances (Hyvarinen, 1996). A white cup sitting on a white table is an example of a low contrast situation. A person with impaired contrast sensitivity function would have difficulty seeing the cup, because its hue and luminance is only faintly different from the table's. Decreased contrast sensitivity can be an early indicator of glaucoma and diabetic retinopathy. It also occurs with many other conditions that cause vision loss, and its assessment should be a part of any vision evaluation.

Clinical observations that may indicate poor contrast sensitivity include:

∎ inability to accurately identify colors of similar luminance and hue
∎ difficulty in pouring liquids without spilling
∎ decrease in performance when in dim lighting.

As with measurement of acuity, contrast sensitivity function should be measured at distances in which the person is required to perform functional tasks. Assessment tools for contrast sensitivity include the Pelli-Robson test and Lea Symbols Low Contrast Visual Acuity Test. The person's ability to recognize letters or symbols will determine which test is the most appropriate. There is also a grating test, the Cambridge Low Contrast Gratings, for those individuals who are not able to match or name letters/symbols.

One method the occupational therapist can use to determine if a client is experiencing contrast sensitivity dysfunction is to have the client perform a task in bright light and then perform the same task in dim lighting. The task can be as simple as matching colored pieces of paper. If the client is able to accurately match the colors in bright light but not dim light, a problem with contrast sensitivity is indicated. The therapist should ensure that the client's eyes have had time to adapt to the decrease in light level before performing the second portion of the observation. If the therapist is able to see the difference in the color of the paper prior to when the client can perceive it, this may be an indication that the client's eyes are deficient in their ability to adapt to changing light levels.

Visual Field Deficits

Visual field deficits are most commonly caused by postchiasmal pathway lesions, occipital lobe lesions, anoxia, central retinal artery occlusion, and glaucoma. The loss of visual field can cause changes in oculomotor behavior such as irregular and inaccurate saccades and changes in visual exploration of the environment (Warren, 1996). These changes result in many functional problems involving mobility and activities of daily living.

Evaluation of visual field losses include the quantification of the deficit and assessment of the functional problems that may result. Decreased performance during daily living tasks can provide the first evidence that a client has sustained a visual field loss. Observations that may indicate this type of vision loss are provided at the end of this chapter.

The occupational therapist can perform a confrontation test to screen clients suspected of having a visual field loss. Confrontation testing is a simple procedure that gives a gross approximation of the size and type of visual field loss. The examiner sits in front of the client and has the client fixate on the examiner's nose. The examiner then presents stimuli in opposite visual fields and has the client indicate if he or she can see the objects. Each of the four quadrants of visual field should be tested. If the client does not see the stimulus in any specific quadrant or hemifield, a visual field loss is indicated. The stimulus used is often the examiner's hands/fingers. However, other objects can be used, such as pencil toppers or brightly-colored dots affixed to tongue depressors. Confrontation testing should be used only in conjunction with careful observation of the client during daily living tasks since confrontation testing alone is only useful as a gross indication of the presence of a visual field deficit. This type of testing may miss more subtle visual field losses.

The most accurate method of testing for visual field loss is the use of computerized automated perimetry (Warren, 1993). If a therapist does not have an automated perimetry device in his or her clinic, referral to an ophthalmologist or optometrist can be made. In this type of testing, the person places his or her chin on a chin rest and fixates on a central target inside a bowl-shaped device. As the person fixates on the central target, lights are displayed inside the bowl. The person is asked to respond each time he or she sees the light by pushing a button. Perimetry evaluation can be of the kinetic or static type. In kinetic measurement, the test spot moves from the side toward the center of the visual field until it is noticed by the client. In static measurement, points of light are flashed in specific spots in the visual field, and the client indicates whether he or she sees them.

Some persons with developmental disabilities may not be able to be reliably tested with automated perimetry examination due to motor or cognitive limitations. For these individuals, a tangent screen visual field evaluation could be more appropriate. Tangent screen evaluation can also be performed by an ophthalmologist or optometrist. A tangent screen is utilized mainly for evaluating for the presence of central field scotomas, but can also detect the presence of a peripheral field loss. It does not provide results as accurate as an automated perimetry for peripheral field loss, but it is quick and the evaluator can control the pace of the test. In this evaluation, the person is asked to fixate on a central point on a black screen affixed to a wall. The screen measures approximately 57″ × 57″, and testing is performed at a distance of 1 meter. The examiner uses a black wand with a white light on the end and presents it in different portions of the visual field. The person being examined is asked to indicate when he or she is able to see the light. The examiner marks the screen with a pin at the spot where the client first perceives the light. The resulting pattern is an outline of the client's good visual field.

Oculomotor Dysfunction

The purpose of oculomotor function is to keep the image being viewed on the fovea (area of most acute vision) of each eye (Daroff, 1974). The accurate control of the eyes is dependent upon the integrity of the ocular structures, extraocular musculature, the brainstem, cortex, and the cerebellum. Any damage to these structures can cause oculomotor problems.

One common cause of oculomotor dysfunction is trauma. In a study performed by Schlageter, Gray, Hall, Shaw and Sammet (1993), it was found that 59 percent of traumatic brain injuries admitted to an inpatient rehabilitation hospital had problems with oculomotor function. These problems can occur due to damage to the structures of the central nervous system, laceration of an extraocular muscle, or entrapment of a muscle due to orbital fractures (Baker, 1991). Cerebrovascular accidents and vascular diseases such as diabetes, hypertension, and atherosclerosis can damage structures of the central nervous system that control the movements of the extraocular muscles. Other diseases that attack the CNS, such as Parkinson's, Huntington's Chorea, Alzheimer's, and muscular sclerosis can also damage these structures, thus causing paralysis or paresis in one or more of the extraocular muscles.

Paralytic strabismus is often the result of such damage. Strabismus is a noticeable deviation of one eye in relation to the other (Lavich & Nelson, 1993). This deviation can be in any direction, depending upon which extraocular muscle has been affected. Characteristics of paralytic strabismus include diplopia and restriction of eye movement. Some common complaints resulting from strabismus are diplopia, eye fatigue, and headaches after a period of sustained viewing. More clinical observations are listed at the end of this chapter (Appendix C).

The evaluation of oculomotor dysfunction as a diagnostic tool requires experience and skill. It is recommended that if a therapist believes a client has experienced a recent onset of this type of problem, a referral be made to a qualified professional for detailed evaluation. However, the occupational therapist can perform a screening test to determine areas of functional deficits. This screening should determine whether the eyes work together and in what situations the visual system works the best/worst. To answer these questions, the testing should include measurement of eye alignment, range of motion, and the ability to locate and fixate on targets (Warren, 1993). It should be noted at this time that difficulties experienced in performing accurate saccades, pursuit patterns, and localization/fixation tasks could be attributed to visual field loss (central or peripheral), as well as oculomotor dysfunction. Visual field evaluation should be performed if problems are noted with these tasks.

Eye alignment can be measured by observation of the corneal light reflex. This test consists of asking the client to fixate on a pen light and then observing the reflection of the light on the corneas of both eyes. When the eyes are aligned, the reflection will appear in the same location on each pupil. If one eye is deviated inward, the corneal reflection will be located towards the lateral side of the pupil in that eye. If the eye is deviated outward, the reflection will be towards the medial side of the pupil. Vertical deviation will place the reflection toward the bottom or top of the pupil, depending upon the direction of displacement (Lavich & Nelson, 1993). Another screening test for eye alignment is the cover test. The client is asked to fixate on a central target. One eye is then quickly covered, and the examiner observes the uncovered eye to determine if it moves to establish fixation. The test is then performed with the other eye. No movement of the eyes indicates that the eyes are aligned (Warren, 1993).

The purpose of a visual saccade is to place the image of the object being viewed onto the fovea. The individual's ability to accurately and quickly perform visual saccades can be observed by having the client alternate fixation on two objects held approximately 6 inches apart and 16 inches from the bridge of the nose (Warren, 1993). The client should be able to quickly and smoothly shift gaze between the two targets. The examiner should watch for difficulties in initiating the saccade and the accuracy with which the saccades are performed.

Smooth pursuit eye movements can be measured by having the client fixate on a target that is moved through the nine cardinal gaze positions. Observation should be made with regard to speed, coordination, and range of motion of the eyes. The patient's ability to perform convergence movements should also be evaluated at this time. This skill is tested by having the client fixate on a central target that is moved towards the bridge of the nose. The examiner should note at what distance convergence is broken. In persons with normal oculomotor control, the near point of convergence is approximately 3 inches from the bridge of the nose. Insufficiency in convergence can cause increased difficulty in performing tasks that require focusing at close distances.

Finally, the therapist should observe the client during localization and fixation tasks in different visual fields. The examiner should hold up a target in various locations and distances and ask the client to find and look at the object for a period of time. Observations made include the ability of the client to quickly find the object and the ability to maintain fixation on the object.

Adaptation Deficits/Glare Sensitivity

The ability of the visual system to function in different lighting levels can be affected by a variety of conditions and disease processes. Adaptation problems are common among the visually impaired population, as is sensitivity to glare (Lampert & Lapolice, 1995). Both conditions can cause significant functional difficulties, especially in mobility tasks.

The eye's ability to adapt to changing light levels is a function of the rods and cones, cells within the retina that are stimulated by light. Cones function best in bright light and provide color vision. They are more numerous than rods and are concentrated in the macula and fovea. Rods are extremely light sensitive and function best in low lighting situations. They are most numerous in the periphery of the retina (Gardner & Schoch, 1987). When a person goes from a brightly-lit area to an area with dim illumination, the eyes adjust within 10 to 15 minutes. During this time, the cones begin to decrease their activity and the rods respond by increasing theirs. If a person has a condition that has affected the peripheral vision, such as glaucoma, retinitis pigmentosa (RP), or a visual field loss from trauma, his or her ability to adapt to low-lighting situations may be impaired. In some cases, as with RP, the loss of rods is progressive and the end result is night blindness. Persons with this condition have totally lost their ability to adapt to low lighting and essentially lose most vision under low light levels.

Adaptation to an increase in illumination occurs much more rapidly than to decreases in lighting. When a person enters a lighted environment from a dark one, he or she should be able to adapt in about 2 to 6 minutes (Jose, 1983). This adaptation occurs as the cones are stimulated by the increase in lighting level and the rods are bleached out by the same.

Clinical observations that may indicate a problem with light adaptation include:

▮ The person becomes hesitant, trips or bumps into objects when entering an area of decreased illumination.

▮ When outdoors, the person has difficulty ambulating in areas that have alternating shade and sunlit areas and becomes fearful when in dimly lit areas.

▮ The person shields eyes or wants to wear sunglasses or brimmed hat at all times and avoids windows.

Sensitivity to glare, as stated above, is a common complaint among persons with visual system disturbances (Jose, 1983). Glare is generally caused by opacities in the ocular structures anterior to the retina, but it is also a complaint of those persons who have diseases that affect the retina. Cataracts often cause a scattering of light rays that results in a decrease in acuity and color discrimination, as do any corneal or vitreous opacities. Glare also decreases perceived contrast and can cause fatigue and strain. Clinical observations for glare sensitivity are similar to those made for adaptation problems.

TREATMENT OPTIONS

The treatment for visual dysfunction is the same as for any other disability. The goals are to minimize areas of weakness and to maximize strengths. These goals can be achieved through adaptation of the person's environment, through training in compensatory techniques and use of adaptive devices, or a combination thereof.

The effectiveness of any intervention will depend upon the person's ability to understand his or her vision loss, his or her ability to follow directions, to remember instructions, and his or her basic ability to adapt. Whether the person with a developmental disability is living in a group home or with a parent or guardian, it is also vital that the caretakers understand the nature of the vision loss and the resulting functional implications.

The occupational therapists should first look to adapt the person's environment to maximize function, especially when working with an individual with a developmental disability. Three areas of critical importance in evaluating the impact of the environment on the person's ability to function with a visual loss are lighting, contrast, and pattern. After adapting the environment using these principles, magnification devices and training in compensatory techniques can be used if the client is still experiencing difficulties in performing functional tasks. Teaching compensatory techniques such as eccentric viewing or teaching the use of a magnifier may be difficult with this population due to physical and cognitive deficits. General information on treatment options are presented below, followed by specific problems and their possible solutions.

Lighting

The first step that the occupational therapist must take in assisting the person with visual impairment is to assess the lighting situation at his or her work place or home.

The importance of proper lighting cannot be overemphasized when working with persons experiencing vision loss of any type. Central visual field disruption will cause a decrease in contrast sensitivity, and peripheral field loss will cause problems with adapting to dim lighting situations. Increased illumination can stimulate portions of the retina that have a decreased sensitivity to light, thus minimizing the effects of threshold scotomas and improving perceived contrast between objects. Therefore, adequate illumination is critical for maximizing the abilities of the client with vision loss to cope with his or her environment.

There are two categories of lighting that the therapist needs to be aware of: ambient illumination, and directional or task illumination. Ambient lighting is provided by ceiling fixtures, torchiere lamps, table lamps, and so forth, and provides basic room illumination. Some of the light rays from these fixtures are projected directly into the living space, and some bounce off of ceilings, floors, and walls. Proper ambient illumination is critical for mobility tasks. If it is not possible to increase the amount of ambient light by increasing the wattage of the bulbs being used or by adding more light fixtures to the area, changing the colors of the walls and ceiling to a lighter hue may brighten the areas enough for improved function. Task lighting is that which is pointed directly at the activity being performed. This type of illumination is best provided by a directional lamp with a solid shade that has a support that allows for flexibility in positioning. It should be directed over the shoulder of the eye with the best vision or opposite the working hand and close to the work being performed. Care should be taken to ensure that the light does not shine into the person's eyes and that shadows do not fall on the task being performed. Proper task illumination is critical for performance of activities that require detail vision.

The ability to adjust illumination levels is also an important consideration when working with persons with visual impairment. Those individuals with glaucoma experience a "washing out" of images when the light level is too high, and bright lights can cause significant glare problems with persons who have cataracts or corneal scarring. Trauma or diseases that affect the optic nerve such as multiple sclerosis can cause significant sensitivity to light. Persons with macular degeneration, diabetic retinopathy, or field deficits often complain of a "dimming"of images and require extra lighting. Adjustment of the amount of illumination can be achieved through the use of dimmer switches, higher or lower wattage bulbs, and the proximity of the light source to the targeted area.

The control of glare is an important consideration when adjusting illumination. Glare can come from the surface of the activity, reflecting light into the person's eyes, and from the light source itself. If a person consistently complains of glare after all appropriate adjustments have been made to illumination sources, the use of a visor or sun filters may be indicated. These devices will restrict the transmission of light into the person's eyes, thus decreasing the effects of glare.

Contrast

As defined above, contrast sensitivity is the ability to discriminate among objects of similar luminances. Many ocular conditions cause a decrease in this ability, resulting in a variety of functional problems. Contrasts that can be perceived by the normally-sighted individual can be impossible for the person with poor vision to see. For the individual with a visual disturbance, enhancing contrast can be a vital component in improving the ability to perform certain tasks. One way to enhance contrast is by increasing the amount of light on the subject (discussed in more detail in the previous section). Changing the color of the background to a hue of higher contrast to the objects in the foreground is another way to assist a person with poor contrast sensitivity. For example, a person may have difficulty applying white toothpaste to a toothbrush with white bristles, especially if this task has a white sink or counter as its background. To improve this individual's ability to accurately perform this activity, a dark washcloth could be placed on the counter or sink to heighten the contrast between the bristles and its background. Taking this concept one step further, red or blue toothpaste can be used to provide higher contrast between it and the white bristles of the toothbrush. The use of yellow filters can also enhance contrast for some tasks, especially reading printed material.

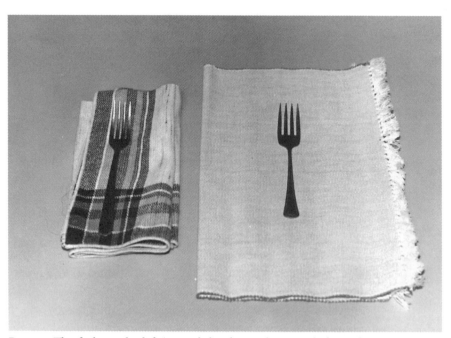

FIGURE 5.1   Pattern: The fork on the left is much harder to distinguish from the patterned background of the napkin than is the fork on the right, which is on a solid-colored napkin

Pattern

The presence of pattern often hinders the ability of the person with vision problems to perform functional activities. Pattern can be described as "background noise" affecting the eyes in ways similar to the way static on the radio affects the ability to hear. Table cloths, placemats, bedspreads, rugs which have printed designs are examples of objects whose patterns may interfere with a person's ability to perform certain activities of daily living (ADL). Pattern tends to "draw objects in" and makes locating foreground items very difficult for the person with visual dysfunction (Figure 5.1). These individuals may have difficulty locating items on their plate or at their placesetting if these objects are presented with a patterned background. The clutter found in drawers and on desks is another example of pattern that makes it difficult to locate needed items. To improve the person's ability to function in their environment, the presence of pattern should be decreased. Solid-colored tablecloths, napkins, and plates can be used at the dinner table to make location of utensils and food items easier. In the workplace, solid-colored placemats, which define the person's work space, can be used if their table or desk has a patterned surface. Organization of drawers and desktops is also important in decreasing the detrimental effects of pattern at home and work.

Magnification and Optical Devices

If the client with poor vision is still experiencing significant difficulties with a particular task after environmental adaptations are made, the use of magnification devices can be considered. The most common detail task that requires magnification is reading. However, some other activities such as crocheting, playing cards, or performing assembly tasks while on the job may also require magnification. There are several types and strengths of magnifiers on the market, each with its own advantages and disadvantages.

Magnification strength is measured in diopters. When light rays pass through a plain plate of glass, the rays travel in a straight line, remaining parallel. However, if that glass is curved, refraction or bending of the light rays occurs. A diopter is a measurement of the light bending power of a particular piece of glass or lens. The diopter number is higher for lenses that have more light bending power (Jose, 1983). As the curve of a magnifying lens increases, so does its strength. Because of this fact, the higher power lenses tend to be smaller and thus provide a smaller field of view. Strengths of convex lenses are given a plus diopter value, and concave lenses are given minus diopter values. The optical devices discussed here all have plus values (adds). To determine the strength of magnification required by the person, one must first measure the best-corrected acuity. The reciprocal of this measurement gives the minimum diopter power needed for accessing details approximately the size of newsprint. For example, if a person's visual acuity is 20/200, first reduce the fraction to its simplest term, in this case 1/10. The reciprocal of this fraction, 10/1, gives the minimum number of diopters needed in a magnifying device to allow the person to see details the size of newsprint. It should be noted at this time that this number is merely a starting point. The activity to be performed may require more or less magnification, depending upon its size and contrast and the lighting situation.

Diopter measurement is converted to "X-power" for most magnifying devices. The exceptions are the headborne magnifiers and spectacles. The "X-power" of a magnifier is written as "3X" or "10X." This is the most common description of a magnifying device's strength at the retail level. To convert the "X-power" into diopters, merely divide the number of "Xs" by four. For example, the diopter strength of a 3X magnifier is 12.

The type of magnification device used by the client is determined by the activity being performed, whether the person requires the use of both hands when performing the activity, and the client's motor, visual, and cognitive skills.

Listed below is an assortment of types of magnifiers and their advantages and disadvantages. Magnifying devices can be purchased at optical supply stores, but the strengths and styles found may be limited. More variety can be found in catalogues that specifically carry low vision supplies. Some of these catalogues are listed in the resource section at the end of this chapter. It is important that the magnifying device used by an individual with low vision is of the proper strength and style. Using an improperly prescribed device can be extremely frustrating. Until the therapist has adequate experience, it is recommended that he or she consult with other professionals who specialize in this area before dispensing magnifying devices.

Headborne Magnifiers/Spectacles (Figure 5.2).   These devices give the widest field of view and allow both hands to be free to perform an activity. They range in strength from + 2 to + 48 diopters. Binocular vision is possible to approximately + 10 if prismatic lenses are used. These magnifiers require a close working distance, to which it is difficult for some individuals to adjust. Some headborne devices can fit over the person's own glasses allowing the person to use his or her own correction plus the magnification power of the device.

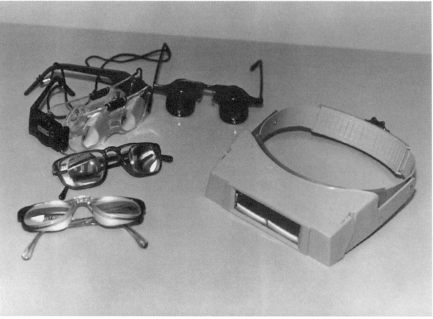

FIGURE 5.2 Examples of headborne devices and spectacles. Visor-style device (on right) can be worn over the patient's own prescription glasses. Note the prismatic–stye glasses on left, in foreground. Prism allows for binocular vision up to +10 diopter in strength. Binocular-style glasses in the rear are used for distance viewing.

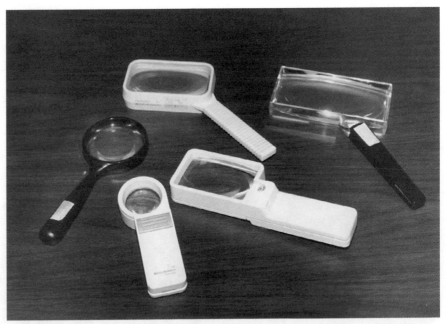

FIGURE
5.3 Handheld magnifiers in foreground have built-in light to illuminate objects being viewed.

Hand Held Magnifiers (Figure 5.3). Hand-held magnifiers are commonly sold in optical shops and retail stores. Some come with a built-in light source. These devices are portable and can be used with the client's own glasses. One hand must hold the magnifier, unless it is used with a mounting device. Prolonged viewing is often uncomfortable and may cause hand/arm fatigue. The person must hold it at the correct focal distance to achieve optimal magnification, and some persons find this distance difficult to maintain. However, these are very good for spot viewing tasks, such as looking at appliance dials, reading prices, or identifying money.

Stand Magnifiers (Figure 5.4). Stand magnifiers are ones that provide a base on which the lens is mounted that holds the lens at the proper focal distance from the object being viewed. These devices are awkward to use on nonflat surfaces, and are most often used for reading. Stand magnifiers can come with their own light source, powered by either batteries or a transformer that plugs into a wall outlet. They can be very strong but provide a narrow field of view. Activities cannot be performed under most designs.

Architect-Style Light/Magnifiers (Figure 5.5). This type of magnifying device has the lens mounted on a flexible or gooseneck-style arm that is set

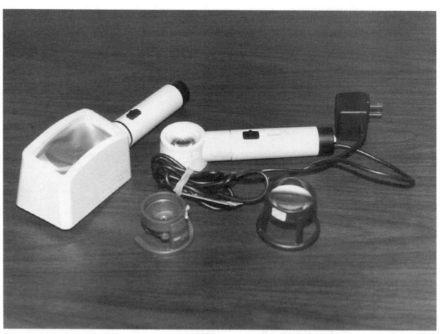

**FIGURE
5.4** Examples of stand magnifiers. Magnifiers in the rear have their own light
sources. Light sources can be powered by a plug-in handle (on right) or a
battery (on left).

into a base or can be attached to a table. These magnifiers sometimes come
with their own light source, often a fluorescent or high-intensity lamp. They
provide a wide viewing area and activities can be performed under them.
Magnification strengths are generally on the low end of the scale (+7 to
+12 diopters). This style of magnifier is most often used with craft activities.

Telescopes.   Telescopes are mainly used for viewing distant objects. These
units are portable and are useful for such spot viewing as street signs and
aisle markers. They may be very difficult to use for a person with low vision
and require extensive training to ensure proper utilization. The field of view
is limited when using these devices, which causes problems in locating the
proper target. Balance problems can also be experienced since peripheral
vision is severely limited during its use.

Compensatory Visual Skills

Training in the use of compensatory visual skills for central or peripheral
field loss may prove difficult for the therapist working with individuals with
developmental disabilities. Success depends upon the ability of the person

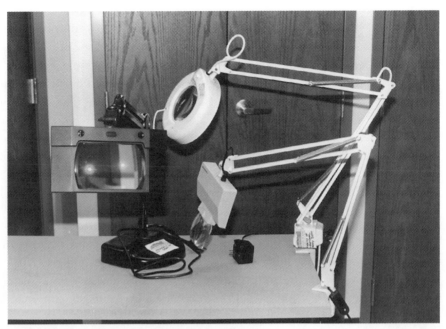

FIGURE
5.5
Examples of architect-style lighted magnifiers.

who has sustained vision loss to cognitively override habits that have been established for a lifetime. The experience and knowledge of the therapist is also critical in achieving these goals. The following descriptions of these processes are meant merely to be introductions to the concepts presented. Therapists who wish to utilize compensatory visual skills training in their work should consult with other professionals who are more experienced in this area or seek further information from the references listed at the end of this chapter.

Central Visual Field Loss.   When a person experiences a central visual field loss that affects the fovea, an eccentric viewing position is naturally and reliably established (Schuchard & Fletcher, 1994). This preferred retinal locus (PRL) is then used to perform visual tasks normally performed by the fovea (Schuchard, 1995). However, the person who experiences this is often unaware of how to quickly and accurately locate the PRL during activities of daily living. The goal of the therapist working with these individuals is to improve the ability of the client to use the PRL in functional tasks.

Observation of the client as he or she is attempting to see an object can assist the occupational therapist in determining where the PRL is located.

A simple screening can be performed by the therapist in this determination. The examiner should sit directly in front of the client and ask him or her to look at the therapist's face. Observation should be made as to which direction the client's eyes move to view the examiner's face. This movement will be in the direction of the established PRL. The client should also be asked if he or she can see the examiner's entire face or if any part looks distorted or dim. Areas of distortion indicate where the field loss or scotoma is located.

Eccentric viewing training teaches the client with central visual field loss to use this PRL during functional tasks. Clients are first asked to locate objects with their PRL in different visual fields and then to maintain fixation as they perform functional tasks. The success of this training depends upon the client's ability to follow directions and the ability to control eye movements. (More information on eccentric viewing training can be found in the LUV Reading Series, distributed by Mattingly International listed in Appendix A.)

Peripheral Visual Field Loss.   The loss of peripheral visual fields greatly affects the person's safety in mobility tasks and ability to locate objects in the environment. These individuals generally use poor scanning strategies and also tend to overlook details in the affected field. When dealing with functional problems, the client should be taught proper strategies to compensate for these deficits in addition to environmental adaptations.

The therapists should first determine where the field loss is located. This can be achieved through the use of a confrontation screening and subsequent perimetry evaluation. Behaviors that use the individual's remaining vision to monitor the missing visual field then should be taught and reinforced through structured activities. The desired behaviors are wider head turns and saccades, faster eye and head movement, the use of an organized, efficient search pattern, and an increase in anticipatory behavior (Warren, 1993). Examples of activities that can be used for reinforcing these behaviors include card matching, searching for objects or colors in the environment, and balloon volleyball.

Specific Problems/Solutions

Eating

Problems.   Difficulties encountered in eating include locating items on the table, identifying foods, cutting meat into bite-sized pieces, eating neatly, and handling certain food items such as peas or salad.

Solutions.   To improve the client's ability to perform these tasks, the therapist should first increase the light level by moving the client close to a window or adding a directional light to illuminate their place setting. Decreasing the background pattern through use of solid-colored tablecloths, placemats, napkins, and plates can also be of assistance. Placing food items in separate dishes can help the client to manage some types of loose foods. Increasing contrast between the food and the dishes can allow the client to more easily see the food. Having the client lean over the plate when bringing food to the mouth can reduce spillage. Knocking over items on the table is a common problem for individuals with both peripheral and central field losses. If the client tends to knock over items when reaching for other objects, teach him or her to "trail" the fingers over the surface of the table when reaching. Using this technique, if an obstacle is encountered, the client will hit the base of the object instead of the top, thus decreasing the chance of knocking it over. Techniques used by the blind can be taught for cutting meat and handling foods if necessary.

Dressing

Problems.   Locating items in drawers and closets is often a problem for persons with vision loss in either the peripheral or central fields. For those persons with decreased contrast sensitivity discrimination of colors can also be difficult.

Solutions.   Add light to the area is possible. Battery-powered wall lights are easily installed in closets, and a directional light placed near drawers can illuminate their contents. If neither of these options is possible, the person may benefit from the use of a flashlight when searching for needed items. Improving the organization of the closets and drawers may also prove beneficial, providing the person is able to maintain the order. Hanging matching clothes together in the closet and the use of dividers in drawers for different colors can help. Clothing items that are similar in color and style can be marked with a simple system using brass safety pins. For example, dark blue pants can be marked with a single safety pin in the waist band while black pants would have none.

Minor Hygiene

Problems.   Putting toothpaste on a toothbrush, locating items needed for minor hygiene tasks, applying makeup, performing hair care and nail care are all tasks that provide difficulties for persons with poor vision.

Solutions.   Once again, the therapist should assess the illumination level of the area in which these tasks are performed. If needed, the therapist can increase lighting by using higher wattage bulbs or adding lighting fixtures. The therapist can decrease the pattern present by organizing the area and using solid-colored placemats/towels as backgrounds for tasks. The contrast between foreground objects and the background can be increased by using light- or dark-colored placemats/towels as appropriate. To improve the client's ability to find personal care items, the therapist can put brightly-colored tape or stickers on them. To improve the client's ability to apply makeup or to shave, he or she can use a magnifying mirror with or without lights. Nail care is very difficult because of the poor contrast between the nail and the skin. Clipping or cutting nails can be dangerous, so the person should be on a regular schedule of filing his or her nails to ensure safety.

Meal Preparation

Problems.   Activities of low contrast, such as measuring ingredients, pouring liquids, and cutting/chopping/slicing food items are often difficult for persons with visual dysfunction. Those tasks that require detail vision such as setting appliance dials and reading instructions or labels are also problem areas.

Solutions.   As in all other areas, the illumination level of the area in which meal preparation is performed should be assessed first. If the light level is low, lighting can be increased through use of extra fixtures or use of a flashlight (for illuminating appliance dials). Contrast levels should also be addressed. Contrast can be increased between the food being prepared and the cooking utensils by using black/white cutting boards when chopping or slicing and using dark cups/glasses when pouring light-colored liquids, and vice versa (Figure 5.6). Measuring can be done more easily if separate, different-sized cups are used instead of a glass cup with measurements marked on the side. Appliance dials can be marked with tactile cues or brightly-colored stickers at the appropriate settings. Magnifying devices can also be utilized to read appliance dials or measuring utensils and to see the food items being cut or sliced.

Functional Communication

Problems.   Reading and writing are often areas that are affected by vision problems. Reading can be classified as continuous and spot. Continuous text reading includes reading magazines, newspapers, and books. Spot reading tasks are those that supply the reader with information about the task

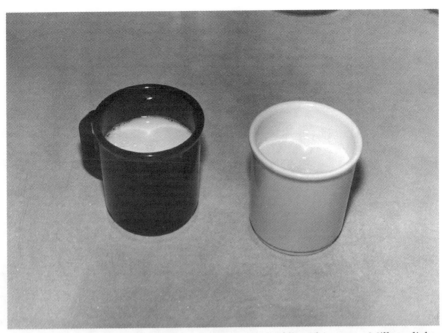

FIGURE
5.6

Use of contrast to improve ability to see the level of liquid in cups. Milk or light colored liquids should be poured into dark cups (left) to maximize contrast between the liquid and its background.

being performed. They include reading food labels, prices, money, telephone numbers, the thermostat, watches, and telephone dials. Writing tasks that are affected by poor vision can be as simple as signing documents or as complex as writing letters.

Solutions.   As with all other problem areas, the lighting level should be assessed initially and appropriate adaptations made. Improvement of contrast levels is often difficult in reading tasks that are preprinted but can be increased in written information through the use of bold, felt-tipped pens instead of pencils or ball point pens. Written communications should also be printed in large letters instead of written in cursive writing.

Enlargement of preprinted materials can assist the client experiencing poor vision access the presented information. Large-print books and magazines are available through many outlets for continuous text reading. Magnifying devices can be used to enlarge printed materials that are not available in large print editions.

Spot reading appliance dials, money, prices in stores, food labels, and telephone dials can be performed most easily with handheld or headborne

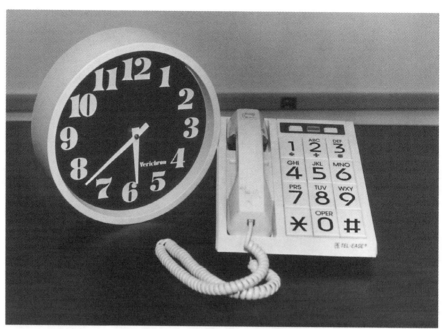

FIGURE
5.7
A large-numbered phone with high-contrast lettering (on right) can make dialing the telephone easier for a person with low vision. The same principles of object enlargement and improved contrast are also used in the clock (on left).

devices. Large numbered telephones are available in retail stores if the client experiences difficulties dialing the phone because of visual impairment (Figure 5.7). There are also adaptive devices with enlarged numbers to attach to existing telephones that can be purchased from low vision catalogues. For time-telling, there are large-numbered digital clocks, talking timepieces, and large bold-faced watches and clock available in many retail stores (Figure 5.7).

Writing tasks can be made easier through a combination of improved lighting, contrast, and enlargement of the task. Task lighting directed at the writing surface should be placed so that the writing hand does not cast a shadow on the page. Increased contrast can be achieved through the use of a bold, felt-tipped pen and bold-lined paper. Headborne devices or magnifying spectacles can sometimes enlarge the material enough to allow for accurate and legible writing.

Distance Viewing

Problems.   Distance viewing problems mainly occur during community activities. Reading bus signs, street signs, seeing street lights, and reading aisle signs in stores are all examples of difficulties encountered by the person with vision loss. Watching television is one of the main concerns of poor distance vision in the home.

Solutions.   Enlargement of the target being viewed can be achieved through the use of a telescopic magnifier. If glare is causing the client problems during outdoor tasks, the use of colored sun filters can reduce this effect thus allowing the client to more clearly view his or her surroundings. To assist the person in seeing the images on the television, headborne devices are available for distance viewing, or the client can simply move closer to the set.

Mobility

Indoor Problems.   Bumping into opened doors, door frames, furniture, and other obstacles are often problems for individuals with vision loss. Difficulties may also be encountered when going up and down stairs, as well as adjusting to varying light levels in different rooms. Decreased contrast sensitivity, poor light adaptation, and peripheral field loss cause most indoor mobility problems in persons with visual dysfunction.

Solutions.   As with all other areas discussed, lighting should be evaluated first. Is the illumination of rooms and hallways adequate for safe ambulation? If not, additional fixtures should be added. As the person goes from one room to another, does the illumination level vary? For example, is there a significant difference in the lighting level of his or her room as compared to the hallway? Persons experiencing problems with light adaptation may find this difference debilitating as they move from one place to another. Lighting should be uniform throughout the environment.

If lighting is adequate, the addition of contrast to the environment should be considered. For example, if a hallway is well-illuminated and the client continues to have difficulties in safely navigating it, a runner that contrasts with the floor as a guide can be installed. Painting the baseboard with a color that contrasts with the wall and floor is another example of the use of contrast to solve this problem. Improving contrast can also make stairways safer for the individual with vision loss. The leading edge of steps can be marked with a nonskid tape that contrasts with their color. This allows the client to more readily see where the steps are located and the number of stairs to be navigated. If the person bumps into furniture, it may be the result of poor contrast sensitivity. A person with poor contrast sensitivity may not be able to see the edges of furniture if the contrast between the furniture and its background is low. If this is the problem, the objects should be marked with a high-contrast material. For example, a brightly-colored towel attached to the arm of a couch or chair can identify its location for the client with vision loss.

The resolution of mobility problems may require the incorporation of compensatory visual skills training in addition to the environmental adaptations listed above. If visual or tactile cues are added to the environment, the person must be trained in their effective utilization. The person may need to scan the environment more effectively and notice details he or she would normally overlook. He or she must then understand the purpose of those cues and how to use them as guides. As mentioned above, these compensatory strategies may be difficult to teach to some individuals with developmental disability.

Outdoor Problems.   Difficulties encountered by persons with visual dysfunction in outdoor mobility include the ability to safely navigate uneven terrain, seeing curbs, safely crossing streets, seeing street signs and stop lights, and seeing signs on busses. These problems can be caused by decreased acuity, poor contrast sensitivity, glare sensitivity, and visual field loss.

Solutions.   The use of sun filters can sometimes improve the person's ability to perceive objects of low contrast such as curbs and subtle changes in the walking surface. Filters can also be used to decrease the effects of glare. Telescopes can provide magnification for reading assorted signs and street lights. If the person will be required to cross busy intersections or perform other tasks that could significantly compromise his or her safety, it is recommended that he or she be referred to an orientation and mobility specialist. These professionals are described below.

PROFESSIONAL RESOURCES

There are many other professionals who can assist the occupational therapist in the evaluation and treatment of clients who have experienced vision loss. Some of these professionals are in the medical community, and others provide services within the framework of the national blindness system. This system is a network of services provided by state, federal, educational, and private organizations. Following are some of those professions and a description of the resources/services they provide.

Ophthalmologists

Ophthalmologists are medical doctors who complete a residency in ophthalmology. They are responsible for diagnosing and treating ocular diseases that cause vision loss. Some ophthalmologists specialize in the treatment of specific types of conditions. For example, there are retinal specialists, glaucoma specialists, and neuroophthalmologists. Most persons with developmental disability are probably under the care of a general ophthalmologist.

Optometrists

Optometrists have a college degree and a doctorate of optometry. Optometrists are not medical doctors but specialize in a variety of areas. An optometrist who specializes in the treatment of low vision can be an important resource for the therapist working with an individual with vision loss. These professionals have experience in evaluation of visual function and training in compensatory techniques and in the prescription of optical devices.

Orientation and Mobility Specialists

Orientation and mobility specialists (O&M) are professionals who have a master's or baccalaureate degree and are trained in addressing the travel needs experienced by the person with vision loss. They work in a variety of settings including schools and private and state organizations. The O&M specialist uses an assortment of methods for teaching safe and effective travel to low vision or blind individuals. These tools include training in the efficient use of visual skills, optical devices, and the use of a long cane, if appropriate. The O&M specialist can be an important resource for consultation regarding a client who is experiencing mobility problems due to vision loss.

Rehabilitation Teachers

Rehabilitation teachers have a college degree and specialize in addressing the functional problems experienced by the person with vision loss in daily living tasks. They utilize adaptive techniques and devices to increase independence in self-care, meal preparation, minor hygiene, and leisure activities. As with the O&M specialist, rehabilitation teachers work in a variety of settings and organizations. They are most often found in residential schools, independent living centers, and state organizations.

REFERENCES

Baker, E. (1991). Ocular motor abnormalities from head trauma. *Survey of Ophtalmology, 35,* 245–267.

Boyle, C.A., Decoufle, P., & Yeargin-Allsopp, M. (1994). Prevalence and health impact of developmental disabilities in U.S. children. *Pediatrics, 93,* 399–403.

Carter, K. (1983). Assessment of lighting. In R. Jose (Ed.), *Understanding low vision* (pp. 403–414). New York: American Foundation for the Blind.

Colenbrander, A., & Fletcher, A. (1992). Low vision rehabilitation: Visual acuity measurement in low vision range. *J. Oph Nursing & Tech, 11(2),* 62–69.

Daroff, R.B. (1974). Control of ocular movement. *British Journal of Ophthalmology, 58,* 217–223.

Dickman, I. (1983). *Making life more livable: Simple adaptations for the homes of blind and visually impaired older people.* New York: American Foundation for the Blind.

Drost, P.J., Archer, S.M., & Helveston, E.M. (1991). Measurement of low vision in children and infants. *Ophtalmology, 98,* 1513–1518.

Fletcher, D.C., Schuchard, R.A., Livingstone, C.L., Crane, W.G., & Hu, S.Y. (1994). Scanning laser ophthalmoscope macular perimetry and applications for low vision rehabilitation clinicians. In A. Colenbrander & D.C. Fletcher (Eds.), *Low Vision and vision rehabilitation, ophthalmology clinics of North America, Vol. 7* (pp. 257–265). Philadelphia: W.B. Saunders.

Gardner, T.W. & Shoch, D.E. (1987). Loss of vision. In *Handbook of ophthalmology: A practical guide* (pp. 39–51). New York: Appleton-Lange.

Gardner, T.W., & Shoch, D.E. (1987). Diseases of the retina, choroid and vitreous. In *Handbook of ophthalmology: A practical guide* (pp. 149–162). New York: Appleton-Lange.

Giatnutsos, R., Ramsey, G., & Perlin, R. (1988). Rehabilitative optometric services for survivors of acquired brain injury. *Archives of Physical Medicine, 69,* 573–578.

Hritcko, T. (1983). Assessment of children with low vision. In R.T. Jose (Ed.), *Understanding low vision* (pp. 105–137). New York: American Foundation for the Blind.

Hyvarinen, L. (1995). Considerations in evaluation and treatment of the child with low vision. *American Journal of Occupational Therapy, 49,* 891–897.

Jose, R.T. (1983). Optics. In R.T. Jose (Ed.), *Understanding low vision,* (pp. 187–210). New York: American Foundation for the Blind.

Lampert, J., & Lapolice, D.J. (1995). Functional considerations in evaluation and treatment of the client with low vision. *American Journal of Occupational Therapy, 49,* 885–890.

Lavich, J.B., & Nelson, L.B. (1993). Diagnosis and treatment of strabismus disorders. *Pediatric Clinics of North America, 40,* 737–752.

Manacker, S.J. (1993). Visual function in children with developmental disabilities. *Pediatric Clinics of North America, 40,* 659–674.

Marx, M.S., Werner, P., Cohen-Mansfield, J., & Hartmann, E.E. (1990). Visual acuity estimates in noncommunicative elderly persons. *Investigative Ophthalmology & Visual Science, 31,* 593–596.

Rubin, G. (1989). Assessment of visual function in eyes with visual loss. *Ophthalmology Clinics of North America, 2,* 357–367.

Rubin, S.E., & Nelson, L.B. (1993). Amblyopia: Diagnosis and management. *Pediatric Clinics of North America, 40,* 727–735.

Schlageter K., Gray B., Hall K., Shaw R., & Sammet, R. (1993). Incidence and treatment of visual dysfunction in traumatic brain injury. *Brain Injury, 7,* 439–448.

Schuchard, R.A. (1995). Adaptation to macular scotomas in persons with low vision. *American Journal of Occupational Therapy, 49,* 870–876.

Schuchard, R.A. & Fletcher, D.C., (1994). Preferred retinal locus: A review with applications in low vision rehabilitation. In A. Colenbrander & D.C. Fletcher (Eds.), *Low vision and vision rehabilitation, ophthalmology clinics of North America, Vol. 7* (pp. 243–256). Philadelphia: W.B. Saunders.

Warren, M.L. (1993). A hierarchical model for evaluation and treatment of visual perceptual dysfunction in adult acquired brain injury: Parts 1 & 2. *American Journal of Occupational Therapy, 47,* 42–66.

APPENDIX A: RESOURCE LIST

Optical Aids/Adaptive Equipment

AFB Product Catalogue
American Foundation for the Blind
Product Center
100 Enterprise Place
P.O. Box 7044
Dover, DE 19903
(800) 829-3299

The Lighthouse Low Vision Products
Consumer Catalogue
36-20 Northern Blvd.
Long Island, NY 11101
(800) 453-4923

LS&S Group
P.O. Box 673
Northbrook, IL 60065
(800) 486-4789

Independent Living Aids, Inc.
Can-Do Products
27 East Mall
Plainview, NY 11803
(800) 537-2118

Mattingly International
Low Vision Products
938-K Andreasen Drive
Escondida, CA 92029
(800) 286-4200

Maxi-Aids
P.O. Box 3209
Farmingdale, NY 11735
(800) 522-6294

LUV Reading Series (Eccentric Viewing)

Mattingly International
938-K Andreasen Dr.
Escondida, CA 92029
(800) 286-4200

UV Filters (Sun/Light Filters)

NoIR Medical Technologies
6155 Pontiac Trail
South Lyon, MI 48178
(800) 521-9746

Visual Function Assessments

Contrast Sensitivity Function

Lea Symbols/Numbers Test
Precision Vision
721 North Addison Rd.
Villa Park, IL 60181
(708) 833-1454

Pelli Robson Chart
Clement Clark
3218-D East 17th Ave.
Columbus, OH 42319
(800) 848-8923

Mattingly International
938-K Andreasen Dr.
Escondido, CA 92029
(800) 826-4200

Acuity Measurement

Colenbrander Meter Combined
    Low Vision Test Chart
Mattingly International
938-K Andreasen Dr.
Escondido, CA 92029
(800) 826-4200

Vision Associates
7512 Phillips Blvd. #50-316
Orlando, FL 32819
(407) 352-1200

LeaSymbols Visual Acuity
    Test System
Precision Vision
721 North Addison Rd.
Villa Park, IL 60181
(708) 833-1454

Organizations

American Foundation for the Blind
15 West 16th Street
New York, NY 10011
(800) 232-5463

Helen Keller International
90 Washington Street
New York, NY 10006
(212) 943-0890

APPENDIX B: RECOMMENDED READING

Dickman, I. (1983). *Making life more livable: Simple adaptations for the homes of blind and visually impaired older people.* New York: American Foundation for the Blind.

Jose, R.D. (Ed.). (1983). *Understanding low vision.* New York: American Foundation for the Blind.

Mangold, P. (1980). *The pleasure of eating for those who are visually impaired.* Castro Valley, CA: Author.

APPENDIX C: VISUAL IMPAIRMENT

Checklist of Pertinent Clinical Observations

ACUITY

Ask the client to read a line of standard size print in a newspaper

_____ complains of print looking fuzzy or blurry
_____ complains of not being able to bring print into focus
_____ continuously adjusts focal length of the page as if trying to bring the print into focus
_____ complains of print being too small or too faint
_____ brings the page of print in very close (less than 16 inches) to try to read it
_____ shifts the page of print to one side of midline (up, down, left, right) to read it
_____ views printed line out of the corner of the eye or by looking above or below the line of print

General Observations:

_____ complains of inability to recognize faces
_____ states can see better out of the corner of eye
_____ states that vision fluctuates throughout day
_____ uses a flashlight to view objects

CONTRAST SENSITIVITY FUNCTION

Ask client to fill a clear glass with water from the tap or a pitcher to within one half inch from the brim of the glass

_____ complains that he or she can't see the level of water as it rises in the glass
_____ over fills the glass
_____ uses tip of finger over the brim of the glass to tactually determine the level of the water
_____ moves in very close to the glass to view it as it fills
_____ tilts the glass back and forth to create movement of the water in order to determine the level of the water in the glass

Ask the client to fill a black cup with milk to within one half inch from the brim of the glass and compare performance.

Observe the client ambulate in environments with low contrast features such as unmarked curbs, subtle changes in the support surface (transition from carpet to vinyl flooring without a significant change in color), areas with poor illumination, furniture that does not contrast from surrounding features, door frames that do not contrast from doors, etc.

    ____ hesitates when approaching curb or subtle change in support surface
    ____ misses curb or does not see it until directly on top of it
    ____ trips when transitioning between support surfaces
    ____ bumps into or comes very close to low contrast obstacles (furniture, etc.)
    ____ uses hands to guide self around an obstacle

General Observations:

    ____ complains of inability to recognize faces
    ____ performance declines in dimly lit surroundings
    ____ complains of inability to see changes in color of light at a stoplight
    ____ unable to accurately distinguish colors of similar hues such as dark blue from black, purple from blue, white from beige, etc.
    ____ requests additional light when performing a task

VISUAL FIELD DEFICIT

Observe the client ambulate through crowded areas with moving obstacles.

    ____ collides or comes very close to obstacles consistently on one side in an unfamiliar environment
    ____ stares straight ahead at the floor immediately in front of him/her
    ____ consistently stares to one side
    ____ stays very close to one side of the wall when ambulating down a hallway
    ____ uses fingers to "trail" wall to tactually guide self
    ____ refuses to take the lead when ambulating—prefers to walk behind others

_____ appears anxious/uncertain in crowded areas

_____ stops walking when passing by another moving person or object until the object/person has passed by

_____ complains of feeling off balance particularly to one side

Ask the client to read a paragraph of 1 m print larger printed on an 8.5 × 11 inch piece of paper.

_____ transposes words when reading by omitting or misreading letters on one side of the word(s)

_____ abbreviates scan to one side when reading a page of print, omitting word(s) on a line

_____ is only able to read print accurately if uses finger to trace line of print

_____ consistently loses place on one side of the page when reading

_____ hesitates when reading words, reads words slowly or misreads a word initially, then corrects self

General Observations:

_____ reads only half of a wide sign

_____ avoids crowds and crowded environments such as shopping centers

_____ transposes numbers

_____ displaces writing to one side when completing a form

_____ handwriting drifts up or down when writing on line or addressing an envelope

_____ complains of being unable to follow what is happening on television particularly when viewing a dynamic sporting event (football, basketball, etc.) or a show with a lot of action

_____ has difficulty accurately dialing a telephone: transposes numbers on dial and presses wrong number

_____ complains of disorientation when riding in a car or a wheelchair

_____ avoids obstacles in familiar environments but collides with obstacles in unfamiliar environments

VISUAL INATTENTION

_____ only comments on objects or visual details on one side of a visual scene

_____ initiates scanning pattern beginning on the right side of an array and scans only right side

_____ hesitant to shift eyes across midline towards left side; inability to maintain fixation on an object placed to left of midline

_____ reluctance to turn towards the left or an avoidance of left turns during ambulation

_____ failure to search the environment for information needed to adapt, such as failure to look at a clock or a wristwatch when asked what time it is

_____ failure to rescan or check work for errors when completing a complex task

_____ reduced effort on tasks

_____ easily distracted by motion occurring on right side

_____ unable to maintain concentration on a task which requires sorting through visual information or attention to visual detail: forgets what he/she is looking for or makes mistakes in identification

COMBINATION OF VISUAL INATTENTION AND VISUAL FIELD DEFICIT

_____ failure to acknowledge or notice persons on one side

_____ failure to pick up or notice an object on one side during a visual search for the object

_____ places only one foot on wheelchair footplate or ear piece of eyeglasses on one ear

_____ shaves or applies makeup on only one half of face or combs hair only one side

_____ eats food on only one side of plate

_____ veers off towards one side when using wheelchair or when ambulating

_____ consistently bumps into furniture or objects on one side in familiar environments

_____ misreads time on a clock and does not correct error

_____ omits or misreads words and does not correct error

_____ complains of clumsiness but uncertain as to reason for clumsiness

_____ places both legs through one hole in underwear or pants

_____ misplaces clothing or toiletry items when getting dressed

_____ becomes disoriented when moving in environment; unable to locate needed landmarks

OCULOMOTOR DYSFUNCTION

_____ complains of double vision, or blurring vision or a shadow when viewing objects: usually varies with focal length or direction of gaze; may be constant

_____ complains of being unable to keep objects in focus when working at a near focal distance

_____ complains of eye fatigue or eye pain (not eye irritation) after a period of sustained focusing on a task

_____ complains that print begins to swirl on a page or move after a period of sustained focus

_____ complains of blurring when changing focus from a near object to a distant object

_____ assumes a consistent and deliberate head position when viewing objects

_____ shuts an eye or turns head when viewing an object up close

_____ squints when viewing objects

_____ complains of onset of headache after a period of sustained viewing

_____ complains of fatigue after a period of sustained viewing

_____ excessive blinking when viewing objects not related to eye irritation

_____ complains of nausea during ambulation or head movement; accompanied by sense that peripheral visual field is in motion

_____ resists change in head position

_____ reluctant to participate in activities presented at a specific focal distance or attempts to change the distance at which the activity is placed (for example: changes focal distance of reading materials)

_____ eye(s) appear to turn in or out when viewing objects

_____ muscle tone in neck or mandibular area increases when head or body is moved

_____ complains of difficulty concentrating on tasks which require sustained focus at a near distance

_____ complains of eye pain with movement of eyes

MISCELLANEOUS OBSERVATIONS

_____ complains of sensitivity to light or keeps eye lids partially closed in brightly lit areas

_____ nystagmus in primary gaze

Reprinted with permission from M.L. Warren.

PART 3

Specific Applications

6

Using a Sensory Approach to Serve Adults Who Have Developmental Disabilities

Bonnie Hanschu, OTR

INTRODUCTION

This chapter will describe how we came to understand the significance of a *frame of reference* and how a sensory oriented frame of reference made the significant difference for adults served by occupational therapy in an institutional environment. The term *frame of reference* refers to a particular clinical perspective that has guiding principles to govern the treatment and evaluation of people who have severe disabilities. A *frame of reference* provides a consistent set of assumptions to direct, control, or judge one's clinical approach. It guides clinical activities, but it does not provide a recipe or formula for action (Mosey, 1981; Reed, 1984). Service providers maintain a responsibility to accurately identify needs and then to adjust what they do according to the effectiveness of programs designed to meet those needs.

Consider several individuals for whom a sensory orientation made a big difference. In each case, viewing the person's responses through sensory oriented eyes helped us to understand that self-stimulatory or maladaptive behavior could reflect a sensory need. If that was appropriate, we were curious to find out what would happen if we were to respond by providing strong, pleasurable sensation. To guide our choice of sensation, we observed what each person sought through his or her own behavior, and we incorporated the results of offering each a variety of sensations to identify those that elicited approach versus avoidance responses. We kept in mind a priority concern that we avoid any sensation a person seemed to not like or to find unpleasant.

Case #1

Before.   A 41-year-old female had a well established history of picking at herself. The picking resulted in broken skin and oozing sores that required medical treatment. This behavior and its progression were documented all the way back to early childhood and remained her priority problem despite attempts to intervene with medications and a variety of intense behavioral strategies. Behavioral attempts included differential reinforcement of alternative or incompatible behaviors and the use of aversives and restraints. Nothing had altered the frequency or intensity of the picking, and this behavior alone was the barrier preventing this woman from moving to a less restrictive setting.

After We Started Using a Sensory Approach.   A program was started in which the woman was given doses of proprioception and pressure touch, for about 10 minutes every hour, on the hour, during her waking hours. Following the dose of sensation, a helper invited her to participate in an activity she was expected to enjoy. Within a period of 6 months, her rates of picking dropped from an average of approximately one pick per minute during her awake hours to only a few picks per several hours. Her team had a goal of finding her a community based placement within 4 years before she began the sensory treatment. Because of the success of the program, she was successfully placed within 7 months in a home-like foster care environment with a couple, their dog, carpeted floors, and live plants. The couple continued the program of sensory doses throughout the woman's transition to her new home, fading the frequency of the doses to only occasional use of the technique in preparation for events that were expected to be more stressful. At the end of the 6-month postdischarge period, the placement was still rated a success by everyone involved, and the picking behavior had not returned (Reisman, 1993).

Case #2

Before.   A 24-year-old female had an established history of recurring episodes during which she became totally out of control. When she was doing well, she had many abilities and was relatively adaptive. She dressed and fed herself. She was continent and took care of her toileting activities with only occasional prompts to flush, use soap, or turn off the faucet. She was good humored and complied with requests. She smiled and showed evidence of pride when helping household staff with routine domestic chores, such as carrying dirty dishes to the sink, wiping the table, or putting chairs in place. Unfortunately, after just a few days like this, her adaptive behavior would disintegrate and she would rapidly escalate to being out of control.

During these times she was incontinent of bladder and bowel. She would not eat and would take only occasional sips of liquid. She whined or screeched almost continuously as if she were in severe distress. She was intolerant of clothing and stripped or ripped her shirts as fast as they were put on her. She ran from one place in the room to another and abruptly flung herself into solid brick walls. Her cheeks were a ruddy bright red from slapping herself. She would throw her mattress and any piece of heavy furniture she could get to, posing a threat to anyone who happened to be in the path. It was impossible for anyone to console or calm her. Month after month she would have 20 or more days like this, spending most of that time being held in a prone position on a thick floor mat to protect her and those around her. The only interventions that helped get her through these episodes were physical containment and heavy sedation.

After We Started Using a Sensory Approach.   She was started on an intensive program of sensation that involved being bounced gently on a trampoline, being held tightly from behind and swayed gently from side to side, being gently stretched in a supine position, and being swung slowly and rhythmically in one direction at a time in either a swing or a hammock. In a matter of several months, she had improved to the point of being able to leave the campus to perform work in the community. She dressed appropriately and made the trips successfully with just her job coach. She ate in public eating establishments, used public restrooms without incident, and carried out a job at a local church, vacuuming the carpets and polishing the pews. She was a changed person.

Case #3

Before.   A 36-year-old female, totally blind since birth, had a terrible time tolerating touch from others. Her physical problems were substantial; her hips disarticulated in a wind-swept deformity. She could not sit without total support and her wheelchair was adapted with cumbersome modifications to assure her comfort as well as her safety. She required total care and had to be handled multiple times a day to meet her most basic needs. Whenever she was transferred, fed, dressed, cleaned up after an accident, or repositioned, she screamed and cried as if someone were tearing her limbs from her body. When she was left alone, she would gently rub a spot on the side of her head, smiling and occasionally making playful sounds. These were the only times she did not seem to be in acute distress.

After We Started Using a Sensory Approach.   She was started on a program that involved transferring her as quietly as possible to a hammock swing and then gently swinging her for several minutes. This was accomplished by using a specially designed *transfer pad* that enabled care providers to move her without touching her. She got the swinging at least three times a day and at least twice in the evenings. After the swinging, she was provided with several minutes of pressure touch to her legs and arms and soft objects were pressed gently into her lap. After the sensory services were started, one of her more consistent direct care providers had an idea. She made the woman a weighted poncho that had a snug fitting hood for her head and heavy fabric that covered most of her body. The woman would smile and relax immediately after the poncho was put on her. The sensory strategies seem to make her much more comfortable, and her team credited them for enabling her to get through morning and evening cares without becoming upset.

Case #4

Before.   A 32-year-old male, blind from birth, displayed no sense of balance when walking and would fall over unless he could hang onto someone's arm or a handrail. He did not tolerate shirts and stripped them off and flung them away as fast as someone tried to put one on. He was typically found sitting on the floor, tailor-fashion. He would rapidly scoot away in the opposite direction when anyone approached. He would not sit in chairs unless someone insisted by pressing him into it and holding him down at the shoulders. When left alone, he made almost continuous clicking noises and displayed almost continuous hands-in-the-pants behaviors.

After We Started Using a Sensory Approach.   He received increasingly intensive sensory services over the course of 3 years. At the end of the 3 years, he was walking on his own with a reciprocal gait rather than a side to side sway. He sat in chairs routinely now and he even liked to get into suspended equipment to swing, something he had refused to do through almost 3 years of encouragement to try. Videotaped "before" and "after" films at 1-year intervals revealed significant progressive structural change, as well as dramatic changes in his behavior and interaction. Initially his legs were severely bowed. By the end of 3 years, his legs had actually straightened. In the third tape, there was a complete absence of clicking noises. He approached care providers on his own and would sit in a chair and interact with someone who talked to him. He accepted help from someone who stood behind him reaching around to guide his hands through a task. This was a kind of close contact he would have no part of before. Throughout his sensory service, his medications were steadily reduced until psychotropic medication was eliminated entirely. This man ultimately moved to a community based group home with three other individuals. He did work-for-pay in a structured day program to which he rode the bus without difficulty. None of this had ever been considered for his plan because goals of this nature were considered to be an unrealistic expectation for him. The time coinciding with the introduction of sensory-based service for him was the first time in the course of his 20 plus years of institutionalization that he showed any progress, let alone the steady trend of progress in all of his active treatment goals.

Figuring Out a Better Approach

These were four people whose lives were stuck in time until they were provided with a treatment approach that met their needs. They are similar to adults with developmental disabilities being served in long-term care settings all over the United States. What we learned about what made the difference for them is the subject of this chapter. The chapter describes the setting where their stories took place and how a conflict arose concerning the prevailing frame of reference. The chapter goes on to detail the search for a more fitting frame of reference and emphasizes that finding a better approach sometimes requires *figuring out* a better approach. The chapter closes with a discussion of the new frame of reference, now being called the *Ready Approach*, and what we learned from developing and implementing an untested sensory approach.

Perhaps the most important lesson we learned from the experience described in this chapter was that, when people are not improving, it may be because we have not yet come up with the right approach to help them. The 1990s have been called the "Decade of the Brain," and brain scientists have discovered that even damaged brains can be remarkably resilient. When they are given even a little bit of help, the results can be stunning.

BACKGROUND

The Setting

Our facility was a placement of last resort for adults with severe developmental disabilities. Some were physically able but severely behaviorally challenged. Others had physical disabilities and problematic behaviors. Still others were totally physically dependent, occasionally also medically fragile. Even some of the medically fragile individuals had challenging behaviors. Every person had complex and profound functional and performance deficits, serious combinations of interdependent problems. Almost all had grossly impaired or absent communication.

Aggression, defensiveness, and self-stimulation were the order of the day. In some households and in many day programs, staff struggled to get through each shift with no one getting hurt. Unless someone was working with them directly, those who were physically able spent their time stripping, engaging in hands-in-the-pants behaviors, mouthing, eating inedibles, and making nerve-racking sounds. Programming was almost at a standstill, and lack of active treatment was a source of recurring multiple citations during licensing surveys.

Most of the people we served had been challenged by brain damage since birth. The rest incurred severe brain damage during their formative years. The damage was usually associated with biological factors such as genetic faults, chromosomal abnormalities, metabolic disturbances, infections, or anoxia; other causes included traumatic injury, disease, and damage from chemical or toxic agents. Regardless of the cause, each person ended up with devastating brain damage. The vast majority had lived in an institutional environment since infancy or childhood. As a result, they had developed additional secondary problems associated with sensory deprivation, lack of opportunity, and all the other depersonalizing factors that are so hard to eliminate in large institutions.

No matter what teams identified as priority needs, the ever present stereotypic, self-stimulatory, and self-injurious behaviors continued to demand attention. Staff made concerted efforts every day to focus on "positive programming," where the goal was to develop new skills or abilities. However, those attempts were derailed every day by the need to control, or at least manage, problem behaviors. It eventually occurred to us that those behaviors reflected the significance of unmet sensory needs, but it was hard to think "sensory" when we were so focused on behavior.

The Prevailing Approach

Behaviorism was well established as the predominant frame of reference at our institution. There were at least two good reasons for that. First, it was well known that people who have mental retardation sometimes learn new skills best when they are trained with highly structured, consistent reinforcement of positive responses. Second, many people served in our institution faced significant obstacles to community based opportunities and less restrictive placement because of maladaptive behavior. Therefore, behavior modification was a top priority.

It was appropriate for a treatment facility like ours to have a wide range of behavioral expertise available and it did. In addition to a well staffed behavioral psychology department, every team had its own behavior analyst. The roots of behavioral thinking went even deeper, because people with behavioral expertise were also the team leaders, the supervisors, the managers, and, in general, the people most influential in all programmatic and organizational decisions.

No one questioned whether behaviorism had an important place in the treatment of people with developmental disabilities. An approach does not become the predominant view, recommended by experts around the world as the premier choice, unless there is good evidence it has merit. Behaviorism has a long, well documented history of producing results with hundreds of thousands of people who have severe disabilities.

Because behaviorism was *the* frame of reference in our organization, other alternatives were not considered. Yet, social changes were leading to legislative initiatives, such as the required downsizing of our institution's population from 2,000 to a few hundred. When we got to 400 clients it was clear that behaviors were the greatest barrier to community integration. As we approached 200 residents, it had become urgent for staff to figure out more effective ways to deal with challenging client behaviors so people remaining in the institution could be served more safely and transitioned into community settings with more success.

We began to see that there were several indications that a behavioral frame of reference was not the best alternative for the remaining group we were trying to serve. Yet, behaviorism had been the predominant approach in settings like ours for so many years. It was hard to break away from behavioral thinking.

The Conflict for Occupational Therapists

Occupational therapists, as well as other therapists, in our setting, frequently experienced conflicts in such a behaviorally oriented setting. Everything about the people we served needed to be described in behavioral terms so its frequency, intensity, or duration could be observed or tested using objective means. Therapists were even cautioned about how to discuss muscle tone or other sensorimotor issues in their reports and admonished to focus on observable behaviors that could be improved, for example,

■ how far a person could reach
■ how many seconds a position could be held
■ how many objects a person could move to a specified location.

Therapists understood the need to operationalize desired outcomes by describing them as something that could be observed or measured. How else could we obtain objective and reliable data upon which to make decisions? However, describing behaviors is different from applying a behavioral frame of reference, and that difference was not always understood. Many therapists consequently felt pressured to abandon their sensorimotor orientation in favor of a behavioral perspective, an outcome that severely compromised the value of having therapists on interdisciplinary teams in the first place.

It was their sensorimotor frame of reference that helped therapists recognize the inappropriateness of people with significant postural and motor control problems being *conditioned* with edibles or other *reinforcers* to improve their task performance. Such training often took place at mealtime for people

■ who could not sit in chairs
■ who had no stable base of proximal support
■ who had insufficient motor control to grade muscle actions
■ whose inadequate integration of primitive reflex patterns made it difficult for them to control extraneous movements.

In rare instances, aversive behavioral procedures were used to get people to open their mouths to receive food, completely missing how much difficulty they had coordinating their suck-swallow-breathe patterns. Everyone knows better now, but these examples show that when we do not understand the nature of a need we can make well intended, but potentially harmful, decisions.

Therapists also questioned another implication of behavioral approaches—the tendency to view everything a person does as adaptive or maladaptive behavior. Human nervous systems are truly remarkable in their capacity to protect us from what we cannot manage. From a sensory perspective, it is possible to argue that some maladaptive behavior might actually be a clever compensation on the part of a nervous system struggling to keep a person safe, comfortable, or free from demands that are beyond the person's ability. In such instances, behavior called maladaptive might actually be quite adaptive (Reisman & Hanschu, 1992).

We see lots of behaviors in an institutional setting that, from a behavioral perspective, need to be modified. From a sensory perspective, those same behaviors provide evidence of just how much pressure we are putting on someone's nervous system. Misinterpreting such behavior could result in adding to, rather than decreasing, the amount of stress on someone's nervous system. That could explain why there was mounting evidence provided by ongoing programmatic data that our people were not improving, and their behavior seemed to be getting worse in some cases.

Behavioral training did not seem to be working. In fact, medical and program records of the people remaining in our care indicated that, if behavioral interventions had ever worked, there was only a temporary gain, and there was evidence a person could actually regress after intensive behavioral intervention. This observation in our setting was consistent with the results of multiple studies reported in the psychological literature that short-term success in eliminating or decreasing maladaptive behaviors may be achieved, but targeted behavior sometimes returns with a vengeance, or new, more troublesome behaviors emerge in its place.

Unfortunately, when there is little or no improvement, especially with adults, care providers, including therapists, sometimes attribute lack of progress to limited potential for change, citing limitations associated with age, severity of disabilities, or disabilities being well established over so many years. They may emphasize the need to maintain abilities the person already has, believing it is unrealistic to expect improvement. We now have reasons to view that line of thinking as erroneous for many individuals (Bidabe, 1991). It is also easy to blame lack of progress on administrative issues such as staffing or funding, especially when there is frequent organizational upheaval associated with downsizing. With so many possible explanations for lack of progress, there is little reason to suspect that it might be most directly related to the program's prevailing frame of reference.

The Power of Management

We might have continued on the same course indefinitely, if not for a licensing survey that prompted a change in our top management. Along with the new leadership came a mandate to provide effective service or prepare for the consequence, which was assumed to be closure. This executive agenda cut through months (potentially) of discussion and got us in a much more united effort to solve overall programmatic problems.

In occupational therapy we saw the management change as a significant opportunity to help make a difference. We were even guardedly optimistic that program philosophies more compatible with our view might be considered. We had been using the *Model of Human Occupation*, a frame of reference that helps occupational therapy practitioners use a uniform approach and terminology to identify functional abilities and life tasks that need attention. This model helped us isolate functional and performance deficits, but we were still left with basic questions. What were the underlying causes of the person's functional deficit? How much improvement in function could we expect? What needed to change for the function to improve? We had to apply more specific clinical frames of reference for answers to those questions.

In addition to behaviorism, neurodevelopment and sensory integration are frames of reference commonly applied by occupational therapists in the field of developmental disabilities. These last two seemed to be particularly important for therapists who serve adults with multiple handicapping conditions and severe sensorimotor problems. As therapists, we had tried applying them separately, and then we tried mixing and melding ideas from each. No matter what we tried, we kept coming to the same conclusion. Each alternative explained many things we observed and each offered methods and techniques that helped in some situations, but none quite matched our clinical experience. They were useful, but we still did not have a clinical perspective that was consistent with our experience.

Meanwhile, the situation for people being served remained intolerable. We finally concluded that we would not be able to rely on an existing frame of reference and that we would instead have to figure out, at the very least, a variation of an existing approach. We needed a way to describe our people that would enable us to make a greater—and more predictable—therapeutic impact. In view of the pressure from licensing, finding that way became our number one challenge.

THE SEARCH FOR A BETTER WAY

Despite our efforts, we could find no one approach that provided the answer for our situation. We had to figure out how to do things better, but we were not even sure what "better" involved. Our only remaining option was to review our clinical reasoning and to evaluate our own clinical observations and experiences.

We knew that the major problem for all people in our care was brain damage, and as occupational therapists we believed that was significant. Therefore, we reasoned that we should know more about the relationship between brain damage and the performance problems displayed by the people we served. Since behavior was so frequently the focus of a person's program, we felt it was especially important for us to look at challenging or excessive behaviors as a possible reflection of what goes on in the brain. These lines of reasoning took us directly to a sensory perspective.

We decided to see what would happen if we were to interpret the challenging behaviors as evidence of a priority sensory need (Reisman & Hanschu, 1992). Relying on sensory integration and neurodevelopmental principles to guide us, we proceeded to introduce individual programs with strong sensory elements. We started to emphasize the importance of heavy work and taught staff how to safely give therapeutic "doses" of sensation, including direct compression or stretch at joints, and pressure touch to backs, arms, and legs to provide stronger body sensation. We got equipment into household and day program areas so that people could swing before challenging events or major transitions. We even organized therapy staff to provide direct service in the work areas, scheduling extended blocks of time according to the number of people with sensory needs in the area. We also figured out how to incorporate strong sensation at strategic times in the daily routine, namely, during transitions, mealtimes, morning care, and medical appointments.

Benefits became evident almost immediately, but we still were not sure how to explain or predict what was happening. We believed the improvement had something to do with increased opportunity to get strong sensation because nothing else had changed. Enhanced sensation was simply structured into the person's experience. As clients began to look more comfortable and more "settled," they became more initiating, indicating what sensory activity they wanted and when. Rather than frantically going for vigorous sensation or engaging in insistent self-stimulation, they looked like they were comparing choices and selecting what they preferred. Although we often controlled their choices, being able to choose from alternatives made it more possible for them to "lead" us, rather than our controlling the interaction. This was quite a new development for many of them.

We were encouraged by results associated with sensory techniques, but we did not yet have a frame of reference, consisting of logically connected ideas, that we could support with scientific evidence. Sensory integration theory, which in many ways was so helpful at getting us closer to the nature of the need, actually held us back a bit. It did not easily or fully explain what we were doing or seeing. We spent a lot of time and effort trying to reconcile our experience with the theory before we began to realize that a different theory might be more applicable. Explanations that fit our population did not start to emerge until we got beyond sensory integration to the more generic concept of sensory processing and until we started to delve into what scientists were discovering about the neurobiology of behavior. Until then, we were trying to get a theory about sensorimotor function to explain behavior, as if sensorimotor function and behavior were one and the same. The limitations were not in sensory integration theory; they were in how we were trying to use it. Nevertheless, sensory integration theory got us started in the right direction: thinking sensory.

Thinking sensory was one thing; trying to reconcile a sensory perspective with the prevailing behavioral view was another. We immediately encountered conflicts and inconsistencies that made it difficult to use the two approaches together. For example, the behavioral approach for designing individual programs took no account of neurology, that is, the brain damage experienced by the people we served (Crick, 1994; Edelman, 1992). In contrast, sensory approaches were dependent on an understanding of neurohabilitative considerations. Another conflict was that behavioral approaches relied heavily on learning theory, while sensory theory suggested the possibility that learning might be blocked.

The discrepancies between the two approaches magnified our concern that behavioral thinking might actually result in significant misunderstanding or misinterpretation of behaviors displayed by many of the people we served. This concern had been raised even by prominent behavioral psychologists who were starting to acknowledge sensory explanations for some behaviors (Durand & Crimmins, 1988; Lovaas, Newsom, & Hickman, 1987). We envisioned a future where teams might need to choose one approach over another, but we realized their task would be formidable unless we could offer clearer explanations of the sensory issues and defend what we said. That got us searching the neuroscience literature, particularly what it had to say about the neurobiology of behavior.

Closing in on Priority Issues

Many authorities on the nervous system describe how behavior is dependent upon sensation coming into the brain and being *processed.* Different authors offer different perspectives of the processing involved, such as anatomical (Brodal, 1992) and biochemical (Rahmann & Rahmann, 1992; Shepherd, 1988). Although there are still many questions about how the brain processes sensation, scientists believe they are getting much closer to the answers. What is known provides us with possible, if not probable, explanations for how the brain registers and integrates sensation and for how sensation influences emotion, awareness, cognition, and behavior (Chopra, 1989; Churchland, 1993; Gazzaniga, 1988, 1992, 1995; Goleman, 1995; Kandel & Schwartz, 1991, 1995; Kotulak, 1996; LeDoux, 1996; Masters & McGuire, 1994; Nuland, 1997; Pearsall, 1996; Ruden, 1997; West, 1991). In general, *processing sensation* enables the brain to do several things related to experience: make sense of it, organize responses to it, and form memories of it (Kandel & Schwartz, 1991, 1995; Kotulak, 1996; Ruden, 1997). This raises another question about behavioral approaches: if someone's brain is unable to comprehend the meaning of experience, how would reinforcing aspects of that experience promote learning? How can one learn something that makes no sense? Perhaps there was a neurobiological explanation for why the most carefully designed, consistently applied behavioral interventions might have no lasting effects, as was the case for the people in the remaining group at our institution with whom such interventions had been tried over and over again for a period of many years.

Neuroscientists also tell us that most of a person's sensory processing involves neural activity in lower centers, such as the brain stem, cerebellum, and limbic structures—centers that work well below the level of consciousness (Kotulak, 1996; Masters & McGuire, 1994). This processing enables humans to do all kinds of complex tasks automatically, without any thought, often without awareness of doing them. Those of us who have cars and routinely drive back and forth between two familiar locations, such as work and home, can probably relate to the experience of finding ourselves at one of the locations with no memory of having driven there. Our brains can do extremely sophisticated tasks for us, such as driving a large piece of expensive equipment through heavy traffic, calling for our attention only if something unusual occurs. Adequate sensory processing frees people to live full lives, to give their conscious attention to what most interests them. Some people actually make a nice living capitalizing on highly efficient sensory processing, for example, professional athletes.

There is obviously a wide range along the continuum between functional and dysfunctional sensory processing. That range made us all the more aware of the degree of disordered sensory processing in our clients who did little that was automatic, unless it also involved strong emotion. Then they could move in a flash. Otherwise their actions often seemed delayed and deliberate, as if they were paying attention to every detail. We also saw the problem of experience apparently not being stored in memory. Numerous direct contact staff reported the observation that "if we've done it once, we've done it a million times, the same way, every time; yet, it's always like it's the first time." Neuroscientists tell us memory does not store confusion.

Given such observations and seeing how our clients responded in various situations, it seemed highly likely that their sensory processing was significantly disordered. Not only did their sensory processing seem insufficient to support the development of a repertoire of automatic responses, it was also too disordered for most clients to get enough meaning out of their experience to form adequate memory of that experience. We now know much more about memory mechanisms and how they influence behavior. Joseph LeDoux's work clearly differentiates emotional memory from something we could call rational memory (LeDoux, 1996). Emotional memory is thought to be fully functional at the time of birth, laying in memory circuits that can be, as Daniel Goleman describes it, tripwired to provide immediate, strong emotional reactions in the presence of just a few stimuli that trigger the memory (Goleman, 1995). In contrast to emotional memory, rational memory is not fully functional until around the age of 2. Rational memory is provided by circuitry that enables the brain to interpret experience, to understand what is happening, to provide a context for what one may be feeling. That we recognize a face is a product of rational memory; that we have feelings about the person with that face is a product of emotional memory. The day-to-day reactions of our clients seem to perfectly illustrate emotional memory dominating responses without the benefit of rational memory's mediation. Other factors may have contributed, but we certainly could argue that disordered sensory processing probably made it difficult for our clients to form rational memories of their experience. How could anyone's brain interpret what it experienced and mediate that person's response to experience, if it could neither get the meaning nor store memories of the experience?

The more we came to understand how the chemistry and circuitry of the brain influence behavior, the more we had to rethink assumptions about several aspects of the people we served. However, our ability to rethink assumptions was still complicated. We had lots of new ideas and we were excited about how perfectly they seemed to fit our clinical observations, yet we still lacked a cohesive set of consistent and compatible assumptions to guide our clinical reasoning. When we tried to use sensory integration theory to explain the needs of our group, we ran into limitations. For example, experts on the topic emphasize that sensory integration requires *active* participation to plan, organize, and generate *adaptive* responses (Ayres, 1972; Fisher, Murray, & Bundy, 1991). How could we justify, as a treatment technique, giving strong sensation to someone who remained essentially passive? This, according to the sensory integration experts, was nothing more than sensory stimulation (Fisher, Murray, & Bundy, 1991). Some sensory integration experts also stress that effectiveness of sensory integration is reflected by sensorimotor ability (Ayres, 1972; Fisher, Murray, & Bundy, 1991). Therefore, we had trouble explaining how some individuals could have so many functional, performance, and behavior problems, yet the quality of their *sensorimotor* ability could seem quite intact. How could they move with ease and finesse, when they wanted to do so, if disordered *sensory integration* was a fundamental problem?

We faced another conflict in our ability to rely on sensory integration theory when we got the Wilbarger explanation of *sensory defensiveness.* According to Patricia and Julia Wilbarger, defensiveness can occur in anybody at anytime (Wilbarger & Wilbarger, 1991). If faced with circumstances that severely tax the protective mechanisms managed by the brain's limbic structures, any of us, even as adults, can develop sensory defensiveness according to the Wilbargers. The idea that defensiveness can occur in anyone at anytime is also consistent with Joseph LeDoux's explanation of fear responses in his book *The Emotional Brain.* Yet, according to experts on sensory integration theory, sensory integration dysfunction includes tactile defensiveness (Royeen & Lane, 1991) and results from damage to lower brain centers *early in the life of the brain,* usually before the age of three (Fisher, Murray, & Bundy, 1991). This tactile problem seemed to be the same tactile defensiveness that the Wilbargers had described as the most common form of sensory defensiveness, with sensory defensiveness being *a condition that can arise anytime in the lifespan.*

It seemed we needed to figure out if sensory defensiveness might more appropriately be viewed as a separate and distinct problem. Our need to figure this out became even more compelling when we saw the degree to which the distinction influenced our diagnosing. Using the Wilbarger explanation, we saw defensiveness all around us in our adult population. If we viewed defensiveness as one aspect of sensory integration dysfunction and followed the criteria advocated by Fisher, Murray, & Bundy, the problem was less rife. However, we also found that the treatment protocol developed by the Wilbargers achieved more significant improvement, much faster, than any of the other sensory strategies we had tried. This presented still another conflict in trying to explain sensory defensiveness as an aspect of sensory integration dysfunction because, according to the Wilbargers, *if necessary, you impose* the treatment. Yet, imposing strong sensations is considered to be inappropriate from the perspective of sensory integration theory.

It was becoming increasingly obvious to us that we probably could not rely solely on sensory integration theory to explain the needs of, or plan an appropriate intervention for, our adult population. In addition, it looked like any frame of reference we developed would have to be able to explain sensory integration and sensory defensiveness as two distinct aspects of a more generic brain mechanism or activity. For adults served in an institutional environment, we decided the more generic activity, *sensory processing*, was the issue on which to focus our attention.

Sensory Processing and Neural Plasticity

Neural plasticity was another well documented aspect of brain activity that captured our interest. *Neural plasticity* accounts for a person's ability to recover from a stroke as well as the ability to learn increasingly complex information and skills. *Plasticity* is the capacity of the human brain to improve its circuitry for better communication among various neural networks (Aoki & Siekevitz, 1988; Brodal, 1992; Churchland & Sejnowski, 1993; Kandel & Schwartz, 1991, 1995; Kotulak, 1996; Kuno, 1995). *Plasticity* even enables the brain to repair or modify circuitry that becomes damaged (Levitan & Kaczmarek, 1997; Nicholls, 1994; Rahmann & Rahmann, 1992; Shepherd, 1988). This highly dynamic, ongoing process helps the brain achieve and maintain maximal efficiency. It is known to be present in the human brain, even damaged brains, for the whole of the lifespan.

We were fascinated by the phenomenon of neural plasticity because of our observation about sustained improvement in the adults with whom we were using sensory techniques. There were indications, in many of the individuals who improved, that the improvements were stable. We observed this stability in more and more people the longer we continued to use sensory techniques. We found, for example, that, with some people, there came a time when we could fade the frequency and intensity of service without seeing any regression. Now, after years of experience with this approach, we find this same "permanence" in the progress made by many children who are treated for sensory processing problems. We think the relatively permanent change results from improved circuitry that helps the brain become more efficient in its ability to adapt to varied situations. It seems to be a manifestation of *neural plasticity* in action. This is not to imply that there is never regression, but even in the adult setting, where some of our people were in their 50s, those receiving sensory services could sometimes have three medication reductions before displaying any signs of regression. When regression did occur, it was relatively minor and a short period of more intense sensory service would help the person recover a more adaptive level of performance. Our conclusion: sensory strategies and enriched sensory experience appeared to be facilitating sensory processing *and* neural plasticity. This was very exciting indeed!

Brain stem Sensations

Changes associated with plasticity are known to involve the brain's chemistry and circuitry. Both are influenced by experience, but both are influenced first and foremost by brain stem sensations. Brain stem sensations "wake up" the nervous system and help it become "ready" to support increased neural activity associated with our being alert and doing something. Brain stem sensations are important to maintain responses like

- muscle tone
- equilibrium reactions
- physical sense of self
- modulated arousal
- focused attention (Brodal, 1992; Kandel, & Schwartz 1991, 1995).

Brain scientists tell us that about 80 percent of what we do is managed for us by lower brain centers, processing sensations and generating adaptive responses automatically, without our having to give a single conscious thought to what we are doing. That 80 percent relies directly on efficient processing of brain stem sensations. When sensory processing is disordered, one of the first things that gets compromised is the ability to do things automatically, to act adaptively without having to think about what we are doing. The 80 percent starts to become the 20 percent. That is what happens in people who have disordered sensory processing.

Of all the sensations coming into the brain, the brain stem relies most on three types of sensation to help it know when to activate and turn-up the firing in multiple central nervous system mechanisms. They are

- tactile or touch sensations
- proprioceptive or joint sensations
- vestibular sensations from movement of the head and the pull of gravity.

Patricia Wilbarger calls these the *power sensations* because they have such an enormous influence on all aspects of brain activity. These are the same three sensations that occupational therapy practitioners have found to be so effective in their sensory techniques. For over 30 years, inspired by the likes of Margaret Rood, A. Jean Ayres, and Lorna Jean King, occupational therapists have been making it a specific point to incorporate these sensations into various treatment programs.

If you ask a hundred people to name the basic senses they will probably name touch, taste, smell, vision, and hearing.

Many science textbooks do the same. Even therapists may forget to include proprioception (joint sensations) and vestibular sensations (detection of gravity and movement). Yet, we have experiences everyday that point out how important movement and joint sensations are. Think about lying back in a recliner to take a few moments to rest after a busy day. You are likely to find that you quickly become drowsy. The next thing you may notice is a voice in your head telling you it is important to get out of the chair before you fall asleep, but when you finally decide to get up you find it is impossible to move. Your brain decided that since you were going to rest you would not need muscle tone. Consequently, it significantly reduced the messages to muscles that tell them to maintain a tonal ready state. Why should the brain expend effort to provide something you do not need? When you decided to get up, you momentarily caught the brain off-guard. Muscle tone was needed and the brain was not prepared. Your alternative was to rely on *cortical mediation*, activity in the higher centers of the brain that involve awareness, thinking, and intention, so you could do something that would otherwise have been automatic, namely, moving. This may be akin to the experience our clients have when they have to use cortical mediation for responses that are normally automatic. It would explain their seriousness, the intensity of their concentration, their deliberateness, and their slowness to respond.

When you finally got out of the recliner, you probably discovered that, by the time you got to where you were going, you felt wide awake. In the process of moving, your brain got the strong brain stem sensation it needed to increase your alertness naturally—sensation from muscles and joints and from the vestibular apparatus in each ear. General alertness relies much more on brain stem sensations, than on vision and hearing. Visual and auditory sensations are processed by higher brain centers that analyze and interpret the meaning of what you experience. To compare the difference between brain stem sensations and sensations that are processed primarily in higher brain centers, we can contrast the difference between being awake and alert versus *knowing* exactly where we are and what is happening once we are awake and alert. The *knowing* part of the equation comes from vision and hearing.

Experience has shown that sensory techniques using powerful brain stem sensation are extremely helpful with many individuals. Authors from many different fields attest to the benefits of strong brain stem sensation (Brockle-hurst-Woods, 1990; Grandin, 1992; Iwasaki & Holm, 1989; McGimsey & Favell, 1988; Pearsall, 1996; Reisman, 1993; Rosenthal-Malek & Mitchell, 1997; Silver, 1993; Tomporowski & Ellis, 1985; Trott, 1993; Watters & Watters, 1980). Providing brain stem sensation takes advantage of how the human brain naturally uses sensation. Therefore, sensory techniques are relatively safe when used by someone who understands the principles of neurohabilitation. Occupational therapists have a natural treatment alternative with the potential to achieve impressive results without being intrusive or expensive. With so many benefits, one might expect a sensory approach to be embraced with open arms by service providers, especially in situations where nothing else seems to be working. That such eagerness may not be present is an example of how lower brain centers can also influence the human response to any prospect of change.

THE CHALLENGE OF CHANGE

When occupational therapists in our institution started advocating a sensory perspective as an appropriate "primary" frame of reference for everyone, they had in mind the benefits of viewing clients first and foremost in terms of sensory needs. Knowing how effectiveness of sensory processing influences everything a person does, therapists reasoned that sensory needs could be a barrier to every person's ability to benefit from other services. Therefore, it made sense to therapists for teams to know when sensory needs were likely to be something to take into consideration.

Of course, that implied that everyone on the team accepted the legitimacy of a sensory perspective. As it turned out, this was not the case. We were advocating something many involved did not support or even understand. Therapists were not only asking strongly behaviorally oriented treatment teams to make a significant shift in their thinking; they were actually asking the whole institution to make a monumental change in how it operated. Taking sensory needs into account as a primary consideration meant that responses previously assumed to be learned behaviors might have to be interpreted in a different light. That created the possibility that intervention plans might need to be significantly modified, and that led to the strong possibility that team members might need to interact with clients in a new way. Allowing for primary sensory needs presented the possibility of major change for many levels: individual service providers, teams, design of individual programs, as well as probable overhaul of the whole organizational program. For such a major shift to occur, teams, supervisors, managers, and administrators had to make many tough, sometimes unpopular decisions. The fact that it was a large organization, with a multidecade history of doing things one way, did not help. Even if it is not working, there can be something reassuring about doing what is most familiar.

We knew it would take time and careful planning to have minimal disruption of essential services. We knew our roles and responsibilities could change dramatically, and we were apprehensive about managing the increased demand on our time, attention, and expertise. We were also working in an organization that was dealing with recurring periods of downsizing. As the number of staff decreased, we had to keep collapsing and reconfiguring groups which meant reorganizing staff and program locations. Downsizing also meant periodic closure of older buildings so major relocations were needed more than once. It was a complicated and challenging work environment, not the best of circumstances for encouraging people to think about significant changes in program philosophy. Consequently, even though we understood and believed in the benefits of making the necessary changes, we, who were therapists, had our own trepidations to overcome.

Meanwhile, it was decided that the therapy department should proceed, person by person, to redesign individual program plans to take sensory needs into account. Fortunately, almost as fast as redesigned programs got started, positive results became evident. Seeing the benefits for clients so quickly certainly made it easier for people to consider a sensory frame of reference with a more open mind. The case examples at the beginning of this chapter illustrate why, despite the upheaval associated with all the changes, many people were quite positive about the new sensory perspective. Even the skeptics contributed to the effort by forcing us to answer questions and figure out solutions we otherwise might have overlooked.

Eventually, we had the opportunity to see the benefits of a fully integrated sensory model. With the change came tremendous improvement in clients, well beyond anything we would have predicted. The benefits of the change could be seen in other aspects of the institution's operation, as well. For example, instead of getting citations on every standard in the licensing regulations as before, once the sensory orientation was fully in place, the program got no citations; it actually got commendations! The mask of sensory issues that made it so difficult to see the abilities and potential of the people we served had finally been removed and people evaluating our services were as enthused and impressed by the change as we were.

THE READY APPROACH

In retrospect, it is evident that we were on our way to developing a new frame of reference. In the years to follow, the ideas that started to emerge from our experience in that adult program have become more crystallized. They are now assembled in a frame of reference called the *Ready Approach.* Advances in the brain sciences continue to refine our understanding of the neurobiology of behavior and how sensation can be used to influence that neurobiology. That information has helped us to further refine the theory that underlies the approach we developed for the institutionalized adults. We now know from first-hand experience that the *Ready Approach* can make a dramatic difference for adults and children, even those who have the most severe sensory processing problems. Even though the approach still needs to be formally tested, it has been introduced with positive results in programs for people of all ages, in all kinds of settings, all over the United States. Service providers are hungry for an approach that works, especially with adults who have severe behaviors. The *Ready Approach* appears to be a promising alternative that is worthy of consideration.

The frame of reference that made such a difference turned out to be a sensory perspective based on a set of assumptions rooted primarily in both sensory integration theory and what neuroscientists tell us about the neurobiology of behavior, cognition, emotion, and consciousness. It provides an organized approach that enables service providers to consistently and systematically

1. determine priority needs
2. make appropriate recommendations to treatment teams
3. get visible or measurable improvement
4. predict how soon and to what degree those changes are likely to appear.

It seems to be especially well suited for children or adults who have the most challenging behaviors, but therapists are reporting that it enhances progress in many other individuals as well. It is believed that the approach helps by enhancing the ability of a person with disordered sensory processing to respond more adaptively. It helps the disorganized or struggling nervous system to become *ready* to respond, *ready* to interact, *ready* to catch on to what is happening and what it means. Giving people time and sensation that bridges the gap between being ready and just being expected to respond seems to be a key difference. It is not unusual to see the benefits of the approach in a single interaction, showing up as more adaptive behavior, social interaction, or task performance.

Positive changes associated with the approach that are typically observed or reported first include improvements in

- alertness
- ability to regulate arousal
- interest and attention
- sleep related behavior
- eating habits and mealtime behavior
- willingness and ability to dress or stay dressed
- initiation of interaction with others.

Individuals served with this approach often start to look happier and more comfortable. Over time, they are likely to spontaneously express new, relatively complex skills that familiar care providers describe as "amazing" and "something the person was never taught." We used the techniques associated with this approach with a man in his 30s who was blind and who would never wear shirts. He became upset if attempts were made to put one on him and would frantically strip as soon as someone succeeded in getting one on him. One day, the certified occupational therapy assistant who worked with him handed him a T-shirt and asked him to put it on. He took it, faced it in the right direction, and put it on correctly with no assistance whatsoever. A colleague reported her experience with a man in a different institutional environment. He had frequent toileting accidents and never used the toilet without maximal assistance and prompting. He had never removed his pants or put them on by himself during toileting or any other time. One day, he just went to the bathroom without prompting, undressed to use the toilet, finished and redressed, flushed the toilet, and came out to wash his hands. All this with no assistance. The staff who worked with him could not believe the change in his degree of independence.

These are not unusual reports, nor are they isolated examples. Direct contact staff working with people getting this approach in our organization frequently reported new abilities in the daily log that they described as "incredible," something "never seen before." They described clients who for the first time approached them for positive interaction, brought them a piece of sensory equipment, like a brush, and indicated they wanted sensation. They described people who had always avoided peers, who suddenly seemed to want to be with other people. Medical and dental personnel reported that someone tolerated an examination without medication and that they arrived for the appointment on their own with just one escort to assist. They found this change particularly remarkable in individuals who had been unable to tolerate examinations, who typically had needed several escorts, sometimes as many as six or seven, to get them to the appointment, at which time they would be medicated to relax or sedate them.

The ideas that now define the *Ready Approach* made a profound difference in our institutional setting. Many of the people we served made remarkable progress; their lives changed for the better in ways we would never have imagined possible. After years of no progress or regression, everyone started to improve. Our institution went from being threatened with decertification, which would have meant forced closure, to being identified as a model program. On every index, from personnel issues, such as sick leave use and Worker's Compensation claims, to measurements regarding the progression of medication reductions and the success of community based placements, our numbers improved (Reisman & Hanschu, 1993).

Today, many organizations are still downsizing, creating recurring episodes of havoc for people who live or work in large institutions. In states across the country, political changes are altering the philosophies and financial priorities for public and private agencies, sometimes necessitating sweeping changes that drastically affect how adults are served. For years, many people have believed that it is not realistic to expect major progress in adults with severe, long standing, well established problems. It turns out that this kind of thinking may have a devastating consequence for the people we serve, limiting what we see as possible and, therefore, limiting what we are willing to try.

Ironically, studies reported in the *Autism Research Review International*, Vol. 11 (1), suggest that movement out of institutions into community settings may not be the best alternative for everyone. Nevertheless, the days of large institutions seem to be coming to an end. For service providers and the people being served, these can be difficult times, when funding and politics can make our work a discouraging and frustrating experience. In the face of all that, the *Ready Approach* offers hope for people who have seemed unreachable. It is an alternative that can remind us all of the remarkable resilience of the human brain and its ability to recover from and rise above its experience, even when that experience is less than ideal. Occupational therapy practitioners who participate in the process are likely to find that working with adults who have the most challenging problems turns out to be an exciting, rewarding, and most enjoyable experience, regardless of the environment in which the adults are served. Our experience is also a reminder that, when we get it right, people can accomplish amazing progress. One of the great pleasures of being an occupational therapist is the opportunity to witness such improvement; but even better, we help make it happen.

A NEW WAY TO VIEW OLD PROBLEMS

The sensory processing perspective that underlies the *Ready Approach* is simply a frame of reference, an alternative way to view the needs of people with complex handicapping conditions associated with developmental disabilities. As a frame of reference, it influences what we see, how we describe it, what we identify as important issues, and what we consider to be an appropriate course of action. As is the case when we use any frame of reference, nothing about the person actually changes. All we are doing is looking at the same old problems in a new way. This section will describe the view from the perspective of the *Ready Approach*. In the *Ready Approach*, the concern is whether or not someone's sensory processing is effective enough to enable the person to respond adaptively. We could say the *Ready Approach* makes the difference between instinctive reactions and conscious responses. The crucial questions become: is the person *ready* to respond, *ready* to interact, and *ready* to do something that has meaning to that person?

We have established how *readiness* is compromised by disordered sensory processing. But sensory processing is also compromised by lack of *readiness*. The brain takes in sensation. That is how everything enters the brain, as sensation. Normally, various brain mechanisms then go to work to decode and translate the sensations into recognizable perceptions. The perceptions become information that enables the brain to catch on to what is happening, to get the meaning of what the person is experiencing. When the brain has trouble recognizing the relevance of specific sensations within the full range of sensations we experience, when certain sensations are given too much importance and other sensations are not given enough, then the brain *computes* a flawed set of perceptions. Meaning computed on the basis of faulty perceptions will invariably be flawed itself. This meaning, however flawed it may be, gets stored in memory for future reference. Then, when similar stimuli are present in the future, the brain decodes the sets and patterns of the stimuli from that flawed perspective and the stage is set for a vicious cycle of disordered sensory processing.

Readiness Is the Ability to Respond

Responding occurs after the brain has analyzed the sensations coming in, computed the meaning of what we are experiencing, weighed options, considered consequences based on prior learning, and then figured out an organized response based on all it wants to accomplish through what we do. *Responding* is a form of *replying* to one's experience. It is hard to *reply* to something if the brain's attention is diverted to other matters. This is the problem for people who are not *ready*. Their brains miss important information to be gleaned from the present experience, because 80 percent of brain activity and attention is riveted to safety, survival, comfort, being free of pain or confusion, and feeling in control. Consequently, the brain disregards other information that would be relevant, and the person becomes increasingly stuck on safety and comfort needs.

Reacting is not as adaptive as *responding* in everyday circumstances. *Reacting* is important when we are in danger, so we do not waste time thinking and analyzing. Instead, our actions are *triggered* by the sensory stimuli in the situation. This gets us out of harm's way quickly, sometimes before we are even aware of being at risk (Goleman, 1995; LeDoux, 1996). *Reactions* are driven by the most primitive, pleasure seeking, pain avoiding brain centers. These centers do not think before they do; they do not weigh options and consider the consequences. They just fire off strong urges, moving us toward or away from specific stimuli. That is fine in emergencies, but in everyday, routine situations *reactions* are clumsy and incomplete, like pieces of *responses*. The incompleteness makes them less than adaptive.

Since everything coming into the brain enters as sensation (Ruden, 1997), *Ready* proponents believe the key to facilitating more adaptive responses, to enhancing *readiness*, is to improve the effectiveness and efficiency of sensory processing by influencing the sensation a person takes in. This brings us to two basic goals for helping people who have disordered sensory processing. They amount to either taking something away or adding something in, to influence the sensory intake equation at any particular time.

Goal #1: Lower Demands on a Struggling Nervous System

This involves changing the environment. One option is to move someone to an environment that is already structured to lower sensory demands.

Another option is to modify how people experience time, space, interactions, and activities in their present environments. Pressure on a struggling nervous system will be lowered if there are fewer distractions and interruptions, if there are more cues available to help the person predict what is going to happen next, and if there is plenty of time to settle and get reorganized before being asked to respond again. Implementing environmental changes that take sensory needs into account can sometimes make enough difference, all by itself, to bring about more adaptive behavior (Duker & Rasing, 1989; Merrill, 1990). We have observed this over and over again.

Goal #2: Provide Sensation to Enhance Brain Efficiency

People who have disordered sensory processing need increased opportunities to obtain direct, strong doses of helpful sensation. When it comes to the fundamentals of sensory processing, the most helpful sensations are brain stem sensations, like touch, proprioception, and vestibular sensation. These are the sensations that activate helpful brain chemistry, that nurture and nourish neural circuitry, that enhance the computation of meaning by giving context and perspective to the brain's interpretation of what it is experiencing.

Enhanced opportunities to get strong brain stem sensations can be provided to someone through three alternatives:

- hands-on techniques, such as pressure touch to body surfaces or compression or stretch to joints
- activities with natural opportunities to move, exert, or have physical contact, such as doing heavy work
- activities set up or structured to incorporate strong brain stem sensation, such as going through an obstacle course.

The most powerful results are achieved when therapists are skilled in a) determining and treating the nature of someone's specific sensory needs, and b) designing enriched sensory diets. Ideally, services are designed to achieve both sensory goals, that is, decrease pressure on a struggling system and provide helpful sensations. Since so much can safely be accomplished by providing an enriched sensory diet, we will consider that option first.

Enriched Sensory Diets

The term *sensory diet* refers to the kinds of sensory opportunities and experiences available to a person as part of that person's daily routine (Wilbarger

& Wilbarger, 1991). Sensory diets can be influenced by modifying the environment to simultaneously add opportunities to get strong brain stem sensation while removing excessive pressure on a struggling system. People with sensory processing problems need *enriched sensory diets*, meaning that someone has taken special care to structure the natural day to maximize sensory benefits. Diets are especially likely to include opportunities to get large doses of helpful sensation at strategic times of the day. Some individuals get enough benefit if they just have periodic opportunities to do heavy work, that is, physical exertion using the large muscles of the body. For example, to provide heavy work opportunities *at strategic times*, one might structure an opportunity to stack furniture or carry books to a storage site shortly before going to the cafeteria for lunch. In the extreme of severity are people who are so overwhelmed that they have gone into a relatively permanent state of *shutdown*. They need sensory diets that start out being much more subdued. Until they can tolerate more sensation, such individuals may need to be served in quiet environments where the lights can be dimmed, where there are no distractions or interruptions, where someone approaches them gently or not at all.

Enriched sensory diets almost always need to be planned on an individual basis, but many enriching opportunities can be shared by more than one person in a particular setting. It is important to remember that *all* human nervous systems benefit from opportunities to get strong brain stem sensation, so sensory opportunities structured to help one person often benefit everyone in a group.

Successful Treatment Depends on Effective Evaluation

Clinical reasoning is always required to match treatment choices correctly with treatment needs. In the *Ready Approach*, clinical reasoning begins with the ability to interpret behavioral indicators of the effectiveness of someone's sensory processing. Many therapists use the *Sensory Integration Inventory for Individuals Who Have Developmental Disabilities* to get a profile of sensory indicators (Reisman & Hanschu, 1992). The *Inventory* can usually be used with anyone over the age of 2, but the therapist who interprets the results must be able to rule out indicators that can be explained by something else. Behaviors can look like sensory indicators but actually be symptoms of a motor control problem, an attempt to communicate, an attempt to achieve comfort from physical or emotional distress, a learned response, or a frank pathology, such as Down's Syndrome.

Even if someone does not have a fundamental sensory processing problem, the person may still benefit from sensory techniques based on the *Ready*

Approach or sensory integration theory. It is important to not call something a sensory processing problem if there is another explanation that explains the symptoms nicely. It is also important to remember that, whenever we use any clinical frame of reference, whether it be behaviorism, neurodevelopment, or a sensory approach, our interpretations and conclusions can be no more than our best educated guess. The fact is, no one knows the full picture of what may be influencing someone's behavior at a particular time. We deal in possibilities and sometimes probabilities, but rarely in certainties.

It is good to know as much as possible about different clinical frames of reference, so we do not overlook the significance of a particular interpretation because of our own ignorance. Considering how often functional problems manifest as maladaptive, excessive, or challenging behaviors, it is wonderful that so many people are becoming more knowledgeable about how brain chemistry and circuitry influence behavior, especially since that influence typically affects behavior in ways that are well beyond the person's understanding or control. When we understand better, we automatically take a lot of pressure off their systems.

Recognizing Four Sensory Processing Problems

It is possible to differentiate four distinct sensory processing problems. Each relates to separate and discrete neural mechanisms involving how sensation is detected, filtered, interpreted, and incorporated into the brain's computation for *readiness*. Disorder in one mechanism can greatly influence or create disorder in other mechanisms. A person can have one or more of the four problems at the same time, but it seems that optimal results are usually obtained when problems are treated in this order:

1) sensory defensiveness
2) disordered sensory modulation
3) inadequate sensory registration
4) sensory integration dysfunction.

Sensory Defensiveness

There are two characteristics of someone's response that increase the probability that the person has sensory defensiveness. The first is an exaggerated avoidance of specific sensations that is out of proportion to the situation. The second is the element of surprise. Most defensive people have periodic episodes of *unpredictable* dramatic behavior. No one can provide an explanation for the reaction, including the person who reacted. The reaction seems so illogical that people who spend time with the defensive person may feel they need to be on their toes at all times in order to avoid anything that might "set the person off."

Most of what we know about defensiveness is based on the work of two occupational therapists, Patricia and Julia Wilbarger, a mother and daughter team who have collaborated in studying the issue of sensory defensiveness for many years. Patricia Wilbarger was a partner of Jean Ayres and, with Dr. Ayres, cofounded Sensory Integration International. Patricia is considered by most to be the premiere occupational therapy expert on the issue of defensiveness, having devoted the main part of her career to this single specific condition.

Joseph LeDoux's book, *The Emotional Brain*, provides an interesting take on defensiveness from the perspective of primitive memory mechanisms responsible for what he calls fear reactions (LeDoux, 1996). His insights, combined with those of the Wilbargers, are enabling therapists to understand, recognize, and treat defensiveness as never before, in people of all ages and functional abilities, around the world.

Defensiveness is a serious disorder that can affect anyone at anytime in their lifespan. It seems to be a crucial piece of the sensory puzzle, because it is both a *common* and a *serious* problem. In some environments, where people with severe sensory processing problems are served together in groups, the incidence of those displaying evidence of defensiveness can approach 75 percent or higher. Defensiveness to touch is by far the most common, present in about 80 percent of defensive individuals, according to the Wilbargers (1991). Their estimate is certainly consistent with our observations.

People can also be defensive to movement (vestibular sensations), oral sensations, sounds, and even to visual stimuli and odors. It is not unusual to work with people who are defensive to more than one type of sensation. As far back as the 1970s, Barbara Knickerbocker, the occupational therapist who gave us the term *sensory defensiveness*, was already reporting dyads and triads of sensation, especially the triad involving touch, sounds, and olfactory sensations (Knickerbocker, 1980). She had observed that, if the children she served displayed an aversion to one of the sensations in the triad, they were likely to display some degree of aversion to the other two. Many people with developmental disabilities find movement unpleasant or even frightening. Individuals who display defensiveness or an aversion to movement or postural changes, like those who are defensive to touch, tend to be hypervigilant or too preoccupied with the potential for the offending sensations to give adequate attention to other matters. Thus, defensiveness alone can create the appearance of significant sensory processing problems which may disappear once the defensiveness has been treated.

It is not hard to see how defensiveness creates a major barrier to a person's ability to interact freely and benefit from other treatments. Occupational therapy practitioners should be familiar with the diagnosis and treatment of sensory defensiveness because this processing disorder is easy to miss, especially in its more subtle forms. Given what we know now, it is difficult to justify defensiveness remaining in someone's system when the Wilbarger protocol can be such an effective treatment.

Disordered Sensory Modulation

This is a significant problem affecting self-regulation of arousal. In some settings, it is likely to be as, or even more, common than defensiveness. Sensory modulation problems usually show up as overarousal (hyperactivity), attentional problems (distractibility), or shutdown—a paradoxical problem of looking underaroused when you are actually so overly aroused your brain dampens sensation to keep you more comfortable. Disordered modulation can also show up in the form of fluctuating arousal and underarousal, where someone has difficulty maintaining sufficient alertness to even remain awake or aware of the environment. Overarousal and distractibility often go hand-in-hand. People with both are likely to engage in stereotypic behaviors, especially persistent self-stimulation. In general, self-stimulation can be evidence of other problems, but when it is present in people who also have difficulty with transitions, it is important to consider the probability that the person has disordered sensory modulation.

Inadequate Sensory Registration

This is a problem that can involve heightened as well as diminished detection of specific sensations, either having the potential to cause significant secondary problems. An example of overregistration would be the person who fixates on visual stimuli in the ambient field. When we focus attention on one type of stimuli, registration of other stimuli is dampened (Hobson, 1994). Hyperfocusing can lead to an imbalance in how stimuli in a particular sensory channel are registered. Registration problems, however, show up most commonly as underregistration of vestibular sensation (movement) that tends to make the person uninterested in moving. The subsequent lack of movement can lead to something akin to sensory deprivation, with secondary underregistration of proprioception (joint and muscle sensations) that, in turn, can lead to inadequate physical sense of self, directly compromising someone's ability to get the meaning of what they experience (Damasio, 1994; Greenspan, 1997). Impaired tactile discrimination, another form of inadequate registration, often improves on its own as registration of vestibular and proprioceptive sensation improves, again showing that problems registering sensations in one system can lead to impaired registration of other sensations. Adequate vestibular processing does seem to be a basic need. It is important for all movement, for bilateral abilities, perceptual abilities, and for most task related responses. We frequently see individuals whose inadequate vestibular registration severely compromises their overall functional skill and independence. Fortunately, this is a problem that seems quite amenable to treatment and the main challenge for the therapist is to recognize when it is present.

Sensory Integration Dysfunction

Sensory integration involves the ability of the central nervous system to take in sensations from different sensory channels at the same time; to filter, organize, and sort the sensations, in order to discern their meaning; and then to use the sensation and its meaning to generate an adaptive response. The differentiating feature of sensory integration and sensory registration is the difference between processing multichannel sensation entering the nervous system at the same time (integration), and the ability to discriminate aspects of specific stimuli entering through one sensory channel (registration).

Sensory integration is the most sophisticated aspect of sensory processing, in that it requires effective communication between lower and higher brain centers to assure that responses are well suited to the situation, well planned and well executed. It is difficult for sensory integration to be adequate if one or more of the other sensory processing mechanisms is disordered or inefficient. Nevertheless, unless sensory integration is itself disordered, improvement in the other aspects of sensory processing almost always leads to direct improvement in sensory integration. Therefore, it is wise to withhold judgment about someone's sensory integration until all other sensory processing problems have been treated.

Therapists who specialize in the application of sensory integration theory have much to offer individuals whose sensorimotor difficulties are more subtle. For example, children with learning disabilities or attention deficit disorders often benefit greatly from sensory integration therapy designed to improve their gross and fine motor abilities. One of the most common referral requests for children with sensory integration dysfunction, for example, is the need for help to improve handwriting ability. The child's behavior and general responses may seem relatively appropriate, but motor tasks requiring rapid and precise adjustments may be difficult. Sensory integration dysfunction can be present in people whose behavior may seem adaptive. This can be contrasted with people who have defensiveness, sensory modulation, or sensory registration problems, where evidence of a problem manifests as too much, too little, or inappropriate *behavior.*

Sensory integration has been regarded by many therapists as something of an umbrella ability, with modulation and registration considered to be aspects of sensory integration. Our severely challenged adults taught us that it is important to differentiate them as separate problems in order to treat them as separate problems. Treating the problems separately yields much faster and much bigger improvement, especially in people with severely disordered sensory processing.

This does not diminish the importance of diagnosing and treating sensory integration dysfunction. Sensory integration is likely to be a higher priority concern in people who have more adaptive behavior, than those who benefit most from the *Ready Approach.* If sensory integration is disordered and left untreated, it invariably leads to secondary social and psychological problems, even in people who appear to be quite capable. Nevertheless, in adults who have the most severe sensory processing problems, there were usually higher priority needs to address, related to defensiveness, and modulation or registration problems. Sensory integration is usually the least of our initial concerns.

Following Through Based on the Sensory Profile

Once there is evidence of priority sensory needs, the next step is to formulate a hypothesis about how much each of the four sensory processing problems is a factor for the person. Sorting out the nature and relative effectiveness of different sensory processing mechanisms is important, because it is easy to do too much too fast. Donna Williams is an incredibly articulate woman who struggles on a daily basis with severe sensory processing problems. In her remarkable book *Autism: An Inside-Out Approach,* she describes the kinds of sensory challenges faced by many people with autism and explains how using a sensory integration approach may be an example of trying to do too much, too soon (Williams, 1996). We have ample clinical evidence that doing too much, too fast, overwhelms many struggling nervous systems, compromising the results we can achieve. People with the most complex and severe sensory processing problems find it much more helpful to take things in order, one step at a time. When this is done, the brain is much better able to keep up and benefit from the sensory opportunity, forming improved circuitry, including memory circuits, which make it easier for the brain to build on what it is learning. Rather than slowing down the rate of progress, taking things more slowly and in order helps the brain keep up and improve its efficiency faster, which, of course, translates to faster improvement in adaptive behavior as well.

Transdisciplinary Teamwork

It is clear that the more fully a sensory perspective is integrated into a person's ongoing experience, the better and faster the results. There simply is no substitute for everyone being able to respond whenever sensory needs arise, and needs can arise anytime, anywhere. Therefore, when a sensory processing perspective, such as the *Ready Approach*, becomes the frame of reference for a treatment program, everyone involved needs to understand sensory processing disorders and how to help. The more they understand, the more likely they will automatically start working together more closely in a transdisciplinary team model. In such a model, specialists shift some of their focus from direct client service to educating and collaborating with coworkers. Such a shift can be hard for teams and parents to support (unless they have experienced its benefits) especially if their experience has been one of dwindling service associated with *consultative* models.

Transdisciplinary teamwork is not about consultation; it is about working side-by-side to get the job done. When therapists participate in a transdisciplinary model, they do not relinquish responsibility for sensory services. To the contrary, they maintain accountability even as they strive to share and exchange roles with team members to facilitate fuller integration of services.

People who have sensory processing problems *and* developmental disabilities have, what the general systems theorist, Russell Ackoff, calls a *MESS* of problems: multiple, complex, and interdependent. People with *messes* of problems rely on us to provide services that fit their needs. That means our services are organized and delivered by team members whose efforts are well coordinated and supportive of each other. Using a sensory approach can create challenges for team members and organizations who are not accustomed to taking sensory needs into account; but a successful effort can transform lives.

Frequency of Service in the Ready Approach

Over the several years in which we were sharpening our understanding and skills related to sensory issues, one thing was always clear: the more sensory service we provided, the better the results we got. When the sensory services were started, therapy time was not integrated into the daily routine. Treatments were provided in isolated clinics; sessions typically lasted about 30 minutes, usually scheduled twice a week. Almost everyone served at the facility got occupational therapy because it was assumed that giving everyone some therapy was better than giving some individuals more and others none.

It was soon apparent that results from sensory services warranted more therapy time, so two decisions were made. One was that therapy services would be reorganized to provide more intensive treatment to fewer individuals. The second was that therapy staff would stop providing any service that could be provided by someone else. This would enable therapy staff to concentrate their efforts solely on sensory matters and intensify services for those who were considered the highest priority cases. A few receiving intensified service were seen as much as twice a day, sometimes for 45 minutes at a time, but this contact continued to occur in isolated clinics, rather than in the clients' typical environments.

Once again, results indicated that more service was warranted. Progress was so evident with the sensory oriented efforts. People were improving fast, in big ways, and everyone wanted to capitalize on the momentum. So, therapy staff were reorganized once again. This time, in an attempt to bring the therapy service into the natural setting, therapy staff members were scheduled for blocks of time in different work areas where several people with priority sensory needs were served. Again, people receiving more sensory services improved faster and more dramatically, and teams wanted even more intensive sensory service.

Finally, the largest day program of the institution, involving 90 clients, was restructured under the direct supervision of the therapy staff. To facilitate this change, it became more difficult for people who were not served in that day program to receive occupational therapy, although essential support services, requiring someone with occupational therapy expertise, continued to be available on a consulting basis. For people in the subject day program, however, the change meant being immersed in a totally sensory oriented routine. There were no pull-out services, no isolated clinics, and therapy staff with sensory expertise were influential decision makers for all aspects of the program.

Each of the previous changes to intensify sensory services had yielded faster and bigger gains in the people served, but none of these results was anything like the gains achieved when the sensory service was fully integrated into someone's overall program. The full sensory orientation clearly resulted in the most impressive improvement for the largest number of individuals. In fact, after comparing what could be achieved through fully integrated service versus supportive or consulting service, all clinics and therapy equipment were given up to program areas where there was a commitment to using sensory approaches, even with minimal support from occupational therapy.

Summary of What We Learned While Working With Adults

1. **All Behavior Must Be a Product of Sensory Processing.**   If that were not the case, why would there be such a direct correlation between improved behavior and intensity of sensory oriented service?

2. **Sensory Approaches Foster Positive Dynamic Interactions.**   Among the many changes that occurred as we shifted to a sensory frame of reference was increasingly positive interactions among the people associated with the programs: staff and clients. Staff became more client centered, more gentle and responsive with clients. Where relationships had formerly been characterized by the need to control, staff became much more accepting and respectful of client preferences and choices. Staff also became more respectful with each other, and some clients began to approach others for positive interaction.

3. **People Achieve So Much More When They See the Value of What They are Doing.**   People who have severe sensory needs do not have time for team members to argue about territorial issues or matters of control. They need people working on their behalf who know how to share and release aspects of their expertise with and to other team members. Service providers who move from one place to another, seeing many different settings and people, have a very different experience from those who provide continuous service to the same group in the same setting, day after day. As therapy staff, we had never understood that as much as we did after we

were assigned responsibility for a whole day program unit. There is no substitute for being in the shoes of someone else, nor for on-site priming, that immediate feedback, correction, or compliment one provider can share with another in the real work situation. What we accomplished in the tenth year, despite the layoffs and reorganization necessitated by downsizing, was truly incredible, something that would never have been possible if the majority of staff had not been similarly committed to making it work. The difference had to be related to their belief that we were finally on the right track, "in it together," doing something that made sense, and getting results that made the effort worthwhile. By the tenth year, most of the staff were quite familiar with what we understood about meeting sensory needs. No matter how much positive feedback we had provided, no matter how much administration recognized employees for outstanding achievement, no matter what kind of supervision they received, the real change in staff occurred when they saw, first-hand, the results *they* could achieve with sensory strategies.

4. Sensory Approaches Show Respect for Differences.   Interpreting the behavior of others from one's personal point of view is fraught with problems. The terrible toll of misunderstanding or misinterpreting someone's response, especially missing the sensory implication, is evident all around us (Masters & McGuire, 1994), and is poignantly described by those who can tell us what it feels like to be misunderstood, for instance, Anne, the narrator of the film *Learning about Learning Disabilities.*

It seems inconsistent to appreciate the power of the human brain without recognizing the effort it will expend to do things right. Those who have the most severe problems sometimes have the most remarkable abilities, abilities that we may not be able to see because they are hidden behind a mask of sensory issues. Meanwhile, their behavior may be so challenging that we fight exhaustion to get it changed. It is ironic that those who have the most severe problems do not stay awake at night trying to figure out ways to make our lives difficult, yet, when we do not understand, we may stay awake at night unintentionally figuring out ways to make their lives difficult by focusing on how to change their behavior. If our inclination is to interpret the behavior of others as something they do with motives we ascribe to them, then we will invariably put even more pressure on a nervous system that is already struggling. We would never insist that a paralyzed person in a wheelchair walk up a flight of stairs; yet, we may do something comparable to people whose symptoms of sensory processing problems we do not understand.

In their wonderful book about appreciating people who are different, Anne Donnellan, a behavioral psychologist, and Martha Leary, a speech and language pathologist, remind us that behavior does not automatically need to be changed just because it is different. They ask us to imagine what happens if we try to put ourselves in the other person's place, and they predict that we will "begin to see the person as quite remarkable. Remarkable because this person may be struggling to stay in an interaction, to contain a behavior, or to keep from disturbing a situation with involuntary movements. With such a perception we begin to see our relationship to that person very differently. This is a person to learn from as well as to teach. This is a person to work with, not to work on. This is a person who has likely found strategies to accommodate for his or her differences, and to keep *disturbance* to a minimum. Our job is to help expand and extend those strategies, not *for* the person, but *with* the person" (Donnellan & Leary, 1995, p. 57). For us to respect differences in people, we must accept that there are differences, differences we may not understand. Such acceptance helps us to interact with the person from a perspective that does not, in and of itself, become a limiting factor for us and one more barrier for those who are different from us.

When we use sensory approaches, instead of judging someone's behavior, we take into account that the responses we see may well be beyond a person's control. With a sensory perspective, we are much more likely to *respond to* the person, rather than *act on* the person. With sensory oriented eyes, we use a gentle approach, one that encourages, invites, and entices, rather than one that demands, coerces, or controls. Imagine the relief that brings to a struggling nervous system!

5. Behavioral Technology is Different from a Behavioral Approach. Behavioral technology helps us to be objective, collect reliable data, operationalize what we say to make it clearer. It is a must for monitoring progress and making valid treatment decisions. However, behavioral technology is not the same as using a behavioral approach. The first helps us to evaluate the results of our services. The latter is a clinical perspective that influences how we view people. By posing restrictions on our consideration of why behavior might be occurring, behaviorism becomes somewhat arbitrary. Why would anyone serving people with behavior related needs not want to consider other explanations for the behavior, especially if behavioral interventions are not yielding results? Even if behavioral interventions get results, the issue may be less the results and more the cost of those results. What does the change in behavior mean for the person whose behavior was changed? What if the behavioral view turns out to be too limited, as asserted by two Nobel Laureates, Gerald Edelman (1992) and Francis Crick (1994)? What if there is more to behavior than just learned responses?

6. There Is No Single Clinical Perspective that Is the Answer for Everyone.   Interdisciplinary teams, serving a wide variety of individuals, should be able to evaluate several options and alternative views to find what works best for specific individuals. Someone may do best by starting with services based on one approach, but, as improvement occurs, there may come a time when another approach will be more helpful. It is important to select the approach on the basis of the person's need, rather than expect the person to fit the available or prevailing approach.

7. Programs That Try to Provide Something for Everyone are Likely to Diminish their Effectiveness with Anyone.   There are multiple ways to organize services and configure groupings for large numbers of people. Optimal results come with services that are focused to target specific kinds of needs for specific kinds of individuals. It is difficult and impractical to provide for several alternatives when groups are small, but when many people are being served, a single large program can be organized into several different subprograms to provide access to more specialized service.

8. Being a Good Therapist, Whatever Approach You Use, Involves Being a Good Problem Solver.   That means recognizing the difference between problems and solutions. We eliminate problems by figuring out appropriate solutions. If we figure out wonderful solutions, but have not correctly identified the problem, we may not get the results we seek. Program planning, like treatment planning, can be only as effective as the accuracy with which one identifies needs.

SUMMARY OF IDEAS RELATED TO THE READY APPROACH

Ideas from the Neurosciences

1. All behavior is fundamentally a product of the neurobiology of the brain.
2. Brain efficiency is dependent upon the effectiveness of various neural mechanisms involving brain centers and the neural circuitry and neurochemistry that enables them to communicate with each other.
3. Strong brain stem sensation has a profound and pervasive influence on brain chemistry and subsequently on the circuitry that enables multiple brain mechanisms to function properly.
4. Neural plasticity makes it possible for the brain to improve its own efficiency for the whole of its lifespan.

5. Disordered sensory processing may compromise the brain's ability to take full advantage of its many varied sensory opportunities.

6. The human brain thrives on sensation, particularly touch, movement, and body sensations. If it does not get enough of these important sensations, it may drive a person to engage in behaviors that produce the desired sensations.

7. The human brain does not drive a person to engage in self-injurious behavior or persistent self-stimulation unless there is something seriously wrong.

Ideas that Parallel Sensory Integration Theory

1. We can draw inferences about the efficiency and effectiveness of sensory processing by interpreting, from a sensory perspective, the products of brain activity, for instance, behavior, emotion, cognition, and motor responses.

2. Keeping in mind that everything the brain takes in is sensation, we can influence the efficiency of the brain by influencing what sensation the brain experiences.

3. The ultimate goal for efficient sensory processing is adaptive participation in functional activities that are meaningful to the person. There is no substitute for what can be achieved to improve brain efficiency through purposeful engagement in appealing activities and interactions.

Ideas Specific to the Ready Approach

1. There Are Four Different Sensory Processing Problems.   Each should be considered a separate problem, although some people display evidence of multiple problems, sometimes secondary to one or more that are primary. Primary problems should be treated first, and, in the presence of more than one primary problem, there is a specific order in which the problems should be treated to achieve optimal results.

2. Readiness Is a Bridge Between Sensory Processing and Adaptive Behavior.   Being ready to respond means the brain is able to catch on to what is happening, generate adaptive responses, and keep up with new situational demands. When the brain has achieved a *ready* state, the person can participate in functional activities and interactions with *just right chal-*

lenges without becoming overwhelmed, confused, or distressed. When the brain is not *ready*, any sensory demand can be too much.

3. Sustained Optimal Arousal Eliminates Sensory Driven Behaviors. Small recurring doses of helpful sensation increase the probability that a challenged person will be able to maintain readiness and benefit from other available services without having to engage in sensory driven socially maladaptive behaviors.

4. Adaptive Behavior Is Acquired in Natural Routines.   Sensory strategies, designed to enhance readiness, should be delivered in the context of the natural routine, provided that the setting is *sensory sensitive*, modified to lower sensory demands for overly challenged individuals. Nothing improves behavior, performance, interaction, or learning like the opportunity to participate in functional activities that have purpose and meaning for the individual—if the individual is *ready*.

5. Everyone Benefits.   All humans benefit from enriched sensory diets, not just people with disabilities, and everyone benefits when anyone with disordered sensory processing improves. The payoffs include more efficient use of resources and more productive and happier people—clients, family members, care providers, and service administrators.

The case examples at the beginning of this chapter illustrate the difference sensory approaches made for some of the adults served in one large state-operated institution. Every person in the examples had a primary diagnosis of profound mental retardation. All had been served at the same institution for at least 15 years. All had grossly impaired communication, with no reliable means of communicating and no consistent reliable responses to what was communicated to them. Severe behavior problems were well documented for each of them and a variety of intensive behavioral interventions had been tried without success. Each person also had been prescribed a variety of strong medications, sometimes in combinations. None had a history of seizures. All had shown little or no progress for many years. Since 1990, hundreds of adults have been served with sensory programs based on what is now being called the *Ready Approach*. This work has occurred in different states and involved multiple service providers in varied service settings. Many of the individuals served have improved in comparable ways to the case examples, some with even more dramatic results. Our experience with the *Ready Approach* has been encouraging, to say the least.

Successful intervention based on a sensory processing perspective requires an understanding of

1) how the brain responds to sensation
2) the neurobiology of behavior, emotion, and consciousness
3) the four sensory processing problems
4) the power sensations and how they influence the brain
5) how the power sensations can be used to enhance the neurobiology of the central nervous system.

This requires advanced expertise and keeping pace with the findings of brain scientists who are making new discoveries at an exponential rate. There is still much to be learned. In the last 10 years alone, scientists have learned more about the brain and how it influences and is influenced by experience than was known in all the years prior to that time (Kotulak, 1996).

With the *Ready Approach*, we are capitalizing on the incredible new insights of these brain scientists. It is possible that, like the imaging that now makes it possible to trace a thought through the brain, there may be some new technology on the horizon that will make the best and most current insights obsolete, just as our understanding today makes us wonder about the wisdom of so many of our practices of the past. However, for now, everyone involved in sensory oriented services needs to understand how human brains need and use sensation to increase their efficiency. Without such understanding, it is difficult to make appropriate situational judgments related to what sensation is needed, how much, and how to provide it.

Issues related to sensory processing disorders are complex, and the details of the *Ready Approach* and how it works are beyond the scope of this chapter. Occupational therapy practitioners, however, can learn this approach and have access to advanced sensory related expertise in a variety of ways. Most therapists are introduced to sensory integration theory in their basic training. That becomes an important foundation upon which to build, but the evaluation and treatment of individuals who have severe sensory processing problems requires advanced specialist training.

Increased knowledge and technical proficiency related to sensory services can be obtained by working with therapists who are skilled in using sensory approaches. When looking for mentors, we must bear in mind that the measurement for success is in the outcome for clients. Impressive results are much more important than impressive programs. Many service providers welcome qualified therapists for work–study or mentorship programs. Continuing education activities can include formal courses in colleges and universities, and courses designed and sponsored by organizations, such as the

American Occupational Therapy Association, which offers several innovative and flexible choices to accommodate different learner styles and preferences. Several continuing education sponsors concentrate their efforts on training and on publications for those who are specifically interested in sensory issues, and there is an increasing number of Internet sites that enable people with this interest to network, share ideas, and learn from each other. The companies listed under *Continuing Education Resources* are especially concerned with sensory oriented subject matter. Several publications are listed in the *Related Reading* section at the end of this chapter. Any one of them can be a good place to start.

CONCLUSION

In this chapter, we have talked about the challenges and potential benefits associated with viewing adults who have developmental disabilities from a sensory perspective. The development of a specific sensory oriented frame of reference was described and several examples were provided to illustrate the kinds of issues service providers might face, if they were to introduce a sensory processing frame of reference into a long-term care program. It was shown that the specific sensory oriented approach advocated for adults with severe behavioral challenges is based on, but different from, sensory integration theory. It was also shown that new information available in the neurosciences provides the scientific rationale for many features of the approach that builds on current understanding about the neurobiology of behavior, emotion, awareness, and cognition.

Sensory strategies associated with the *Ready Approach* can be an efficient, effective, and relatively permanent treatment for many adults who have not responded favorably to any other intervention alternative. Occupational therapy practitioners have a unique advantage in using the *Ready Approach* for two reasons: a) their neurohabilitative background makes it possible for them to make differential diagnoses related to sensorimotor problems; and b) they are experts at modifying and adapting environments and activities to match special needs. No one has background and training better suited for identifying sensory needs and designing intervention strategies, including sensory diets that take sensory needs into account. What a perfect match: occupational therapy practitioners and adults with developmental disabilities!

ACKNOWLEDGEMENTS

I referred to "we" throughout this chapter because of the many people who contributed to the evaluation of the *Ready Approach,* but I particularly want to acknowledge our consultant, mentor, and colleague, Judith Reisman, PhD, OTR, FAOTA, who opened our eyes and taught us how to see.

REFERENCES

Aoki, C., & Siekevitz, P. (1988, December). Plasticity in brain development. *Scientific American, 56–64.*

Ayres, A.J. (1972). *Sensory integration and learning disorders.* Los Angeles: Western Psychological Services.

Bidabe, L. (1991). *M.O.V.E. curriculum for mobility opportunities via education program.* Bakersfield, CA: Kern County Schools.

Brodal, P. (1992). *The central nervous system.* New York: Oxford University Press.

Brocklehurst-Woods, J. (1990). The use of tactile and vestibular stimulation to reduce stereotypic behaviors in two adults with mental retardation. *American Journal of Occupational Therapy, 44,* 536–541.

Chopra, D. (1989). *Quantum healing.* New York: Bantam Books.

Churchland, P. (1993). *Neurophilosophy: Toward a unified science of the mind/brain.* Cambridge, MA: MIT Press.

Crick, F. (1994). *The astonishing hypothesis.* New York: Charles Scribner's Sons.

Damasio, A. (1994). *Descartes' error: Emotion, reason, and the human brain.* New York: G. P. Putnam's Sons.

Donnellan, A., & Leary, M. (1995). *Movement differences and diversity in autism/mental retardation* (p. 57). Madison, WI: DRI Press.

Duker, P. C., & Rasing, E. (1989). Effects of redesigning the physical environment on self-stimulation and on-task behavior in three autistic-type developmentally disabled individuals. *Journal of Autism and Developmental Disorders, 19,* 449–461.

Durand, V. M., & Crimmins, D. B. (1988). Identifying the variables maintaining self-injurious behavior. *Journal of Autism and Developmental Disorders, 18,* 99–117.

Durig, A. (1996). *Autism and the crisis of meaning.* New York: New York State University Press.

Edelman, G. (1992). *Bright air, brilliant fire: On the matter of the mind.* New York: Basic Books.

Fisher, A., Murray, E., & Bundy, A. (1991). *Sensory integration theory and practice.* Philadelphia: F. A. Davis.

Gazzaniga, M. (1988). *Mind matters: How mind and brain interact to create our conscious lives.* Boston: Houghton Mifflin.

Gazzaniga, M. (1992). *Nature's mind: The biological roots of thinking, emotions, sexuality, language, and intelligence.* New York: Basic Books.

Gazzaniga, M. (Ed.). (1995). *Cognitive neurosciences.* Cambridge, MA: MIT Press.

Goleman, D. (1995). *Emotional intelligence.* New York: Bantam Books.

Grandin, T. (1992). Calming effects of deep touch pressure in patients with autistic disorder, college students, and animals. *Journal of Child and Adolescent Psychopharmacology, 2*(1), 63–72.

Greenspan, S. (1997). *Growth of the mind.* Reading, MA: Addison Wesley.

Hobson, J. (1994). *Chemistry of consious states: How the brain changes its mind.* Boston: Little Brown.

Iwasaki, K., & Holm, M. (1989). Sensory treatment for the reduction of stereotypic behaviors in persons with severe multiple disabilities. *Occupational Therapy Journal of Research, 9,* 170–183.

Joseph, R. (1993). *The naked neuron.* New York: Plenum Press.

Kandel, E., & Schwartz, J. (1991). *Principles of neural science* (3rd ed.). New York: Elsevier Science Publishing.

Kandel, E., & Schwartz, J. (1995). *Essentials of neural science and behavior.* Stamford, CT: Appleton and Lange.

Knickerbocker, B. (1980). *Holistic approach to the treatment of learning disorders.* Thorofare, NJ: Slack.

Kotulak, R. (1996). *Inside the brain: Revolutionary discoveries of how the mind works.* Kansas City: Andrews and McMeel.

Kuno, M. (1995). *Synapse: Function, plasticity, and neurotrophism.* New York: Oxford University Press.

LeDoux, J. (1996). *The emotional brain.* New York: Simon & Schuster.

Levitan, I., & Kaczmarek, L. (1997). *Neuron: Cell and molecular biology.* New York: Oxford University Press.

Lovaas, I., Newsom, C., & Hickman, C. (1987). Self-stimulatory behavior and perceptual reinforcement. *Journal of Applied Behavior Analysis, 20,* 45–68.

McGimsey, J. F., & Favell, J. E. (1988). The effects of increased physical exercise on disruptive behavior in retarded persons. *Journal of Autism and Developmental Disorders, 18,* 167–179.

Masters, R., & McGuire, M. (1994). *Neurotransmitter revolution: Serotonin, social behavior, and the law.* Carbondale, IL: Southern Illinois University Press.

Merrill, S. (1990). *Environment: Implications for occupational therapy practice.* Bethesda, MD: American Occupational Therapy Association.

Mosey, A. (1981). *Occupational therapy: Configuration of a profession.* New York: Raven Press.

Nicholls, D. (1994). *Proteins, transmitters and synapses.* Cambridge, MA: Blackwell Science.

Nuland, S. (1997). *Wisdom of the body.* New York: Alfred Knopf.

Pearsall, P. (1996). *Pleasure prescription.* Alameda, CA: Hunter House.

Rahmann, H., & Rahmann, M. (1992). *Neurobiological basis of memory and behavior.* New York: Springer-Verlag.

Reed, K. (1984). *Models of practice in occupational therapy.* Baltimore: Williams and Wilkins.

Reisman, J., & Hanschu, B. (1992). *Sensory integration inventory-revised for individuals with developmental disabilities: User's guide.* Hugo, MN: PDP Press.

Reisman, J. (1993). Using a sensory integrative approach to treat self-injurious behavior in an adult with profound mental retardation. *American Journal of Occupational Therapy, 47*(5), 403–411.

Reisman, J., & Hanschu, B. (1993). Using the consultative model to introduce sensory integration services for adults with developmental disabilities. *Occupational Therapy Practice, 4*(4), 38–46.

Rosenthal-Malek, A., & Mitchell, S. (1997). Effects of exercise on the self-stimulatory behaviors and positive responding of adolescents with autism. *Journal of Autism and Developmental Disorders, 27*(2), 193–202.

Royeen, C., & Lane, S. (1991). Tactile processing and sensory defensiveness. In A. Fisher, E. Murray, & A. Bundy (Eds.), *Sensory integration theory and practice* (Chapter 5). Philadelphia: F.A. Davis.

Ruden, R. (1997). *The craving brain.* New York: Harper Collins.

Shepherd, G. (1988). *Neurobiology* (2nd ed.). New York: Oxford University Press.

Silver, L. (1993). *Dr. Larry Silver's advice to parents on attention-deficit hyperactivity disorder.* Washington, DC: American Psychiatric Press.

Tomporowski, P. D., & Ellis, N. R. (1985). The effects of exercise on the health, intelligence, and adaptive behavior of institutionalized severely and profoundly mentally retarded adults: A systematic replication. *Applied Research in Mental Retardation, 6,* 465–473.

Trott, M. (1993). *SenseAbilities: Understanding sensory integration.* Tucson: Therapy Skill Builders.

Watters, R. G., & Watters, W. E. (1980). Decreasing self-stimulatory behavior with physical exercise in a group of autistic boys. *Journal of Autism and Developmental Disorders, 10,* 379–387.

West, T. (1991). *In the mind's eye: Visual thinkers, gifted people with learning difficulties, computer images, and the ironies of creativity.* Buffalo: Prometheus Books.

Wilbarger, P., & Wilbarger, J. (1991). *Sensory defensiveness in children ages 2–12: An intervention guide for parents and other caretakers.* Santa Barbara, CA: Avanti Educational Programs.

Williams, D. (1996). *Autism: An inside-out approach.* Bristol, PA: Jessica Kingsley Publishers.

RELATED READING

Ayres, A. J. (1979). *Sensory integration and the child.* Los Angeles: Western Psychological Services.

Baars, B. (1997). *In the theater of consciousness: The workspace of the mind.* New York: Oxford University Press.

Baron-Cohen, S. (1995). *Mindblindness: An essay on autism and theory of mind.* Cambridge, MA: MIT Press.

Bauman, M. (1991). Microscopic neuro anatomic abnormalities in autism. *Pediatrics, 78:* 791–796.

Bauman, M., & Kemper, T. (1995). *Neurobiology of autism.* Baltimore: Johns Hopkins University Press.

Cataldo, M. R., & Harris, J. (1982). The biological basis for self-injury in the mentally retarded. *Analysis and Intervention in Developmental Disabilities, 2,* 21–39.

Churchland, P., & Sejnowski, T. (1992). *Computational brain.* Cambridge, MA: MIT Press.

Comings, D. E. (1990). *Tourette syndrome and human behavior.* Duarte, CA: Hope Press.

Courchesne, E., Yeung-Courchesne, R., Press, G.A., Hesselking, J.R., & Jernigan, T.L. (1988). Hypoplasia of cerebellar vernal lobules VI and VII in autism. *New England Journal of Medicine, 318,* 1349–1354.

Davis, J. (1997). *Mapping the mind: The secrets of the human brain and how it works.* Secaucus, NJ: Birch Lane Press.

Grandin, T. (1992). An inside view of autism. In E. Schopler & G. Mesibov (Eds.). *High-functioning individuals with autism* (pp. 105–126). New York: Plenum Press.

Grandin, T. (1995). *Thinking in pictures.* New York: Doubleday.

Greenspan, S. (1995). *Challenging child: Understanding, raising, and enjoying the five "difficult" types of children.* New York: Addison Wesley.

Hallowell, E., & Ratey, J. (1995). *Driven to distraction: Recognizing and coping with attention deficit disorder from childhood through adulthood.* New York: Touchstone.

Hartmann, T. (1993). *Attention deficit disorder: A different perception.* Grass Valley, CA: Underwood Books.

Hartmann, T. (1995). *ADD success stories.* Grass Valley, CA: Underwood Books.

Irlen, H. (1991). *Reading by the colors: Overcoming dyslexia and other reading disabilities through the Irlen method.* Garden City Park, NY: Avery Publishing Group.

Kinnealey, M., Oliver, B., & Wilbarger, P. (1995). A phenomenological study of sensory defensiveness in adults. *American Journal of Occupational Therapy, 49,* 444–451.

Ratey, J., & Johnson, C. (1997). *Shadow syndromes.* New York: Pantheon.

Reisman, J., & Gross, A. (1992). Psychophysiological measurement of treatment effects in an adult with sensory defensiveness. *Canadian Journal of Occupational Therapy, 59*(5), 248–257.

Sacks, O. (1970). *The man who mistook his wife for a hat.* New York: Harper & Row.

Sacks, O. (1995). *An anthropologist on Mars.* New York: Knopf.

Williams, D. (1992). *Nobody nowhere.* New York: Times Books.

Williams, D. (1994). *Somebody somewhere.* New York: Times Books.

Williams, M., & Shellenberger, S. (1994). *How does your engine run? The alert program for self-regulation.* Albuquerque, NM: Therapy Works.

CONTINUING EDUCATION RESOURCES

The following organizations have offerings that are specifically geared to adults:

Developmental Concepts

(Courses, publications, and consultation related to the *Ready Approach.*)
P.O. Box 31759
Phoenix, AZ 85046-1759
Phone: (602) 482-0572
1 (888) 287-3239 or 1 (888) AT READY
Fax: (602) 482-9851
E-mail: atready@bitstream.net

Future Horizons

(Courses, conferences, and publications, including video and audio tapes, all related to autism.)
422 Lamar Boulevard East, Suite 106
Arlington, TX 76011
Phone: 1 (800) 489-0727
Fax: (817) 277-2270
E-mail: edfuture@onramp.net

Professional Development Programs and PDP Products

(Courses, including defensiveness; publications, including the *Inventory;* and products, all related to serving people with severe developmental disabilities. PDP's annual symposium is considered a must by many therapists working in the area of developmental disabilities.)
14398 North 59th Street
Oak Park Heights, MN 55082
Phone: (612) 439-8865
Fax: (612) 439-0421

7

Structurally-Based Manual Therapy Leads to Improved Function

Lynn D. Simpson, OTR/L

Adults with mental retardation are often not considered for therapeutic intervention in the same light as other populations because many of the dysfunctional behaviors displayed by them have been labeled "mental retardation" and are presumed, therefore, to be untreatable. Such labelling tends to preclude examining other reasons for these behaviors, such as physical or physiological. Traditionally, in this population dysfunctional behaviors are viewed as being fixed, systemic, and psychologically-based entities in which the behaviors themselves are treated rather than their causes.

In this chapter, dysfunctional behaviors—motor, self-injurious, perceptual, and social—will be regarded as symptoms of structural dysfunction. Structural dysfunction refers to a disruption in the normal balance of the body's framework of bones/joints, muscle, and fascial connective tissue. Structurally-based therapy (Greenman, 1989; Mitchell, Moran, & Pruzzo, 1979; Upledger & Vredevoogd, 1983; Weiselfish & Kain, 1990) will be presented and discussed here as a means to improve functional performance. The premise of this therapeutic approach is that structural, biomechanical stresses within the body framework interfere with function and establish a pattern of maladaptive behaviors (Simpson, 1996) based on lowered tolerances to stimuli. To alleviate these stresses and improve one's potential for function, manual therapy techniques are employed. These techniques will be briefly described, and the structural approach will be differentiated from traditional functional approaches, such as sensorimotor therapies. To elucidate the underlying theories and concepts of structurally-based therapy, four case histories will be presented of adults diagnosed with mental retardation and other developmental disabilities.

It is important to consider that dysfunctional behaviors may be signs and symptoms of structural dysfunction that place the individual at a disadvantage to respond or react to his or her environment. Recognizing the interplay between structure and function (Barral, 1991; Greenman, 1978, 1989; Heinrich, 1991; Korr, 1978; Mennell, 1992; Upledger, 1987; Upledger & Vredevoogd, 1983) is necessary so an individual can receive the best therapeutic intervention to optimize function. The specific goal of manual therapy is to realign and rebalance the neuromusculoskeletal systems. Employing these therapy techniques results in enhanced movement and ameliorated tolerances to internal and external stimuli and, consequently, maximizes functional performance.

MANUAL THERAPY

What is Structurally-Based Manual Therapy

Structurally-based manual therapy is a part of manual medicine—osteopathy—an approach to health that views the nervous, muscular, and skeletal systems as major components of both physiological and physical/structural health. These three systems can be considered together as a unit (the neuromusculoskeletal system), or two of the systems can be considered together (neuromuscular and musculoskeletal). The evaluation and treatment processes use the therapist's hands to manually assess, through palpation, the function and dysfunction of different body tissues—arthrodial, muscle, and fascia—that constitute the neuromusculoskeletal system. It is possible to have impaired structural balance within a single tissue, such as a muscle spasm, or to have imbalance between different tissues, such as fascial adhesions interfering with muscle function. Further, a disruption in the balance of the neuromusculoskeletal system has the potential to disrupt function in other systems and vice versa (Barral, 1989, 1991; Barral & Mercier, 1988; Upledger & Vredevoogd, 1983). For example, the passage of the subclavian vein (circulatory system) around the clavicle and first rib (neuromusculoskeletal system) in the thoracic inlet may lead to compromised blood flow if the clavicle is depressed and impinges upon this vein (Figure 7.1).

Structurally-based manual therapy is established on a dynamic perspective that views the body as a biomechanical entity whose "lever and pulley system" must be in good working order for the individual to function well. This implies that there is an optimal structural/postural alignment that allows for maximal functioning. Any departure from this alignment produces an

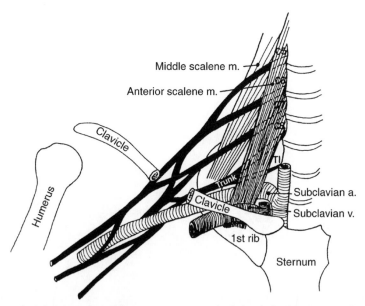

Middle scalene m.

Anterior scalene m.

Clavicle

Humerus

Trunk

Clavicle

T1

Subclavian a.

Subclavian v.

1st rib

Sternum

The thoracic inlet is vulnerable to neuromusculoskeletal dysfunction with subsequent problems in, for example, the circulatory system (see text for more detail).

Source: Goldberg, S. (1991). *Clinical anatomy made ridiculously simple.* Fig. 12-14 (134). Copyright 1991. MedMaster, Inc. Reprinted with permission.

imbalance in the system and creates stresses throughout the total structural framework. Such stresses result in a chain reaction of adaptive responses (compensations), as in a complex system of interconnecting levers and pulleys; the body does, however, reach a point at which it no longer has any reserve to compensate—it is decompensated (Figures 7.2, 7.3).

Overall, then, manual therapy assesses structural integrity: postural alignment, articular balance of both bony and soft tissue interfaces, and mobility. According to this perspective, and in order to achieve maximum benefit from therapy, namely, to fulfill possibly untapped potentials, one needs to look first at structure and then at function.

Structurally-Based Manual Therapy Treatment Techniques

General Considerations

The techniques addressed in this chapter are:

- muscle energy
- myofascial release
- visceral manipulation
- neurofascial release

- craniosacral therapy
- cranial osteopathy
- strain and counterstrain
- zero balancing.

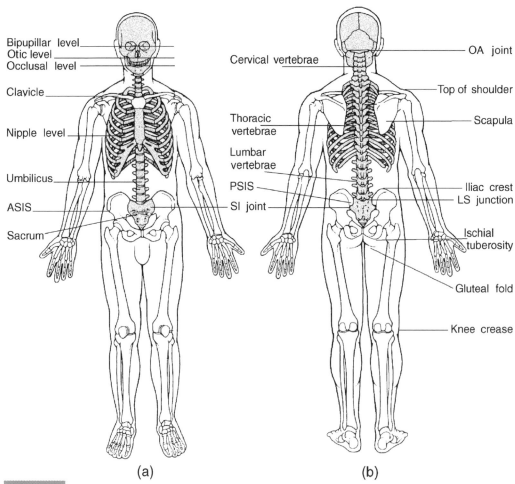

Bipupillar level
Otic level
Occlusal level
Clavicle
Nipple level
Umbilicus
ASIS
Sacrum

Cervical vertebrae
Thoracic vertebrae
Lumbar vertebrae
PSIS
SI joint

OA joint
Top of shoulder
Scapula
Iliac crest
LS junction
Ischial tuberosity
Gluteal fold
Knee crease

(a)   (b)

FIGURE 7.2 (a)(b) Normal posture in which structural alignment in the coronal plane is assessed by comparing the height or level of a) anterior structures, such as the eyes, ears (otic level), and the anterior superior iliac spine; and b) posterior structures, such as the iliac crests, the tops of the shoulders, and gluteal folds. Alignment in a transverse plane is assessed by comparing some of the same structural landmarks but relative to anterior-posterior displacement. ASIS: anterior superior iliac spine. LS junction: lumbosacral junction. OA joint: occipitoatlantal joint. PSIS: posterior superior iliac spine. SI joint: sacroiliac joint. Continued next page (c).

Source: Hole, J. W., Jr. (1993). *Human anatomy and physiology* (sixth ed.) (Fig. 7.2a & b, Fig. 7-18, p. 186). Copyright 1993. Wm. C. Brown Publishers. Reprinted with permission.

Each technique has its own view of function/dysfunction, assessment protocol, and required, specialized treatment skills. All, however, are concerned with alleviating hypomobility and its effect on health and well-being.

Certain techniques are known to be more effective for treating certain tissue dysfunctions than others: myofascial release (Greenman, 1989; Weiselfish &

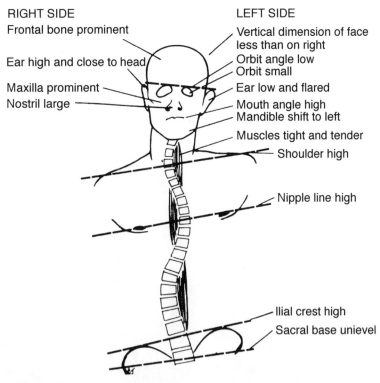

RIGHT SIDE
Frontal bone prominent

Ear high and close to head

Maxilla prominent
Nostril large

LEFT SIDE
Vertical dimension of face less than on right
Orbit angle low
Orbit small
Ear low and flared
Mouth angle high
Mandible shift to left
Muscles tight and tender
Shoulder high

Nipple line high

Ilial crest high
Sacral base unievel

FIGURE 7.2 (c)

c) Abnormal posture.

Source: Royder, J. O. (March 1981). Structural influences in temporomandibular joint pain and dysfunction. (Fig. 7.2c, Fig. 2, pp. 465/65). *Journal of American Osteopathic Association.* 80(7). Reprinted with permission.

Kain, 1991) and neurofascial release (Davidson, 1992) for fascial restrictions; visceral manipulation (Barral, 1989, 1991; Barral & Mercier, 1988; Kain, 1996; Weiselfish, 1996) for fascial restrictions interfering with visceral position and mobility; muscle energy (Breuer, 1989, October & November; Greenman, 1989; Mitchell, Moran, & Pruzzo, 1979; Summerfelt, 1991; Weiselfish, 1994) for articular imbalance at joints and for muscle spasms; strain and counter-strain (Jones, 1981) for both peripheral protective muscle spasm and central hypertonicity (Weiselfish, 1994; Weiselfish & Kain, 1993); craniosacral therapy (Upledger, 1987, 1990; Upledger & Vredevoogd, 1983) and cranial osteopathy (Hruby, 1994, 1995) for cranial suture restrictions, and for intra-cranial and spinal dural membrane tensions; and zero balancing (Brown, 1993, 1994; Smith, 1986, 1996) for energetic restrictions in the bony skeleton. All techniques screen the entire body because the site of pain may not be the origin or cause of pain. Pain is often referred, and habits of movement and positioning that are taken on to avoid initial pain(s) may set up areas of secondary pain that eventually may be stronger.

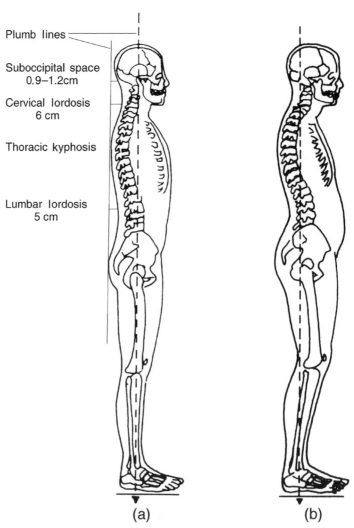

Plumb lines

Suboccipital space
0.9–1.2cm

Cervical lordosis
6 cm

Thoracic kyphosis

Lumbar lordosis
5 cm

(a)   (b)

FIGURE 7.3

a) Normal posture in which structural alignment in the sagittal plane is assessed by evaluating the degree of deviation of the spinal curves (cervical, thoracic and lumbar) from a posteriorly placed plumb line; the distances in centimeters give the normal distances in different areas of the spine. The body should touch the plumb line at the occiput, thoracic kyphosis, and buttocks. There is another plumb line which is drawn to be slightly anterior to the lateral malleolus of the ankle, posterior to the hip joint, and in line with the shoulder joint and external acoustic meatus of the ear. From this latter plumb line, one can observe, for example, placement of the head over the trunk, retraction or protraction of the shoulder, and anterior or posterior tilt of the pelvis. b) An example of undesired structural alignment in which postural compensations are made in order to maintain the eyes parallel to the ground: exaggerated cervical, thoracic and lumbar curves, anterior tilt of pelvis, flexion of hip and knee, dorsiflexion of the ankle, forward head posture (decreased suboccipital space), shortened anterior neck muscles, depression of the jaw, and flattened sternum and rib cage.

Source: Darnell, M. W. (September 1983). A proposed chronology of events for forward head posture. *CRANIO: The Journal of Craniomandibular Practice, 1*(4), (Figs. 1 and 2, p. 50). Reprinted with permission.

To avoid confusion for those who may further explore these techniques, it is necessary to clarify "structural" versus "functional" techniques. In this chapter, I refer to all the above-mentioned techniques as structurally-based manual therapy techniques because they all look for postural and musculo-skeletal bases of structural imbalance. In distinction, functional techniques (Weiselfish & Kain, 1990) view the performance of an activity and focus on improvement in function without focusing on the causes of malfunction. However, in formal presentations and in the manual therapy literature, "strain and counterstrain" is considered a "functional" technique. This is done in order to differentiate between direct and indirect ("functional") technique styles within the field of manual therapy itself. To find out more about the distinction between structural and functional manual therapy techniques, refer to Greenman (1989, p. 101) and Tehan (1980, pp. 94–96).

Based upon my experience working with adults and children with develop-mental disabilities, muscle energy is the most challenging technique for achieving success because the client needs to perform isometric muscle contractions. However, the muscle energy protocol also provides the strong-est foundation to begin to understand structure and the significance of disruption of structural balance.

Muscle Energy

The muscle energy protocol (Greenman, 1989; Mitchell, Moran, & Pruzzo, 1979) assesses postural balance and biomechanical dysfunction (articular balance). Bony landmarks, such as tops of shoulders, iliac crests, anterior superior iliac spines, and soft tissue landmarks including nipple level, gluteal and knee creases, are assessed for alignment and symmetry (Figures 7.2, 7.3). Along with this static assessment of postural alignment, movement is assessed for range of motion and quality of motion. Then it is determined if postural malalignment is due to muscle weakness and/or structural dys-function.

Treatment for muscle weakness enlists isotonic contractions, while treatment of structural dysfunction uses isometric contractions. Isometric contractions along with specific and graded positioning of the appropriate body part reduces the tone of hypertonic muscles. Relaxation of tone allows the muscle to lengthen and, consequently, allows realignment of the skeletal framework.

Strain and Counterstrain

This assessment (Jones, 1981; Jones, Kusunose, & Goering, 1995) examines movement and determines the presence of tender points. (These tender points are different from Travell's trigger points [Ramirez, Haman, & Worth, 1989], which are located in muscle, tendon, ligament, or fascia.) They are areas that are edematous and hypersensitive to touch, and they indicate the presence of articular (joint) compression or protective muscle spasm. Protective muscle spasm and articular compression may develop from chronically shortened muscles as in long-standing poor posture or from reflexive muscle strain. In both poor posture and reflexive strains, the neuromuscular reflex that reports muscle tension to the central nervous system is maintained in an abnormal state of hyperactivity and thus perpetuates the strain and poor posture (that is, shortened state of muscles).

To simplify an explanation of how tender points develop, I will avoid the use of the words *agonist* and *antagonist* to describe muscles and will spell out the different types of strains encountered when using strain and counterstrain as a frame of reference.

Tender points can develop from a number of different situations (Jones, Kusunose, & Goering, 1995; Jones & Wendorff, 1994):

▮ trauma
▮ repetitive motion (overuse syndrome)
▮ panic reaction
▮ high load effort (such as lifting something too heavy for oneself)
▮ emotional stress
▮ chronic poor posture (Weiselfish & Kain, 1993).

What is important to know and to keep in mind is that the tender point develops in a muscle that is a) shortened and chronically maintained in this state, or b) shortened, then abruptly stretched, then reflexively shortened.

Let us look at a situation that is likely to occur in adults with developmental disability. The example is one in which a client with poor head control is being assisted in feeding. The client's chin rests down towards the chest, thus shortening the anterior neck muscles and stretching the muscles in the back of the neck. The well-intentioned aide abruptly lifts the head to position it for feeding. This "lifting,".because of its suddenness, strains (=stretches) the anterior neck muscles, which then causes the muscles to rebound back to a shortened state. This sudden and abrupt stretch effectively acts like stretching a rubber band that, when released, rebounds to a shortened state. The suddenness of the stretch starts a series of reflex responses by the nervous system placing the anterior muscles in protective muscle spasm and triggering the development of tender points. If, however, the muscles had been slowly or methodically stretched, a reflex reaction would not be forthcoming and tender points would not develop.

Strains are produced by

∎ overstretching
∎ long-standing stretch (i.e., postural strain)
∎ *excessive* and *long-standing* tension in a shortened muscle
∎ sudden unplanned stretch to a shortened muscle (e.g., panic reaction).

In the language of strain and counterstrain, there are two different types of strain: "real strain" and "false (reflexive) strain." In the above example, the muscles that were originally maintained in a stretched position are those that develop real strain; they are the muscles at the back of the neck, stretched because the head hangs down on the chest. The shortened anterior neck muscles that were abruptly stretched and then rebounded are the ones that develop false strain. It is in these latter muscles that the tender points develop. Although the abrupt stretch (=false strain) is released, the nervous system continues to report it as strain and, thus, the reason for referring to it as "false." The strain of "strain and counterstrain" refers to the false, reflexive strain.

The muscles that were abruptly stretched, then released, and reporting the false strain acquire an abnormally shortened resting length because they are in protective muscle spasm. Therefore, movements that normally would not stretch these muscles—which are now in spasm—perpetuate false strain. This situation results in limitation of range of motion, and pain.

Thus, pain is due to three conditions:

∎ real strain (e.g. long-standing stretch)
∎ articular compression
∎ false strain (i.e., movement away from the abnormal resting length)

Pain of a tender point is pain that one is aware of only upon palpation.

Treatment focuses on the alleviation of false strain by turning down the hyperactive neuromuscular reflex. This results in muscle relaxation, thus allowing the muscle to return to its normal resting length and relieving articular compression. Following these changes, range of motion of the joint normalizes and pain subsides. To achieve muscle relaxation during treatment, the client's body is passively positioned to maximally shorten the muscles reporting false strain; this position is called "counterstrain." By passively shortening the muscles and then returning the body *slowly* to a neutral position, the muscle spasm is relieved. Counterstrain is a position of comfort, whereas any movement in the opposite direction that abruptly stretches the muscle reporting false strain results in pain.

Both muscle energy, and strain and counterstrain rely on neuromuscular reflexes based on gamma and alpha motor nerve outputs to explain muscle hypertonicity and the return of muscle to its normal resting length following treatment.

Myofascial Release

Myofascial release (Greenman, 1989; Weiselfish & Kain, 1991) assesses structural balance by observing static and dynamic posture as does muscle energy. When imbalance is found, the next step is to determine if fascial dysfunction is a contributing factor. Fascial mobility (Upledger & Vredevoogd, 1983; Weiselfish & Kain, 1991) is assessed in areas of postural imbalance, and then myofascial mapping (Weiselfish & Kain, 1991) is performed to locate more discrete areas of fascial dysfunction (=malalignment and inflexibility). Fascia responds to stress by remodelling and realigning (Silver, 1987). If stress is applied therapeutically in appropriate directions and planes, then realignment of fibers occurs and fascial dysfunction resolves. This helps to normalize structural and postural balance (Figure 7.4).

Neurofascial Release

Neurofascial release (Davidson, 1992) is another fascial release technique. Whereas the focus of myofascial release is local, the focus of neurofascial release is global. After detecting a local area of stress where range of motion is limited, the therapist palpates the body's fascial network to find the "key lesion." The key lesion is the area of fascial dysfunction, the fulcrum, around which the tissues have compensated. This fulcrum can be at a distance from the area of stress initially assessed because the fascia is continuous throughout the body. Ranges of motion are assessed prior to treatment and afterwards to assess effectiveness.

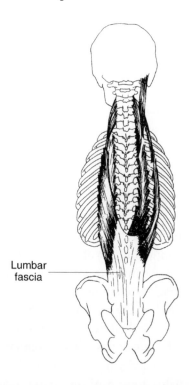

Lumbar
fascia

**FIGURE
7.4**

An example of fascia.

Source: Calais-Germain, B. (1993). *Anatomy of movement*. (Fig.: Intermediate back and neck muscles, p. 69). Copyright 1993. Eastland Press, PO Box 12689, Seattle, WA 98111. Reprinted with permission.

A note of caution: there are other authors who have similarly named their techniques, but these differ in the way they treat the fascial tensions.

Visceral Manipulation

Visceral manipulation (Barral, 1989, 1991; Barral & Mercier, 1988) is a fascial release technique that focuses on the specialized fascia surrounding the organs of the cranial (brain), thoracic (for example, the lungs and the heart), and abdominal (for example, the pancreas and the liver) cavities. In simple terms, this fascia suspends the viscera within the skeletal framework. Visceral manipulation evaluates the movement or mobility of viscera in response to gross motor movement and also assesses the inherent motion of the organs themselves. Gross motor movement has an effect on and is affected by visceral mobility because all fascial sheaths of the body are interconnected. This reciprocal relationship exists because visceral fascia is attached to the bony skeleton (for example, the pleura surrounding the lungs to the ribs), and directly or indirectly to the musculoskeletal system (for example, suspensory ligament of the duodenum to the crus of the diaphragm to the anterior longitudinal ligament of the spine). In this arrangement free mobility of the viscera accommodates bending and twisting of the skeleton, and free mobility of the skeleton accommodates the changes in size and shape of the visceral organs (for example, the full stomach or bladder, or the pregnant uterus). Treatment entails applying small, gentle forces with the hands to improve mobility of the visceral fascia and thereby improve gross motor movement.

Craniosacral Therapy and Cranial Osteopathy

Progressing from treating biomechanical dysfunction (muscle energy) and muscle strain (strain and counterstrain) as muscle hypertonicity, to treating fascial dysfunction (myofascial and neurofascial release, visceral manipulation), we arrive at central nervous system tissues and their role in structural dysfunction. Craniosacral therapy (Upledger, 1987, 1990; Upledger & Vredevoogd, 1983) and cranial osteopathy (Hruby, 1994, 1995) take advantage of the small but palpable, inherent, ongoing movement of and between the cranial and sacral bones. This movement, very broadly and loosely, characterizes the cranial rhythmic impulse also known as the craniosacral rhythm. The specialized fascia of the central nervous system, the dura mater (dural membrane) in particular, is attached to the cranial and sacral bones. Thus, if the normal pattern of movement of any of these bones is distorted, then normal tensions of the dura mater are disturbed. The dura mater is a part of the total body fascial network because it connects with the fascia outside the central nervous system via the spine at the intervertebral foramen. Therefore, abnormal tensions of the dura mater can effect fascial tensions in the rest of the body and ultimately distort structural/postural balance. This is a reciprocal relationship, where body fascia can translate tensions to the dural membrane. The assessment protocol evaluates, through palpation of the cranial (Figure 7.5a) and sacral (Figure 7.2a,b) bones, several parameters of the craniosacral rhythm:

■ rate or cycles per minute (normal is 6 to 12)
■ rhythm or symmetry
■ amplitude or range of motion
■ vitality or energy that describes the quality of the rhythm.

Assessment scrutinizes the distorted movement to differentiate between sutural (bony) (Figure 7.5b) and membranous (dural membrane) restrictions. Also assessed is the mobility of the total body fascial network with particular attention paid to the transverse diaphragms (the cranial base, the hyoid

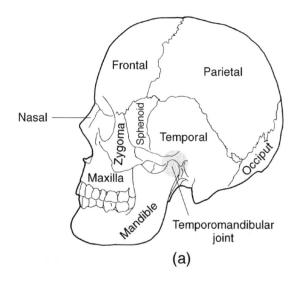

(a)

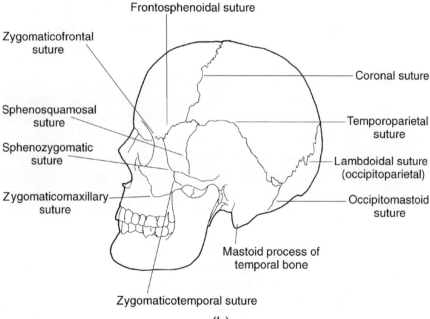

(b)

FIGURE 7.5 a) External cranial and facial bones, and b) some of their external articulations (sutures). These are components of the craniosacral system which are evaluated to determine their mobility, and their contribution to the symmetry, rate, and energy of the craniosacral rhythm. In addition, because of muscle and fascial attachments to these bones, and because of the nerves and vessels which pass through their foramina, their alignment and mobility contribute to head/neck movements, to oral-motor skills, and to visual and vestibular functions, to name a few.

Source: Upledger, J. E., & Vredevoogd, J. D. (1983). *Craniosacral therapy* (Fig. 6-20, p. 78). Copyright 1983. Eastland Press, PO Box 12689, Seattle, WA 98111. All rights reserved.

complex, the thoracic inlet, and the respiratory and pelvic diaphragms) that can impede fascial mobility.

Fascial and dural mobility may also be influenced by emotional stress (Upledger, 1990). Emotional stress, related to physical or emotional trauma, is internalized, and the area of the body affected becomes dysfunctional. Very broad analogies can be made to a headache or an ulcer that are the body's response to internalized emotional stress. During craniosacral therapy the areas of structural dysfunction triggered by the emotional stress may release. As the tissue tensions in the area normalize, the client may again experience the original emotional content of the trauma (MacDonald, 1992; Upledger, 1983). The release of this emotion is called *somatoemotional release* (SER) and is taught as a specialized treatment technique.

Craniosacral therapy and cranial osteopathy treatment techniques mobilize sutural, dural membrane, and fascial restrictions to normalize the cranial rhythmic impulse and structural balance in general.

Zero Balancing

Zero balancing (Smith, 1986) recognizes that structural dysfunction is often due to disruptive forces at the interface of energy and structure in the body. Energy, defined as movement or vibration, is a distinctive force in the body. The assessment protocol requires observation and evaluation of movement. This movement is of two types: gross motor and energy. When assessing gross motor movements one looks for distortions in movement patterns and any disruption in the flow of energy. When assessing energy movement one palpates for energy blocks at the level of the joint. The end point of motion of a joint (the end feel) is where the energetics of the joint can be assessed; this is bone energy that is the primary focus in zero balancing. Structural dysfunction may develop or persist because energetic knots interfere with structural/postural balance. A muscle spasm or an "idea" (mental content) is viewed as held energy in the context of zero balancing. Treatment focuses on releasing energy blocks to promote the health of both structure and energy flow and also to allow for a balanced relationship between the two at their interface.

Wide Range, Systemic Effects of Manual Therapy

The structural approach as described in the following case histories provides a) alleviation of dysfunctions (depression, head banging, hyperactivity) and

b) improvement of functions (for example, gross motor and visual regard). One may ask why focusing on one area or structure of the body has such a wide effect. The structural approach treats the neuromusculoskeletal system, and dysfunction in this system has the potential to disrupt function in other systems (Barral, 1989, 1991; Barral & Mercier, 1988; Davidson, 1987, 1992; Greenman, 1989; Korr, 1978; Mennell, 1992). When assessing structural symmetry, mobility and articular balance of the joints, elasticity/flexibility of fascia, and muscle tone, each are considered both individually and as they relate to each other (Greenman, 1989; Weiselfish & Kain, 1991, 1993) and to other physiological systems (Barral & Mercier, 1988; Davidson, 1987, 1992; Korr, 1978).

If you think of a system of "levers and pulleys," then you can envision that the binding of a joint, a muscle, or fascia has the potential to disrupt the function of distal, as well as local structures. For example, because the fascia envelopes nerves, muscles, and organs and is continuous and interconnected throughout the body, then, if it is binding (=reduction in flexibility), it can cause wide ranging systemic effects.

Taking a second example, muscle dysfunction can also have a wide range of effects. Muscle spasms (a dysfunction) are considered examples of a "facilitated segment" (Korr, 1978; Upledger, 1987, 1990; Weiselfish, 1994; Weiselfish & Kain, 1993). A facilitated segment is a particular level of the spinal cord that, because of long-standing sensory input, becomes hyperresponsive to stimuli and leads to hyperactive motor output. The hyperactive motor output (a function of the central nervous system) will increase the responsiveness of the corresponding level of the sympathetic nervous system. The sympathetic nervous system will, in turn, affect specific visceral and/or peripheral functions. For example, if the fourth thoracic level is facilitated due to protective muscle spasm of the intercostal muscles, then heart function, via the sympathetic nerves, may be altered. Thus, facilitated segments have the potential to affect target organs of the sympathetic nervous system. In this case, treatment of a muscle spasm can, therefore, also effect the circulatory system.

"Levers and Pulleys": Illustration of Wide Range Effects

Now that we have addressed anatomically-based examples of the wide range effects of manual therapy, let us examine a therapy-based example that further illustrates these effects. Let us look at a behavioral problem, inattention to task, where the focus of treatment will be the dropped head posture.

One can develop a treatment plan based on an assessment of structure. The assessment may reveal:

- significant malalignment of four cervical vertebrae
- hypertonicity of the right sternocleidomastoid (Figure 7.6) and left scalene (Figure 7.7) muscles thus maintaining the head in flexion and left rotation
- restriction of the fascial sheaths at the thoracic inlet.

This assessment has now identified three structures—vertebrae, muscle, and connective tissue—that are responsible for the individual's dropped head posture. The structures identified as dysfunctional are viewed as singular links in a chain or web of interconnecting links (Barral & Mercier, 1988; Greenman, 1989; Upledger & Vredevoogd, 1983; Weiselfish & Kain 1991, 1993), which when dysfunctional, have the potential to set off a domino effect resulting in dysfunction in other structures or systems. For instance, the hypertonic left scalene muscles that insert on the ribs may, over time, limit the expiratory mobility of the rib cage (Greenman, 1989, p. 186). Eventually, this may interfere with breathing (respiratory system), endurance, or upright posture (musculoskeletal system) because the rib cage is now hypomobile on the left. In addition, the restriction of the fascia at the thoracic inlet may compromise the function of the vagus nerve (nervous system) to a point that the individual complains of gastric upsets (digestive system) (Barral, 1991, p. 104). The attachment of the sternocleidomastoid muscle to the temporal bone (Figure 7.6) may affect its mobility and thus interfere with temporal bone function resulting in identifiable visual motor disturbance (sensorimotor systems) (Upledger & Vredevoogd, 1983, p. 210). Through manual therapy treatment, needed structural changes can be achieved, and consequently an individual's ability to function changes. These changes may affect motor, social, and perceptual behaviors, as well as physical well-being. In our example—inattention to task—this would be respectively: head/neck movements, visual regard, spatial orientation, and sensation (gastric pain or discomfort).

How Does Structurally-Based Manual Therapy Differ from Traditional Sensorimotor and Other Functionally-Based Therapies?

A goal of rehabilitation is to improve an individual's ability to function in some aspect of his or her life. There are a number of classical approaches

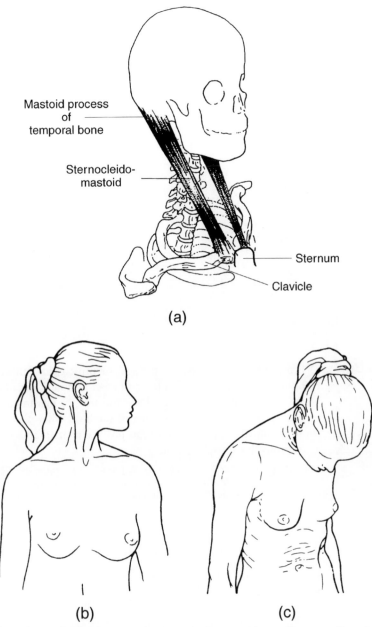

Mastoid process
of
temporal bone

Sternocleido-
mastoid

Sternum

Clavicle

(a)

(b)   (c)

**FIGURE
7.6**

a) Protective muscle spasm of the sternocleidomastoid muscles can affect the function of the shoulder girdle, and the respiratory and craniosacral systems because of their attachments to the sternum and clavicles, and to the temporal bones. b) Contraction of the right sternocleidomastoid muscle produces right sidebending (not shown) and left rotation of the head when the thoracic cage is fixed. c) Contraction of both the right and left muscles produces flexion of the head when the thoracic cage is fixed. These muscles contribute to dropped head posture if maintained in a shortened state, as in protective muscle spasm.

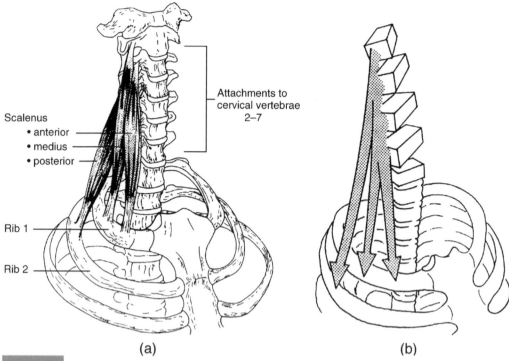

Scalenus
  • anterior
  • medius
  • posterior

Attachments to
cervical vertebrae
2–7

Rib 1

Rib 2

(a)   (b)

**FIGURE
7.7**

a) Protective muscle spasm of the scalene muscles can affect the function of the respiratory system, thoracic inlet, and head and neck because of their attachments to the cervical vertebrae and ribs. b) Contraction of the right scalene muscles produces right sidebending of the head when the ribs are fixed. These muscles contribute to dropped head posture if maintained in a shortened state, as in protective muscle spasm.

Source: Fig. 7.7a: Calais-Germain, B. (1993). *Anatomy of movement*. Fig.: Scalene muscles (p. 77). Fig. 7.7b: Calais-Germain, B. (1993). *Anatomy of movement*. Fig.: Scalene muscles, middle figure (p. 78). Copyright 1993. Eastland Press, PO Box 12689, Seattle WA 98111. All rights reserved. Reprinted with permission.

in occupational therapy used with individuals with mental retardation and those with developmental disabilities which help to improve their capacity to function:

▪ exercise
▪ assistive technology
▪ environmental adaptation
▪ Feldenkrais
▪ sensory integration and sensorimotor therapies.

These focus on functional aspects of rehabilitation (Weiselfish, 1994; Weiselfish & Kain, 1990). Then there is the structural approach (Greenman, 1989;

Mennell, 1992; Mitchell, Moran, & Pruzzo, 1979; Upledger, 1987; Weiselfish & Kain 1990), which does not immediately aim to augment one's ability to function but rather to unlock one's potential for function.

Traditionally, behavioral "symptoms" have been viewed and treated from two perspectives: behavioral and functional. Using the previous example of inattention to task in an individual with dropped head posture, the treatment by these two approaches will be briefly elaborated and compared to structurally-based therapy. The behaviorist will analyze the task and develop sequential steps of increasing difficulty and/or increased time on task to facilitate improved attention to task; he or she will also consider appropriate approaches to deal with any maladaptive behaviors. The health professional, who views this behavior from a sensorimotor or sensory integrative viewpoint, will notice the dropped head posture and may question the efficiency of righting reactions, vestibular function, and proprioception recognizing their role in the ability to maintain focus. A practitioner using the structural approach, having noted the dropped head posture, will evaluate the structural integrity of the cervical and thoracic spines, the sacrum, and temporal bones, keeping in mind that dysfunction due to some or all of these will affect head/ neck proprioception, vestibular function, and righting reactions. Clearly, all three viewpoints are productive; it is their interplay that expands the possibilities for the individual to achieve maximum functional performance.

Rationale for Using Manual Therapy with Adults with Mental Retardation

The structural integrity of an individual affects the potential for movement, socialization, perceptual acuity, and physiological health. Although functional approaches help to develop these potentials, in order to achieve maximum benefit from therapy, namely, to fulfill possibly untapped potentials, one needs to look first at structure and then at function.

To improve function in adults with mental retardation, I initially focused on sensorimotor and sensory integrative approaches. The clients' participation was difficult to engage because of sensory defensiveness, hyperactivity, intolerance for interaction, visual inattention, or because it was one more setting that placed demands of participation on them. The changes, although functional, were not easily transferred to other contexts, for example, from the treatment environment to activity of daily living tasks. It seemed as if nothing was happening on a physiological level, from within the person, to facilitate meaningful change that would allow the individual to make choices during the execution of a variety of tasks. Persistent questions arose:

▎ How does the structural/postural framework affect movements, behaviors, and performance?

▎ Is there a biomechanical dysfunction due to joint or myofascial impairment?

▎ How could the individual's structural framework be influencing functional performance?

With these questions in mind, the idea developed to look at adults with mental retardation and other developmental disabilities not purely within the context of their medical/psychiatric diagnoses but also as regards their structural make-up. Structural imbalance or asymmetry is often easy to observe: it includes dysfunctional gait, forward head posture, scoliosis, and facial distortions. In view of these departures from normal posture, the first thing to realize is that as "imbalances" they create stresses throughout the total structural framework. These stresses trigger compensatory responses both in the structural framework and in behaviors, as they would in any population. With structural imbalance, movement will be distorted, and possibly activity levels and tolerances will be influenced, as well as social and other behaviors (Simpson, 1996). For example, forward head posture may interfere with swallowing (Kraus, 1989; Mennell, 1992; Weiselfish & Kain, 1993), or may present as headaches (Mennell, 1992; Rocabado, Johnson, & Blakney 1982–83) or disturbances in equilibrium (Kraus, 1988). Thus, a key question presents itself: How can the structural framework be "normalized" to improve movement function and, possibly, behaviors in general?

To answer this question, a structural rehabilitative approach (Weiselfish & Kain, 1990, 1991, 1993) was decided upon in order to influence essential and basic elements of function. The influence of structure on function has already been clearly documented (Barral, 1991; Greenman, 1978, 1989; Heinrich, 1991; Korr, 1978; Mennell, 1992; Upledger, 1987; Upledger & Vredevoogd, 1983). It is my contention that structural dysfunction can interfere with normal adaptive behaviors (Simpson, 1996) and, thereby, influences the potential of the adult with mental retardation to effectively respond to sensorimotor therapies. The structural approach affords new possibilities for facilitating change, as well as a new way to view and better understand some behaviors.

IMPLEMENTING STRUCTURALLY-BASED MANUAL THERAPY FOR ADULTS WITH MENTAL RETARDATION

Treatment Environment

The following case histories describe four male residents of state group homes that are established as Intensive Care Facilities (ICF). Each home has six to seven residents; one is coed and the other all male; both have 24-hour supervision. All residents participate in vocational day programs.

Because the homes are ICF residences for individuals with mental retardation, they are required by federal regulations (483.430{b}{1}) to provide those services that are deemed essential for the individual and to continue providing those services for as long as the health professional finds it appropriate and necessary. Each home has a multidisciplinary team of health professionals that includes:

- pharmacologist
- psychologist/behaviorist
- occupational therapist
- physical therapist
- speech-language pathologist
- nurse
- social worker/case manager
- dental hygienist
- recreational therapist
- program supervisor.

Quarterly and annual meetings are held for team members to share their particular professional perspectives on each client in order to develop a comprehensive picture of the individual and to evaluate progress towards team goals.

Occupational therapy treatment schedules are influenced by various factors. Clients are seen one to four times a month as I am in each home once a week. On occasion it is necessary to increase the frequency of treatment in order to effect more rapid change in structural dysfunction for safety reasons. Most clients are receptive to a manual therapy approach in spite of the difficulty of staying in one place for a period of time or the difficulty of interacting; they always come and stay for therapy except at those times when illness, fatigue, or just "a bad day" defers therapy.

The treatment sessions are held either in the home's living room or in a bedroom. Sometimes if a client has roommates or if a common bathroom is in his or her bedroom, we opt to use another client's room with single occupancy. Visual and noise distractions are adapted to as needed. All residents have respected the common area used for therapy.

Treatment Session

Length of the Treatment Session

Treatment sessions range from 5 to 90 minutes. Shorter sessions may occur because the individual is not yet comfortable with the therapeutic process (the process of self-discovery and change) or with being treated and "touched." The initial process of developing trust between the client and the therapist may also initially preclude longer sessions.

Trust as Part of the Treatment Session

Trust plays a significant role in all evaluation and treatment sessions. The therapist must trust himself or herself, must trust the client, and must also have trust in the therapeutic process. Likewise, the client needs to trust himself or herself to change and the body to heal, and needs to trust the therapist and the process. I consider myself a facilitator of change. The individual with whom I work needs to want change. He or she is the captain of the ship who directs the therapy; I am the navigator.

At this juncture, one should not become perplexed with the "mental retardation" condition of the client; wanting to change is not exclusively a deliberate decision. There are levels of functioning from which decisions are made that are not based on deliberate thought processes or cognitive function alone. These individuals seek me out for their sessions and I see them come eagerly each week regardless of the discomfort of lying still, the discomfort of interacting with another person, and regardless of any discomfort experienced in the previous week's session. They keep coming. For me, this is a decision they have made, on some level. I must presume that they come because therapy feels good to them, or because they recognize it as doing something good.

Implementation of Treatment Techniques

Once a detailed evaluation has been carried out (see "Evaluation Protocol," following), the manual therapy treatment approach has been decided upon, and the client is receptive, treatment can begin. Some treatment techniques (muscle energy, strain and counterstrain) require the client to follow directions. This can be difficult because of lack of comprehension, or because of muscle guarding that interferes with achieving specific positions. Other techniques (craniosacral therapy, fascial release techniques, zero balancing) require a relaxed supine position. While this position is often a possibility, at times only moments are captured between motor restlessness or constant chatter. Neither of these situations is insurmountable. The initial implementation of a technique might not be textbook style, but one can often apply the principles of a technique using some creativity. If you need someone to take a deep breath (very often not understood), ask him or her to blow and then catch him or her on the inhalation. If you need an isometric contraction, play a game of resistance. If you need quiet, work around the fidgetiness and catch those glimpses of quietude. There have been times when I have used an assistant for distraction or to implement multihand treatment. Instead of supine, use sitting. Often sitting, even while engaged in a task, is initially substituted for the relaxed supine position. Results from treatment obviously take longer to achieve, but the key is, they can be achieved.

Sometimes gentle restraint—using the practitioner's arms, legs, or head—is necessary because of motor restlessness. Some situations are difficult to resolve. If you do not restrain, you cannot implement a particular treatment technique, and if you do restrain, muscle guarding occurs. This has been a persistent situation with "Steve" (see case histories) when trying to release his occipitoatlantal joint. Frequently, the best way I have found to initially address these problems is to use treatment techniques that focus on the energetic component of a structural dysfunction, such as zero balancing, direction of energy or body unwinding (craniosacral therapy, cranial osteopathy), or therapeutic touch (Krieger, 1979). If fidgetiness is encountered during treatment, one needs to assess if this behavior is due to a discomfort of experiencing movement in an area where previously there had been none (structural dysfunction), is due to pain, or is due to an emotional (Upledger, 1990) or energetic component (Smith, 1986) bound up in this area of the body. Finding an answer helps to make a decision as to which treatment technique is more appropriate.

Communication During the Treatment Session

Communication is an essential part of both the evaluation and treatment sessions. Treatment depends on a two-way relationship. It is important to learn to communicate with adults with mental retardation, to read their signs:

■ body language

■ changes in the quality of the voice

■ changes in breathing pattern

■ changes in tolerances

■ the quality of visual regard

■ changes in facial expression.

They often cannot verbally express the subtle or even the large changes occurring within themselves. Treatment cannot progress unless the therapist "hears" what is communicated and respects it. In addition, I talk to them, giving instructions ("Let this tissue soften"), telling them what I am doing, reassuring them, and telling them what they can do when experiencing changes in their body ("Trust yourself and your body to change." "New movements may be scary."). This helps develop their trust in me and, I believe, they understand me, whether through language or touch. And remember: Many have receptive skills even if their expressive skills are negligible.

Adults with mental retardation, in addition to being receptive, are responsive to manual therapy. To see an individual with autism look up at you and smile while experiencing the release of fascial restrictions is heartening. More importantly, it is a confirmation of the benefit of the approach.

It is also important to communicate with group home staff and team members about the structural approach. Initially, it was surprising to experience others' relief at the possibility of finding a reason for maladaptive behavior other than finding fault with the patient's personality, which usually results in labelling the patient "uncooperative." Team members and staff will be more aware of what to look for in a person's behaviors and become better able to make referrals for therapy and to communicate their observations to you.

Ending the Treatment Session

Learning when to stop a treatment session is important so that one does not tax or overload neurophysiological systems (Breuer, 1989, October & November; Brown, 1993, 1994; Smith, 1986, 1996; Upledger & Vredevoogd, 1983), or exceed the client's tolerance. When working with "Larry" (see case histories), I would end the session when he covered his face—a signal of discomfort or possible forthcoming aggressive behavior. Eventually I picked up behavioral cues so sessions could end before his hand went to his face. It is preferable to end sessions on positive notes. One needs, however, to differentiate between discomfort experienced during tissue release, which is often part of the therapeutic healing process, from the discomfort of exceeding someone's tolerance for treatment. The latter may result in maladaptive behaviors.

Amount of Time it Takes for Change to Occur

Both structural and functional objectives are part of treatment plans; structural objectives are the building blocks for functional change. For example: improved biomechanics of the lumbosacral junction (structural) leads to improved sitting balance (functional). In my experience, the easily observable and tangible functional changes take 3 to 12 months to appear (treating once weekly). Large, observable improvements include changes in gait, chewing patterns, balance, and spatial awareness.

Subtler functional changes—such as increased smiling or more relaxed breathing—may appear earlier in treatment if they are the building blocks for larger ones, like improved social interaction, greater tolerance for sitting, or taking walks. However, subtler functional changes can take longer to occur if they are refinements of the larger ones, such as using more of the space around you by building on improved proprioceptive sense—itself resulting from improved pelvic girdle and spinal mechanics.

There are occasions when a structural dysfunction, which is a major component of a maladaptive behavior, is resolved, but the behavior does not change in all settings. In effect, the behavior, which over years has become a learned behavior and is habitual, interferes with its own resolution. I have seen this with "Brian" (see case histories) when the chronic muscle spasms of the temporalis muscles resolved. At this point, all teeth grinding stopped during therapy sessions that were as long as 60 minutes. However, the teeth grinding continued outside the sessions. Final resolution of maladaptive behaviors are often accomplished by functional and behavioral programs developed by the team. Successful implementation of these programs requires group home staff to have higher expectations of the client.

Evaluation Protocol

All individuals are evaluated because of a) observed deficiencies in the quality of their movements: hyperactivity, rigidity, or lack of movement; and/or b) some obvious structural imbalance, such as structural malalignment (for example, facial distortion, increased lumbar lordosis) and/or myofascial restrictions. Evaluation entails two steps. The first step is a general screening followed by the second more formal and detailed assessment of structure.

In the first step, one screens for structural dysfunction by starting with observation. One looks at a broad range of behaviors to determine the presence of function versus dysfunction. These behaviors include:

- gross and fine motor skills
- oral-motor skills
- movement patterns (straight planes, rotation, fluidity)
- gait (toe-walking, heel-toe)
- transitions
- perception (movement in space, body awareness, gravitational security)
- visual regard
- sensation (tactile, proprioception/kinesthesia)
- concentration/attention to task
- primitive developmental reflexes
- maladaptive behaviors (aggression, irritability, depression, hyperactivity, self-injurious and pain behaviors)
- physiological complaints (headaches, spastic colon).

When making these observations, one looks for structural imbalance (postural asymmetry, movement distortion, compensatory movements) (Greenman, 1989; Mitchell, Moran, & Pruzzo, 1979; Weiselfish, 1994; Weiselfish & Kain, 1991, 1993) and maladaptive behaviors (Simpson, 1996). If there is dysfunction, the question needs to be raised: Is the dysfunction due, at least in part, to structural impairment?

As an occupational therapy practitioner, one already has some of the tools needed to consider the influence of structure (structural/postural strains) on function. Our sensorimotor background provides us with significant knowledge about movement and development: mobility developing from proximal stability, and perceptual and cognitive functions developing from a sensorimotor foundation of exploration during infancy and childhood, to name just two. Importantly, this knowledge can be directly applied to a structural frame of reference because it provides a basic understanding of movement (dysfunction) that is the general focus of a structurally-based manual therapy approach. By observing and assessing movement and function, one raises questions about sensory processing. Once sensorimotor and/or sensory integrative dysfunction is identified, one can begin to consider the influence of structural/postural imbalance on sensory processing before proceeding solely with a functional treatment approach. The idea is to take a different look at something familiar and explore additional reasons for it: Maybe the equilibrium system is impaired because there is impingement of neural tissue at the internal acoustic meatus; maybe the head droops because the cervical vertebrae are malaligned.

In the second step, one proceeds to identify specific structural dysfunction by more closely examining the components of structural integrity of the shoulder and pelvic girdles, spine, rib cage, head, and extremities. Because the various manual therapy treatment approaches address either different tissues (for example, muscle or fascia) or different aspects of the same tissue (for example, dural or visceral fascia), it is important to first decide if postural/structural integrity is impaired and then to decide which tissue(s) are involved.

First, static posture (Breuer, 1989, October & November; Greenman, 1989; Mitchell, Moran, & Pruzzo, 1979; Summerfelt, 1991; Weiselfish, 1994) is evaluated. It includes, but is not limited to, noting asymmetry of anatomical landmarks (eyes, shoulders, iliac crests) (Figures 7.2, 7.3) and palpating soft tissue (muscle, fascia—inclusive of the dura mater) for texture, tone, and imbalance. Postural symmetry is evaluated in three planes to give a clear picture of three-dimensional structure and movement: coronal (a view from the front or back of a person), sagittal (a side view), and transverse (looking at anterior/posterior or rotational displacement). Effectively, the practitioner is assessing the height, depth, anterior/posterior displacement, and/or degree of rotation of bilateral bony landmarks. If these features are not equal or level, then structural dysfunction exists. Articular balance is also a part of the evaluation of static posture. Here, one assesses the degree of friction-free mobility of tissue interfaces. These interfaces may be bone to bone (glenohumeral joint), soft tissue to bone (cecum to ilium), or soft tissue to soft tissue (right kidney to duodenum).

Postural deviation in a static pose indicates the presence of structural dysfunction. It is also indicative of movement dysfunction (think: "levers and pulleys"), most notably, hypomobility. Therefore, a dynamic postural evaluation (Breuer, 1989, October & November; Greenman, 1989; Mitchell, Moran, & Pruzzo, 1979; Summerfelt, 1991; Weiselfish, 1994) is carried out to include symmetry of movements, limitation of range of motion, functional strength, dissociation of movements, and compensatory or distorted movements. This dynamic evaluation represents the third part of structural integrity, namely, mobility; the other two parts, alignment and articular balance, have been addressed in the assessment of static posture (above).

The information gathered from the static evaluation is correlated with the limitation of movement(s) assessed in the dynamic postural evaluation. This helps to determine whether the movement dysfunction results from asymmetric muscle strength or pull (shortening, spasm), neurologic compromise (central or peripheral) (Weiselfish, 1994; Weiselfish & Kain, 1993), articular imbalance, or fascial restriction.

At some point during assessment, sensory testing and reflex testing are also carried out. Finally, a differential diagnosis, using the various treatment approaches is necessary. This determines which structure(s) is contributing to the dysfunction: Is it muscle, fascia, or joint biomechanics that is impeding normal movement or interfering with adaptive behavior?

The above evaluation protocol is straightforward; however, it is not always as easy to implement with adults with developmental disabilities. By knowing what to look for, and understanding the implications of postural asymmetry, even if you cannot completely and decisively carry out the postural evaluation, you can at least begin to visually, and sometimes manually through palpation, discern structural impairment. When this happens, it can be useful to prematurely begin cranial, energy, or fascial treatment approaches to initiate tissue releases, while recognizing that evaluation is an ongoing process.

With the person who is developmentally disabled there may be no complaint of pain or the complaint of pain may be considered a "behavior." If there is a lack of postural symmetry, then there is structural dysfunction that is compromising that individual's level of performance and the efficiency with which he or she performs a task, and possibly influencing adaptive behaviors. Is this dysfunction important if there is no obvious complaint of pain or discomfort? In my view, yes, because the dysfunction is now a "pathological" basis from which everything else is performed and a springboard for the development of more and more compensatory habits and maladaptive behaviors. When movement occurs, it is either from a well-balanced musculoskeletal foundation that allows for fluid and efficient movements, or from one that is imbalanced and, therefore, pathological. The body automatically compensates in order to adapt to any imbalance. If the initial imbalance is chronic, then over time the compensation becomes part of the pathological foundation for movement. Compensation becomes one's "normal" way of moving. Eventually, the body's mechanisms of adaptation are depleted and movement becomes inefficient, energy consuming, impossible and/or painful. Tolerances may be lowered to all types of environmental stresses. Therefore, the earlier structural dysfunction is alleviated, the easier it is to achieve well-being.

Treatment Protocol

Treatment is recommended based on the presence of structural dysfunction discovered during the evaluation. A treatment plan is developed to normalize function in areas of hypomobility. Hypomobility may be due to biomechanical stress, protective muscle spasm, inflexibility of connective tissue (fascia, visceral fascia, dura mater), or energetic restrictions. The treatment techniques employed will depend on the practitioner's expertise and comfort with particular structurally-based manual therapy techniques, but optimal results occur when the technique matches the dysfunction (for example, craniosacral therapy for dural membrane restrictions).

Treatment plans have long and short term goals. The short term goals focus on improving the structural dysfunction(s) assessed in the evaluation. The long term goal is usually a functional/behavioral objective. The short term structural goals are the building blocks that permit and support achievement of the functional goal. Once treatment is implemented, progress is monitored by reevaluating hypomobility, symmetry of anatomical landmarks, tissue texture, range of motion, quality of movement (resolution of compensatory movements), status of pain, quality of behaviors (more adaptive), and efficiency in performing activity of daily living tasks. Group home sensorimotor or structurally-oriented programs are often developed to facilitate the integration of structural changes into functional performance and to augment direct therapy, respectively.

Development of a Treatment Protocol: An Example

I will use the case history of "Brian" (see case histories) to focus on the relationship between structural dysfunction and "inadequate chewing" in order to demonstrate a structurally-based manual therapy treatment plan, in this case for improving chewing skills. The static assessment revealed gross postural deviations of the spine, cranial structures, and shoulder and pelvic girdles. These postural strains correlated with limitations of movement (dynamic assessment) of the rib cage, spine, lower extremities, jaw, lips, and tongue. In order to improve oral-motor function, the gross postural strains had to be addressed first because proximal stability (axial structural integrity) is a prerequisite oral-motor skill (Alexander, 1988, September & November). Thus, the first structural dysfunctions to be treated were the pelvic and sacral imbalances, lumbar spine hypomobility, and lower extremity asymmetry (because pelvic dysfunction may be related to the abnormal pull of leg muscles on the pelvis) (Figure 7.8). Muscle energy was used to normalize muscle tone and length; a group home program of muscle strengthening and sensorimotor activity was established to integrate the ongoing structural changes into gains in functional performance. Further, treatment included craniosacral therapy that affects sacral and vertebral mobility via the dural membrane. The status of the membrane's structural integrity ultimately affects head/neck function (oral-motor skills). Myofascial dysfunction of the low back and of the thoracic spine and rib cage was then treated with myofascial release. At this point, improved postural alignment and lower body stability were providing Brian with a much more stable base of support from which to develop oral-motor function. Next, muscle energy, myofascial release, and craniosacral therapies were employed to realign the shoulder girdle and cervical spine because of forward head posture. With the entire vertebral column realigned and the head and neck more appropriately situated over the trunk, stresses due to abnormal pull were lessened on the jaw and extrinsic tongue muscles resulting in improved chewing skills.

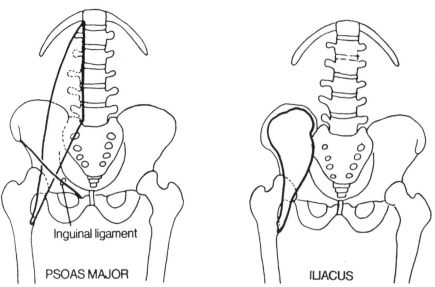

Inguinal ligament

PSOAS MAJOR   ILIACUS

FIGURE 7.8

The figure illustrates an example of leg muscles with their attachments to the pelvic girdle and spine. Because of these attachments, any dysfunction of these leg muscles will not only affect normal movement of the leg, but also that of the pelvis and spine.

Source: Goldberg, S. (1991). *Clinical anatomy made ridiculously simple.* Fig. 4-44, p. 47. Copyright 1991. MedMaster, Inc. Reprinted with permission.

In this example, three types of structural dysfunction that contributed to Brian's poor chewing skills were identified:

- biomechanical (pelvis, vertebrae and hips)
- protective muscle spasm (legs, pelvis)
- soft tissue inflexibility (fascia and dura mater).

Each of the structures identified as dysfunctional (pelvis, vertebral column, hips, and fascia) has the potential to produce an effect resulting in dysfunction in other structures or systems. In other words, structures and functions beyond the primary treatment objective can be affected. In Brian's case, while addressing oral-motor function (primary treatment objective), his breathing pattern (function) matured because structures associated with breathing (ribs, muscles) were directly affected by the structural changes occurring at the spine, and pelvic and shoulder girdles.

CASE HISTORIES USING STRUCTURALLY-BASED MANUAL THERAPY

The following four case histories demonstrate the successful implementation of structurally-based manual therapy with adults with mental retardation. There have been other individuals with whom I have had success, but there have also been those with whom I have had only limited success and some with whom I have been unsuccessful. The reasons are variable. A few individuals, themselves, did not want to change. One woman only wanted somato-emotional release (SER); every time I saw her, she would put my thumb way back on her hard palate and proceed to have an SER. There have been times when I could devise a step-by-step treatment plan but could not implement it. One man was so active and jolly that I could not find "glimpses of quietude" for treatment. And, there have been those with whom I just could not identify a specific structural problem. The following case histories should be read recognizing that manual therapy is a new, important tool for treating adults with mental retardation and that it should be considered as one of a number of approaches for achieving improved function.

The following individuals, all residents of group homes designated as intensive care facilities (ICF), have been receiving occupational therapy services, on average, for 6 years with treatment occurring one to four times monthly.

Larry

Client Background

Larry is a 38-year-old male with a diagnosis of mental retardation with autistic features. Larry is nonverbal with good receptive language skills. He has been treated since June 1990 with a structurally-based manual therapy approach; during a few preceding months he received sensorimotor treatment that was poorly tolerated. An assessment was requested because of rigid hand posture.

Brief Synopsis of Pretreatment Profile

Larry presented with robot-like movements, significant muscle guarding, and severe soft tissue restrictions of the pelvic and pectoral girdles, and along the spine. His gait pattern was a shuffle with toe-walking; he lacked balance reactions, and held his fingers in hyperextension. Autistic behaviors interfered with social interaction and little visual contact was made with people. Initially, treatment sessions were ended because of low tolerance for interaction; this was indicated by Larry putting his hand over his face. Larry did not initiate constructive activities.

Treatment Focus

The broad focus of treatment was to improve soft tissue flexibility in order to facilitate improved motor function. Treatment techniques employed were craniosacral therapy, myofascial release, neurofascial release, visceral manipulation, zero balancing, strain and counterstrain, and sensorimotor.

Major Structural Changes Resulting from Therapy

The primary structural changes that occurred are:

  a) greater elasticity of the fascial sheaths, including the dural membrane system
  b) significant resolution of muscle guarding
  c) alignment of the pelvic girdle
  d) greater mobility of the spine, pelvic and shoulder girdles, especially the scapulothoracic and glenohumeral joints

e) greater mobility of the sacroiliac joints (Figure 7.2a,b)

f) normal expansion of the rib cage

g) release of restrictions at cranial sutures (Figure 7.5b) affording improved mobility of the occipitoatlantal joints (OA) (Figure 7.2b), sphenobasilar junction (Figure 7.9), and temporal and parietal bones (Figure 7.5a). The frontal bone (Figure 7.5a) has released (i.e. increased mobility) and decompression of the lateral cranial base is progressing

h) improved function of the temporomandibular joints (Figure 7.5a)

i) improved mobility of the hyoid complex and of the hard palate (Figure 7.10). Proper functioning (alignment and mobility) of the hard palate (vomer, maxillae, and palatine bones) is important because of its relationship to breathing, oral-motor, and speech functions. This relationship between structure and function exists because of anatomic connections between the hard palate, facial, and cranial bones (Figure 7.5), and because of the relationships among the hard palate, tongue, and teeth.

In addition, following the implementation of the zero balancing protocol in 1995, Larry developed dorsiflexion of both feet, and for the first time there was fluidity of movement of the left hip and ankle; up to that time, muscle guarding at the ankles interfered with movement.

Major Functional Changes Resulting from Structural Changes

Major Motor Changes.   Dissociation of movements and rotation are now present and allow Larry to automatically make transitions through a series of positions (for example, supine-kneeling-standing) rather than simply pushing up from supine to standing. Balance reactions have developed from a new ability to shift weight and dorsiflex his feet. During dressing activities he is able to sit on his bed in a relatively relaxed upright posture in order to put on his pants and socks in contrast to rigidly falling backwards to perform the task. The upper extremities are now able to independently function in manipulatory tasks instead of supporting the lower body during movement or static positioning. Now, instead of using his arms to push himself up out of a chair, he is using his legs. Larry's gait pattern has changed to a normal heel-to-toe progression when walking. Spontaneous head/neck movements involving rotation and sidebending have appeared; the fingers are held in a normal, semiflexed position at rest; and depth of breathing is

246   Structurally-Based Manual Therapy Leads to Improved Function

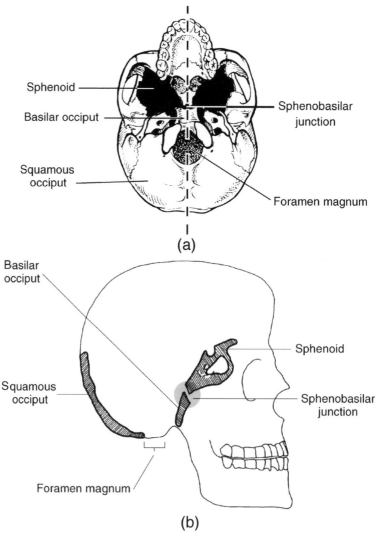

(a)

(b)

Source: Fig. 7.9a: Seeley, R. R., Stephens, T. D., & Tate, P. (1989). *Anatomy and physiology.* Fig. 7-7B, p. 164. St. Louis: Times Mirror/Mosby College Publishing. Reprinted with permission. Fig. 7.9b: Upledger, J. E., & Vredevoogd, J. D. (1983). *Craniosacral therapy.* Fig. 7-19B p. 117. Copyright 1983. Eastland Press. All rights reserved. Reprinted with permission.

FIGURE 7.9

a) Inferior view of the base of the skull to picture the sphenobasilar junction. This is an articulation between the basilar part of the occipital bone and the body of the sphenoid. The dashed line indicates a midsagittal cut. Compression of this junction, along with compression of the occipitoatlantal and lumbosacral junctions, can cause clinical depression. Compression of the sphenobasilar junction may lead to the appearance of one sucking one's thumb, but one is actually pushing up on the hard palate in an effort to decompress the joint. Compression, and lateral and vertical strains can cause a myriad of dysfunctions: pain syndromes, personality disorders, and learning disabilities (Upledger & Vredevoogd, 1983). b) This is a sagittal section through the cranium to view the sphenobasilar junction. Pictured is a vertical strain (a type of malalignment) of the articulation. If the articulating surfaces of each bone were brought into line, thus opposing each other, there would be normal alignment of the junction.

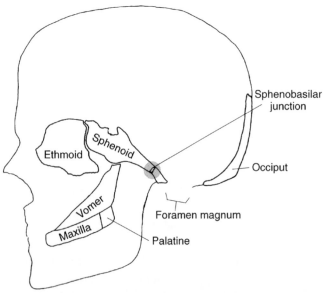

FIGURE 7.10

The bones of the hard palate are the maxillae and palatines bilaterally, and the vomer in the midline. Note the anatomic relationship to the sphenoid and, by extension, to the other cranial bones (see Figure 7.7, which shows the relationship the maxillae have to other facial bones). Proper functioning of the hard palate is important because of its relationship to breathing, oral-motor, and speech functions. (The ethmoid bone is identified to assist orientation).

Source: Upledger, J. E., & Vredevoogd, J. D. (1983). *Craniosacral therapy*. Fig. 9-5 p. 157. Copyright 1983. All rights reserved. Reprinted with permission. Eastland Press. PO Box 12689, Seattle, WA 98111.

greater. At mealtime the lips and temporomandibular joints are functioning with larger and smoother movements. Since 1995, as ankle mobility improved, Larry has learned to hop and to kick a ball using appropriate stance and movements. During some sensorimotor activities Larry can now be described as "loose as a goose" because of improved spinal flexibility; his arms now reach above his head without any resistance due to muscle spasm or fascial tensions.

Major Changes in Other Behaviors.   Tolerance for interaction has changed dramatically with eye contact now regularly made and with increased responsiveness to redirection and to prompts to engage in tasks. He tolerates being touched with no autistic behaviors and responds to interaction with a smile. He is more responsive to his morning routine without aggressive behaviors. We can now hold treatment sessions from 30 to 90 minutes without his hand going to his face, and he often signs "more" when asked if we should stop. Larry now performs tasks using more of the space around him. In addition to seeking therapy, he has begun to seek other constructive activities. When his bedroom is being used to treat another resident, Larry comes in and spontaneously offers his pillow from his bed. He finds me and waits for therapy while I am treating another person.

Brian

Client Background

Brian is a 51-year-old male with the diagnoses of mental retardation, cerebral palsy, autism, rapid switch bipolar disorder, and seizure disorder. He has been stabilized on Tegretol and lithium since 1988. Brian uses language to tell a story but generally not to express needs unless cued. Previous therapeutic intervention consisted of guidelines for eating: the precutting of food and prompting to chew and swallow each mouthful. An assessment was requested to evaluate the appropriateness of his diet prescription. In late 1988 a structural approach to Brian's oral-motor dysfunction was implemented.

Brief Synopsis of Pretreatment Profile

Brian presented significant impairment of postural function: severe forward head posture (Figure 7.3b), flattened and flared rib cage (Figure 7.3b), retracted shoulders with arms maintained against the lateral chest wall, and increased lumbar lordosis (Figure 7.3b). Motorically there was poor dissociation of movements, especially of the lower extremities, and dragging of his right leg when walking; breathing was shallow and primarily diaphragmatic; and he had essentially no adaptive balance reactions. Oral-motor dysfunction presented as: poor lip, jaw and tongue mobility; immature chewing pattern, that is, munching; temporomandibular joint dysfunction (Figure 7.5a), with the mouth opening only 13 mm (normal width is 35–40 mm); reverse swallow with fluids; and exaggerated swallow with solids. His craniosacral rhythm could be described as "stuck in the mud," because movement felt strained.

Brian had significant periods of hypomania and depression, screaming, hyperactivity, and euphoric moods. He also would grind his teeth.

Treatment Focus

A structural approach was implemented to establish more normal postural alignment in order to facilitate improved function of the oral-motor apparatus. Once this objective was attained, treatment focused on achieving greater articular balance to improve sensorimotor function, thereby increasing

Brian's movement repertoire. Treatment techniques used were muscle energy, craniosacral therapy, cranial osteopathy, myofascial release, neurodevelopmental treatment, and other sensorimotor approaches.

Major Structural Changes Resulting from Therapy

The structural changes in Brian's postural profile are:

a) improved alignment of the spinal curves with greater vertebral mobility

b) improved articular balance at the hip and pelvis with relaxation of shortened muscles and normalization of abdominal muscle tone

c) decrease in forward head posture (Figure 7.3b) with realignment of the shoulder girdle

d) improved mobility of the ribs, thus facilitating a mature thoracic-abdominal breathing pattern

e) release of the frontosphenoidal suture (Figure 7.5b), the sphenobasilar (Figure 7.9), OA and lumbosacral junctions (Figure 7.2b)

f) release of the lateral cranial base

g) initiation of the rotary component of movement of the temporal bones (Figure 7.5a)

h) improved elasticity and flexibility of the dural membrane system

i) overall improvement in the craniosacral rhythm

j) improved alignment and mobility of the temporomandibular joint (Figure 7.5a) with the range of motion now 38 mm.

The following quotes are significant. At the time of the release of the frontosphenoidal suture, Brian spontaneously said, "I feel better" while appropriately pointing to his temples. With the release of the sphenobasilar junction he announced, "I'm happy."

Major Functional Changes Resulting from Structural Changes

Major Motor Changes.   Movement capabilities have improved in standing and sitting with the development of lateral weight shift and balance reactions. Function of the lower extremities has improved with greater dissociation between the hip and knee; dragging of the right foot during walking is essentially resolved. Physical stamina and endurance are improved dramatically such that Brian is now able to take walks of 1 to 2 miles and with reported greater stability.

The oral-motor functions that have developed with these structural and gross motor changes are:

- improved tongue mobility and maneuverability
- normal swallow with fluids
- active lip function
- a mature rotary chewing pattern
- better respiratory and oral-motor functions for speech
- better coordination of swallowing with breathing during mealtime.

These changes have allowed uncooked leafy vegetables to be reintroduced into his diet without the risk of choking.

Major Changes in Other Behaviors.   Brian's depressive mood swings have significantly decreased since mid-1991 with the release of the OA, sphenobasilar and lumbosacral junctions (Upledger & Vredevoogd, 1983, p. 141). Since these structural changes, Brian has had no resurgence of increased depressive periods during the past 5 years. Another change in behavior is a reduction in screaming which coincided with the release of the temporal bones. For the 5 months prior to discontinuing therapy, teeth grinding was no longer occurring during therapy sessions. Eye contact with staff and clients has improved, focus on tasks has increased greatly, and Brian is more easily redirected when maladaptive behaviors do occur.

Occupational therapy services were discontinued in 1996. Sensorimotor skills, particularly of the lower quadrant and oral-motor apparatus, had improved significantly because of improved structural integrity. It was felt that Brian's needs could now be better met by regular engagement in gross motor activities to promote and to help maintain overall strength, biomechanical integrity, and overall well-being.

Steve

Client Background

Steve is a 29-year-old male with the diagnoses of mental retardation, attention deficit disorder with hyperactivity, and chronic sinus and ear infections. His medication regimen consists of Beconase and allergy shots, with Sudafed and Tylenol for congestion, headaches, and/or sinusitis. Steve is nonverbal with good receptive language skills. Prior to a manual therapy approach

(December 1990), I attempted a developmental sensorimotor approach to facilitate fine motor skills, but because of severe attention deficit and hyperactivity this was discontinued.

Brief Synopsis of Pretreatment Profile

Steve's hyperactivity consisted of perpetual and vigorous striding throughout the house and/or rocking on furniture; and attention to task was severely limited. He used only peripheral vision to regard objects or people. He indulged in self-abusive behaviors, most notably head banging. He held his thumb in his mouth up against the hard palate (he was not sucking his thumb). Steve was an individual with dysmorphic facies, severe lumbar lordosis (Figure 7.3b) with sacral hypomobility, and rigid neck posture. In supine he avoided flexed postures and often shot into rigid extension especially when his feet were touched. His craniosacral rhythm was barely detectable.

Treatment Focus

The premise for implementing manual therapy was that structural abnormalities, especially of the cranium, were significantly contributing to a feeling of discomfort. In an attempt to rid himself of the discomfort, self-abusive behaviors ensued. It was felt that the head banging was not behavioral in origin, although it may have become learned behavior. To work towards improved structural integrity, the following treatment techniques were employed: craniosacral therapy, zero balancing, and principles of visceral manipulation.

Major Structural Changes Resulting from Therapy

The structural changes that have occurred are numerous:

a) unlocking of the OA joints (Figure 7.2b) and occipital condyles

b) release of the right lateral and vertical strains of the sphenobasilar junction (Figure 7.9)

c) decompression of the sphenobasilar junction

d) release of the frontal bone and associated sutures (Figure 7.5a,b)

e) release of the occipitomastoid suture (Figure 7.5b)

f) decreasing compression of the temporal bones (Figure 7.5a) with symmetrical rotation now present

g) release of the thoracic inlet (Figure 7.1)

h) developing mobility and decompression of the hard palate complex (Figure 7.10)

i) greatly improved elasticity of the intracranial membrane system

j) improved dural tube mobility

k) moderately good craniosacral rhythm in both range of motion and quality

l) overall improved fascial tensions throughout the body

m) pelvic realignment with resolution of the exaggerated lumbar lordosis.

Facial contours have consequently changed. The bump on the right side of the forehead is gone; as a staff person exclaimed: "The egg is gone!" The furrows in the forehead are significantly shallower, eliminating the appearance of scowling, and his eyes do not appear as deeply set under the brow. The corneas went from a dull, yellowish color to white.

Since 1995, treatment has emphasized areas where fascia (including the dural membrane and visceral fascia) and energy are binding. Subsequently, remarkable improvements in mobility have occurred in the following areas: oro- and nasopharynx, right occipitoatlantal joint, right temporal area, hard palate, and the area of the left ocular orbit. With the improved mobility, there has been a significant decrease in Steve targeting his left eye when head banging. Also, since the hard palate became more mobile there have been increased periods of calm both during and outside of the treatment session.

Major Functional Changes Resulting from Structural Changes

Major Motor Changes.   There has been a significant decrease in hyperactive behaviors: a) the frequency and intensity of running through the house has decreased; b) when excited, Steve now rarely laughs loudly or waves his hands in front of his face; and c) he is spending more time on tasks and is more focused with greater attention to detail. From May 1991 through 1994, Steve tolerated dental visits without the use of a papoose; the first of these visits immediately followed the release of the frontal bone. However, since 1995, circumstances of the visits have changed—including staff changes— and the papoose has again been used. Beginning in 1992, Steve has tolerated the wait in doctors' offices without head banging. With the implementation of the zero balancing protocol in 1996, Steve is tolerating the lifting of his feet and legs and does not push into an exaggerated extension posture.

Muscle tension has normalized throughout his body, especially at the neck and low back; he now places his head down on the therapy table rather than holding it up.

Major Changes in Other Behaviors.   Steve now gives direct eye contact. Socially, his mother reports him as being a "happier person"; he smiles more frequently and he is more affectionate. A staff person said, "It seemed he never had time before to be cuddled." Since the fall of 1996, Steve has been making uncharacteristic sounds, also reported by his mother. Some of these sounds seem to carry the intonation and rhythm of normal speech patterns. Laughter is more appropriate. The frequency with which he holds his thumb in his mouth has significantly reduced with release of sphenobasilar compression (Upledger & Vredevoogd, 1983, p. 263) (Figure 7.9).

The frequency and intensity of head banging dropped dramatically following improved alignment and mobility of the OA and sphenobasilar junctions and of the temporal bones; this occurred between 8 and 12 weeks after the implementation of a manual therapy approach. Prior to this Steve bucked like a bronco during sessions with arms flailing, but he always came and stayed for the session. Since these releases his motor behaviors have ranged from only twisting and turning to periods of complete calm lasting 5 to 25 minutes. Head banging decreased from a high of 9.7 incidences a month in the last two quarters of 1990 to somewhat over one incidence a month in 1993; but has averaged about three incidences a month during the following 3 years.

Of particular note are changes in a range of behaviors in 1996 that accompanied release of tissue restrictions in the neck, face, and head. Steve is demonstrating increased expressiveness with appropriate grinning, smiling, and laughing. It seems that cognitive function has improved or been unlocked because eye contact is now very strong in response to verbal instructions during treatment, and behaviors are now interactive, such as being coy. In addition, he stops moving and twisting to listen when instructions are given or when I am communicating something about treatment.

In the fall of 1996, we were able to address the chronic restriction of the right OA joint in a more formal manner because of the increased periods of calm. During and following each of two sessions Steve had dramatic treatment reactions. As noted previously, these reactions are called "somato-emotional release" (SER) (Upledger, 1990; Upledger and Vredevoogd, 1983) because accompanying the release of structural tensions is the release of emotion. For the first time Steve was expressing sadness and anger. Group home staff reported "he couldn't sit" and that he banged furniture hard when repositioning it. They reported he appeared very angry and uncooperative (uncharacteristic behaviors). Steve's worksite reported he was pushing staff and stomping his feet. Both the group home and worksite reported him crying uncontrollably (he has never been known to cry). He uncharacteristically hit/ pushed others during transport from work—he has never previously shown any aggression. During therapy he repeatedly slammed his legs down on the therapy table. During the emotional releases he did not attempt to pull my hands off his body nor bang his eye. These behaviors continued for two to three weeks and then stopped. Steve's medical status was reviewed to identify any possible medical problem; none was found. As of this time, the only functional changes discernable following the SER episodes are significantly decreased motor restlessness during therapy, and a calmer demeanor which Steve now brings to therapy.

Henry

Client Background

Henry is a 33-year-old male with diagnoses of mental retardation, chronic undifferentiated schizophrenia, obsessive compulsive disorder (diagnosed in 1994), and a history of seizures. He is presently on a regime of a decreasing dose of Mellaril while implementing a trial of Klonopin for the psychotic disorder, and he is taking Paxil for the obsessive compulsive disorder. During the 7 years I have been working with Henry, psychotropic therapy has varied. The psychotropic drugs had no apparent effect on the quality of motor behavior except when Mellaril was started in April 1992. At that time, motor restlessness subsided following a period of increased maladaptive behaviors. Prior to this, he had not been taking psychotropic drugs for 1 year. It has not been determined if the perioral movements and cogwheel-like rigidity, both inconsistent, have been signs of tardive dyskinesia and/or extrapyramidal signs. Henry is verbal.

Henry was participating in a time on task program when I started to work with him in late 1988. A review of the data showed him successfully meeting the objective of 20 minutes on task many times, but this was inconsistent and dependent on mood; the program was discontinued. I subsequently developed a sensorimotor program to help integrate movements and decrease motor restlessness (King, 1974; Levy, 1974) in order to increase time on task. However, because of Henry's lack of involvement, this program was continued only as a group home program, while direct therapy began implementing a manual therapy approach in mid-1990.

Brief Synopsis of Pretreatment Profile

Henry demonstrated significant motor restlessness (i.e., pacing, rocking) that interfered with task focus and interaction. Movements were rigid with extreme muscle guarding, and he moved as if from within a suit of armor. His gait was bouncy with hip-hiking and toe-walking. Even movement capabilities he possessed (like swinging his arms in a circle) he could not use because of poor body awareness. Spinal curves (Figure 7.3a) were flattened with severe loss of segmental mobility. He had frequent complaints of headaches and stomachaches. Henry exhibited a flat affect, a monotone voice, and minimal facial expression. Breathing was shallow.

Treatment Focus

The focus of treatment was to develop movement capabilities in order to decrease motor restlessness. The supposition was that with more coordinated and fluid movement, motor restlessness would decrease with a release of soft tissue tensions. To address the structural dysfunction, craniosacral therapy, strain and counterstrain, myofascial release, and sensorimotor therapies were used.

Major Structural Changes Resulting from Therapy

The structural changes that have affected improvement in Henry's behaviors and movement capacity are:

a) greater and freer mobility of the entire spine

b) development of scapulothoracic mobility

c) improved mobility of the thoracic inlet (Figure 7.1) and respiratory diaphragms

d) decompression of the sphenobasilar junction with some resolution of a left lateral strain and an inferior vertical strain (Figure 7.9)

e) decompression of the temporal bones (Figure 7.5a) with noted increased rotary motion

f) improved alignment of the temporomandibular joints (Figure 7.5a)

g) significant improvement in craniosacral function

h) improved elasticity and flexibility of the fascia and dural membrane

i) decreased hypertonicity of the anterior neck muscles (Figure 7.3b)

j) significant alleviation of chronic paravertebral muscle spasms along the thoracic and lumbar vertebrae (Figure 7.2b). This latter was due in great part to a group home program of strain and counterstrain that was implemented twice weekly and then as needed.

Major Functional Changes Resulting from Structural Changes

Major Motor Changes.   Motor restlessness abated during the first year of a manual therapy approach with the initial release of the OA joints (Figure 7.2b), improved temporal bone (Figure 7.5a) function, and increased range of motion and vitality of the craniosacral rhythm. Pacing is essentially resolved; Henry even sits down to converse or have a soda. Rocking now tends to occur only with exacerbation of psychotic behaviors. Muscle guarding has essentially been eliminated from his profile, although high muscle tone remains. Dramatic changes are noted in his gait pattern: he is no longer hiking his hip or toe-walking, and arm swing has appeared. When rolling over he now uses segmental rolling patterns. Dissociation of movements between body parts (hip and knee, shoulder and pelvis) now occurs allowing for greater and safer dynamic balance. During activity of daily living tasks arms are functioning with greater ease. Adaptive movements are more spontaneous in response to his environment, and the rotational component of movement has appeared. Along with improved head/neck function, swallowing is easier at mealtime, and thoracic-abdominal breathing has improved with greater expansion of the rib cage.

What stands out since 1995 is a tremendous leap in proprioceptive awareness, contributed to by the decrease in chronic back spasms and subsequent improved vertebral mobility and craniosacral function. Henry is gaining an awareness of movement such that upon request and after a hands-on demonstration, he can perform trunk rotation, head/neck movements, and shoulder movements. He can now balance on one foot. Fluidity of movement and ranges of active motion are greatly improved.

Major Changes in Other Behaviors.   By the end of the second year of a manual therapy approach, the team nurse reported that Henry was essentially without complaint of headaches, and consequently the use of Tylenol dropped dramatically; also, complaints of stomachaches have subsided. Of note are Henry's comments during sessions: "I feel better." "My headache is gone." "Do more." In addition, his facial appearance is more expressive. Like Steve, despite motor restlessness, Henry stays for sessions, some as long as 90 minutes. Like Larry, when asked if therapy should continue or stop for the day, he says "more."

PERSPECTIVE

The functional performance of the adult with mental retardation is clearly improved using a structurally-based manual therapy approach. It can be concluded that at least some dysfunctional behaviors often displayed by these individuals—motor, social, self-injurious, perceptual—are due in part to structural imbalances rather than solely to mental deficiency. This therapeutic approach looks to treat structural causes as a basis of behaviors rather than treating the behaviors themselves as other approaches generally do. The objective is to provide the individual with a healthier structural foundation rather than solely adapting the environment to his or her needs or adapting the behaviors to the environment. Improvement of structural integrity will provide the individual with more options to respond to internal and external stimuli because a healthy structural framework is more adaptive, providing the individual with new potential for response. Thus, manual therapy differs from other approaches in that it is able to uncover underlying potential to support future changes in function because it addresses the relationship between structure and function.

Even if one comes to accept this essential relationship between structure and function, one must still overcome traditional views about adults with mental retardation. These views, unfortunately, foster the sense that these adults, because of inherent limitations, have little ability to change. However, as demonstrated, these individuals do, indeed, have untapped potential, and acknowledgement of this can lead directly to therapeutic intervention.

These ingrained views about mental retardation often interfere with the natural establishment of trust and communication in the treatment environment. Even deftly skilled therapists, when faced with an adult with mental retardation, fall back into "conventional wisdom" and assume there is little or nothing therapy can do for these individuals, or presume that adults with mental retardation cannot participate actively or even passively as we look to others to do. There is no expectation of comprehension. Yet, they come without bias or preconceived notions about therapy and readily perceive tissue movements and changes. They come because they develop trust in the therapist, and from there everything begins. I was lucky when I started learning manual therapy techniques, particularly craniosacral therapy, because I started with this population. I found in many of these clients that craniosacral rhythms were barely palpable. However, fresh from workshops, I applied these new skills and found that change is indeed possible, first structurally and then functionally. When I then started treating the "normal" population, I was clearly surprised because they already had "strong" craniosacral rhythms; they were just there. How could there be anything wrong? What I came to realize is the extreme nature of the dysfunctions with which I work. If I had started working with the "normal" population, I too may have palpated such gross dysfunction in the adult with mental retardation and mistakenly presumed that little could be done.

Stasis, however, is not an acceptable state for one's health and because potential to change is inherent in all individuals, if we find structural dysfunction, then we always have somewhere to begin and a reason to prescribe therapeutic intervention. Potential need not leap out at you, but it may occur in small packets of change. Change is facilitated by the therapist and is dependent on the individual's ability to trust him or herself to change.

Questions need to be shared and answers explored among the different professions to better understand the whole person and his or her needs. Traditionally, behavioral "symptoms" have been viewed and treated from behavioral and functional perspectives. Through a better understanding of the implications of structural imbalance, perhaps we can now facilitate more fundamental changes.

Some common areas of structural dysfunction that I have frequently observed in the adult with mental retardation are: the sphenobasilar junction (Figure 7.9), occipitoatlantal joints, sacrum, temporal bones, and frontal bone, (Figures 7.2, 7.5a). Hard palate (Figure 7.10) and pharyngeal space restrictions also appear as often does muscle guarding. The thread that seems to connect all of these is the fascia. The clinical impression is that the normal, balanced elasticity of the fascia and dural membrane system is lacking and that this fascial inflexibility distorts postural, sensory and proprioceptive functions. There is an apparent restriction or lack of internal mobility primarily of the fascial sheaths, the elastocollagenous complex (as proposed by Upledger & Vredevoogd, 1983) that supports locomotion and physiological health. It seems that function is not based solely on the integrity of joints and muscle but more on the integrity of the physical properties of soft tissue. Following the release of soft tissue restrictions with manual therapy techniques there is a potentiating of the internal structural environment which can lead to the (re)establishment of soft tissue mobility. It is presumed that what then follows is an internalized awareness by the individuals of a newly established balance from within which resolves or dissipates internal tissue tensions. They all seem to have a new sense of orientation/groundedness and movement based on this new internal balance. This balance is the mobility of the fascia, inclusive of the dura mater, which is essential for externally produced gross and fine motor movements. Without this flexibility, there is a presumed discomfort with the physical body due to the soft tissue restrictions; these, in and of themselves, may cause pain behaviors, lower tolerances, and result in distortions of responses to stimuli from the internal or external environment. Clinically, following treatment, proprioceptive sense seems heightened as it relates to body and self-awareness, and to spatial awareness and relations.

It is important to consider that the dysfunctional behaviors may be signs and symptoms of structural dysfunction placing the individual at a disadvantage to respond to and react to his or her environment. Manual therapy treatment techniques are able to normalize structural stresses, thereby unlocking latent potential for improved functional performance. This approach is of fundamental importance in the treatment of individuals with mental retardation and developmental disabilities in general.

ACKNOWLEDGEMENTS

I would like to give special thanks to Shirley Breuer, Charles Gilliam, and Marion Eagan for their time and comments on the chapter. And to Marion, for her generosity in sharing with me her knowledge and skills through so many years. To Tracy Simpson—whose excitement with learning has inspired me to look behind the obvious—for his stream of thought-provoking questions and for his assistance beyond any and all reasonable expectation.

Some of the material presented in this chapter is based upon data and interpretations originally presented by this author and published in *OT Practice 1*, 40–45 (November 1996).

REFERENCES

Alexander, R. (1988, September). Oral-motor treatment programming for the infant and young child with neuromotor involvement [course]. Marlborough, MA.

Alexander, R. (1988, November). Rib cage: focus on the rib cage for improvement in respiration/phonation, postural control and movement [course]. Milwaukee, WI.

Banus, B. S. (1971). *The developmental therapist.* Thorofare, NJ: Slack.

Barral, J. P. (1989). *Visceral manipulation II.* Seattle: Eastland Press.

Barral, J. P. (1991). *The thorax.* Seattle: Eastland Press.

Barral, J. P., & Mercier, P. (1988). *Visceral manipulation.* Seattle: Eastland Press.

Breuer, S. (1989, October). Muscle energy for the lower quadrant [course]. Hartford, CT.

Breuer, S. (1989, November). Muscle energy for the upper quadrant [course]. Hartford, CT.

Brown, R. (1993, April). Zero balancing I [course]. Hartford, CT.

Brown, R. (1994, March). Zero balancing II [course]. Hartford, CT.

Davidson, S. M. (1987). *Manual medicine: a primer.* Phoenix, AZ: Practical Publications.

Davidson, S. M. (1992). *Setting the fascia free.* Phoenix, AZ: Practical Publications.

Greenman, P. E. (1978). Manipulative therapy in relation to total health care. In I. M. Korr (Ed.), *The neurobiologic mechanisms in manipulative therapy* (pp. 43–52). New York: Plenum Press.

Greenman, P. E. (1989). *Principles of manual medicine.* Baltimore: Williams & Wilkins.

Heinrich, S. (January 1991). The role of physical therapy in craniofacial pain disorders: an adjunct to dental pain management. *Journal of Craniomandibular Practice, 9*(1), 71–75.

Hruby, R. J. (1994, November). Direct cranial osteopathy, craniosacral therapy—level I [course]. Hartford, CT.

Hruby, R. J. (1995, January). Direct cranial osteopathy, craniosacral therapy—level II [course]. Hartford, CT.

Jones, L. H. (1981). *Strain and counterstrain.* Indianapolis, IN: The American Academy of Osteopathy.

Jones, L. H., Kusunose, R., & Goering, E. (1995). *Jones: Strain-counterstrain.* Boise, ID: Jones Strain-Counterstrain, Inc.

Jones, L. H., & Wendorff, R. (1994, April). Strain and counterstrain, level I [course]. Sturbridge, MA.

Kain, J. (1996, March). Visceral manipulation Ia [course]. Hartford, CT.

King, L. J. (1974). A sensory-integrative approach to schizophrenia. *American Journal of Occupational Therapy, 28*(9), 529–536.

Korr, I. M. (1978). Sustained sympathicotonia as a factor in disease. In I. M. Korr (Ed.). *The neurobiologic mechanisms in manipulative therapy* (pp. 229–268). New York: Plenum Press.

Kraus, S. L. (1988). Cervical spine influences on the craniomandibular region. In S. L. Kraus (Ed.), *TMJ disorders: Management of the craniomandibular complex* (pp. 367–404). New York: Churchill Livingstone.

Kraus, S. L. (1989). Influences of the cervical spine on the stomatognathic system. In R. Donatelli & M. J. Wooden (Eds.), *Orthopaedic physical therapy* (pp. 59–70). New York: Churchill Livingstone.

Krieger, D. (1979). *The therapeutic touch.* New York: Prentice Hall Press.

Levy, L. L. (1974). Movement therapy for psychiatric patients. *The American Journal of Occupational Therapy, 28*(6), 354–357.

MacDonald, R. (1992, October). SER I [course]. Hartford, CT.

Mennell, J. M. (1992). *The musculoskeletal system: Differential diagnosis from symptoms and physical signs.* Gaithersburg, MD: Aspen.

Mitchell, F. L., Jr., Moran, P. S., & Pruzzo, N. A. (1979). *An evaluation and treatment manual of osteopathic muscle energy procedures.* Valley Park, MO: Mitchell, Moran and Pruzzo, Associates.

Ramirez, M. A., Haman, J., & Worth, L. (1989). Low back pain: Diagnosis by six newly discovered sacral tender points and treatment with counterstrain. *JAOA, 89* (7), 905–913.

Rocabado, M., Johnson, B. E. Jr., & Blakney, M. G. (1982–1983). Physical therapy and dentistry: An overview. *Journal of Craniomandibular Practice, 1*(1), 46–49.

Silver, F. H. (1987). *Biological materials: structure, mechanical properties, and modeling of soft tissues.* New York: New York University Press.

Simpson, L. (1996). Seeing the forest for the trees: Treating adults with mental retardation through structurally based manual therapy. *OT Practice, 1*(11), 40–45.

Smith, F. (1986). *Inner bridges: A guide to energy movement and body structure.* Atlanta, GA: Humanics Limited.

Smith, F. (1996, November). Alchemy of touch [course]. Hartford, CT.

Summerfelt, M. (1991, September). Manual therapy for the pediatric patient [course]. Farmington, CT.

Tehan, P. F. (1980). Functional technique: A different perspective in manipulative therapy. In E. F. Glasgow, L. T. Twomey, E. R. Skull, & A. M. Kleynhans (Eds.). *Aspects of manipulative therapy* (pp. 94–96). Melbourne, Australia: Churchill Livingstone.

Upledger, J. E. (1987). *Craniosacral therapy II: Beyond the dura.* Seattle, WA: Eastland Press.

Upledger, J. E. (1990). *Somatoemotional release and beyond.* Palm Beach Gardens, FL: UI Publishing.

Upledger, J. E., & Vredevoogd, J. D. (1983). *Craniosacral therapy.* Seattle, WA: Eastland Press.

Weiselfish, S. (1994). *Manual therapy with muscle energy technique for the pelvis, sacrum, cervical, thoracic & lumbar spine.* West Hartford, CT: ANA Publishing.

Weiselfish, S. (1996, June). Visceral manipulation Ib [course]. Waterbury, CT.

Weiselfish, S. & Kain, J. (1990). Introduction to developmental manual therapy: An integrated systems approach for structural and functional rehabilitation. *Physical Therapy Forum, 9*(6), 1, 3–5.

Weiselfish, S. & Kain, J. (1991, June). Myofascial release [course]. Hartford, CT.

Weiselfish, S. & Kain, J. (1993, December). Manual therapy for craniocervical, craniofacial, and craniomandibular pain and dysfunction [course]. Hartford, CT.

8

Let's Do Lunch: A Comprehensive Nonstandardized Assessment Tool

Susan Bachner, MA, OTR/L, FAOTA

INTRODUCTION

"Let's Do Lunch" is a nonstandardized assessment tool based on mealtime activities. The chapter first relates this assessment tool to the managed care environment, an environment that increasingly dominates the provision of health care and related services. Adults with developmental disabilities or the therapists working with them are not immune to the need for cost-containment and outcomes accountability, hallmarks of the managed care movement.

Next, the sociological attributes of food-related activities, important to the understanding of the "Let's Do Lunch" assessment tool, are described, providing an overview of the thousands of years of culture, custom, attitudes, and values that are intertwined with all aspects of food. This should help the reader understand why lunch, in particular, is employed as the vehicle for this structured observation.

Finally, the "Let's Do Lunch" assessment tool is presented. Although the author recommends reading the entire chapter as presented, some may wish to immediately proceed to the last section ("Let's Do Lunch"—A Tool To Study the Interaction Between Social, Psychological and Biological Determinants) that describes the assessment tool in detail, provides illustrative case examples, and discusses the value of using such a tool (see Appendix A for the task analysis assessment tool).

SERVICE DELIVERY IN A MANAGED-CARE ENVIRONMENT

Managed care, in its various formats, now dominates the current health care market. Managed care, which emerged in response to spiraling costs of health care for industry, government, and the public, has been defined by Inglehart as a system that integrates the financing and delivery of health care through selective contracting with providers who agree to provide comprehensive health care services to enrolled members for a predetermined premium (Inglehart, 1994). An additional feature is the modification of provider behavior by financial incentives to reduce the utilization of and access to services.

Managed care, therefore, places primary emphasis on the value of services delivered and, in effect, defines value as the ratio of quality to costs. At present, the highly competitive and profit-driven managed care marketplace emphasizes cost containment and may be described as a price-driven free-fall. However, growing consumer backlash and government interventions are causing demands for higher levels of accountability and a renewed concern for quality of care.

This renascent quality initiative has merged with several other trends to produce a new interest in health care outcomes management and research. These other trends include

- the work of John Wennberg and his colleagues at Dartmouth University, demonstrating profound variations in regional practice without demonstrable differences in patient outcomes (Wennberg, 1991)
- the studies of David Eddy, demonstrating uncertainty about the value of widely accepted medical therapies (Eddy, 1991)
- the efforts by the RAND Corporation and others, demonstrating high frequencies of unneeded and inappropriate care (Chassin, 1996).

Process and Outcome

These initiatives have culminated in a growing interest on the part of managed care organizations, providers, the academic community, health care agencies (both public and private), and the government to link the structure and process of health care to definable and measurable patient outcomes (Donabedian, 1988; Ellwood, 1988). In this context, an outcome may be considered to be the result of a process or treatment (JCAHO, 1994). According to Rogers and Holm, "the focus on functional outcomes is critical because it targets attention appropriately on the patient" (Rogers & Holm, 1994, p. 871). Rogers and Holm refer to Relman's article in the *New England Journal of Medicine* and share his belief that the public's growing concern over the quality and cost of American health care make this an era of "assessment and accountability" (Relman, 1988, p. 1220). To rephrase in terms of process and outcome, *process* is the attempt to do things the "right way," and *outcomes* emphasize doing the "right thing."

Occupational therapists, like to other health care professionals, must be accountable for what they do, why it is being done, what the outcomes are, and what resources are required.

Outcomes Defined by Different Constituencies

Outcomes may reflect clinical events, patient experience, or administrative or fiscal attributes. An occupational therapy outcome is the functional consequence for the client, resulting from therapeutic actions provided by an occupational therapist. However, in the marketplace at large, it is important to understand that conventional measurements of outcomes have been based on the five Ds:

- death
- disease
- disability
- discomfort
- dissatisfaction.

These categories may be partially mapped to five basic dimensions:

- clinical results
- functional status
- well-being
- satisfaction
- cost.

These dimensions are emphasized differently, depending on the point of reference. Payers tend to focus on cost, practitioners on clinical results, and consumers on functional status and well-being.

In selecting outcomes for clients or patients, occupational therapists need to settle on those that carry a reasonable expectation of change—change that is functional and subscribed to by the individual engaged in the treatment process. "Let's Do Lunch" enables the therapist to observe behavior and understand it (in part, as a manifestation of the underlying performance components), to evaluate behavior within the context of what has meaning and value to the client (as described in sociological and psychological terms), and finally, to arrive at mutually agreeable goals or outcomes. It is easier, perhaps, for occupational therapists to collaborate on goals or outcomes that are meaningful to the client than it is for other medical specialists, because of the profession's emphasis on function. As Wetzler suggests, individuals are concerned with their own functional status and well-being (Wetzler, 1994).

Occupational Therapy Outcomes

With occupational therapy services, the "outcome is the functional consequence for the patient of the therapeutic action implemented by an occupational therapist" (Rogers & Holm, 1994). Within the occupational therapy profession, Forer speaks about occupational therapy evaluation and outcome and notes there is "the temptation of many practitioners to use refined clinical measures, such as range of motion, muscle strength as measured by a dynamometer, endurance, lifting and reaching capacity, rather than measuring the actual functional outcome [that is, independence in activities of daily living, return to work or former lifestyle, quality of life and general health perception—SB]. Although increased ROM, muscle strength and endurance, sensory and motor function, and cognitive and psychosocial function are all important, the key question is what is the patient able to do as a result of these increased skills. Furthermore, if an increase of 10 percent in ROM does not appear to make any difference in a patient's ability to dress or feed himself or herself, then the intervention may not be perceived as cost-effective by those paying for services. Care should be taken in identifying the expected outcomes and measures for occupational therapy" (Forer, 1996, p. 4). "Let's Do Lunch" is a tool to quickly assist the therapist in this process for it

> ▌gives a snapshot of all the performance components working or not working in synergy for adaptive responses

▮ reflects life-long cultural issues

▮ offers a built-in list of appropriate outcome items.

Distinguishing Between Clinical and
Client-Referenced Outcomes

The need and importance of knowing client values and preferences are well documented in the literature and directly influence the likelihood of achieving patient satisfaction outcomes. Concern with quality of life issues is finding center stage. However, it is important to clarify that there are, indeed, two discrete paradigms in the spotlight and each reflects a distinction between clinical and patient-referenced outcomes. In their 1995 presentation in the *Journal of the American Medical Association* of a conceptual model of patient outcomes, Wilson and Cleary describe two different models: one held by clinicians and basic science researchers, and the other by social scientists. "The models of these two academic traditions differ in purpose, methods, and intellectual history" (Wilson & Cleary, 1995). For instance, in the clinical or biomedical paradigm, the focus or outcome is framed in biological, physiological, and clinical measurements. "In contrast, the social science paradigm, or the quality of life model, focuses on dimensions of functioning and overall well-being, and current research examines ways to accurately measure complex behaviors and feelings" (Wilson & Cleary, 1995). These models of health have their foundations in sociology and psychology. However, the concept of quality of life, although related, can be distinct.

Silberman, in "From the Patient's Bed," refers to the patients who are often misjudged by the professionals who "treat" them. "Such misjudgments are rooted in an enormous gulf between the way physicians think about disease and the way patients experience it" (Silberman, 1991). To illustrate the point, he presents the *Merck Manual*'s definition of multiple sclerosis (MS) as "a slowly progressive CNS disease characterized by disseminated patches of demyelination in the brain and spinal cord, resulting in multiple and varied neurologic symptoms and signs, usually with remissions and exacerbations" (Silberman, 1991). The response of someone who has MS is illustrative: "What I experience every day is not the demyelination in the white matter of the nervous system. . . . The ongoing and seemingly relentless diminishment of physical abilities which is surely, but gradually eroding my independence. . . . For me, multiple sclerosis is the constant effort to overcome my body's resistance so that I can carry out the most mundane activities, the frustration of not being able to do the simplest of things, . . . and the anguished uncertainty of a perilous future" (Silberman, 1991).

In listening to this narrative, one is struck by the two-pronged description of multiple sclerosis; yet, the medical definition juxtaposed with the human experience is a challenge occupational therapists face routinely, regardless of the populations served. Occupational therapists come to the marketplace with a studied understanding of the significance of function and independence in daily living as well as a medical orientation. In establishing occupational therapy outcomes, the clinical reasoning process must accommodate both.

Need for Determining a Course of Action for Individuals With Profound and Multiple Developmental Disabilities

In working with adults with developmental disabilities that range from severe and profound to mild, how does the therapist, an agent for change, determine a course of action that produces a functional outcome having relevance to the client, as well as to the other outcome dimensions of

- clinical results
- functional status
- well-being
- satisfaction
- cost?

If the client (who may have significant cognitive deficits) is also nonverbal or hampered by any number of communication impairments, what then? How are we therapists to get a quick glimpse into his or her value system, customs, attitudes, and preferences that are the substratums for quality of care outcomes? Information gleaned from medical histories, physical exams, range of motion, and so forth is readily available. Often, the problem is to identify what constitutes an individual's quality of care and client satisfaction determinants. Assessing that information quickly and accurately is the task.

The Value in Nonstandardized Assessment Tools

Standardized tests for adults with developmental disabilities do not yield the information needed for a variety of reasons. By definition, a standardized test works with criteria and parameters that have been carefully established with rigid rules during test development. In order to determine what it would take in the form of cues to move a client to a higher level of expression and performance, the therapist cannot maintain the testing atmosphere and environment for which the scores were referenced. For example, it might be necessary for a therapist to provide additional cues, adaptations, and time in order to elicit optimal performance; these accommodations would violate the standard procedures and compromise the standard scores. In addition, standardized tests do not allow for individual client expression about the social qualifiers that identify a person's uniqueness.

Caplan and Shecter take the position that there is a critical difference between testing and evaluation: testing is viewed by them as essentially a "mechanical enterprise" (Caplan & Shecter, 1995). "Evaluation is, by contrast, an art applied on an individual basis that involves not only testing skills, but also professional creativity, observational expertise, flexibility, and ingenuity in the service of developing a multidimensional understanding of patients— their abilities and deficits, their emotional state, self-regulatory functions, the impact of environmental variables on test performance, and so forth" (Caplan & Shecter, 1995). In their chapter on "The Role of Nonstandard Neuropsychological Assessment in Rehabilitation: History, Rationale, and Examples," they attempt to enlighten clinicians so as to "avoid this kind of psychometric showdown by viewing the evaluation process in a less con-strained manner." They refer to Lezak's 1983 text that "noted that two particular patient populations, the elderly and 'the severly handicapped patient,' might require special testing procedures" (Caplan & Shecter, 1995). It is of interest that, although they feel that adjustments might appear in the neuropsychological testing procedures, they believe it is still possible to adhere to the essential standardized features of the test. While I personally have not found that to be the case when working with individuals having severe and profound deficits, these and other authors represent that view-point. Perhaps some of the differences in opinion relate to disparate testing and evaluation goals, dissimilar consumer presentations, severity of deficits, or locus of client dysfunction, that is, *impairment* versus *disability*. Rogers and Holm refer to impairment as a "dysfunction at the level of an organ or system," while disability is defined as "dysfunction in task performance." (Rogers & Holm, 1994). Lyzette Kautzmann builds on this conceptualization, stating that symptom status or impairment level problems (performance components) may lead to a disability or disturbance in func-tional status (performance areas) that may, in turn, lead to a handicap or social role disruption, affecting a person's overall quality of life (Kautz-mann, 1997).

"Let's Do Lunch": A Model for Combining Quality of Care, Client Satisfaction, and Payer Acceptance

Why concentrate on mealtime in an occupational therapy screening or evaluation? When one considers some of the inherent qualities that begin with the ability to understand the human biological drive for food, as well as the large cultural domain that reflects complex systems of significance, rituals, and meaning, the answer becomes clear. People, indeed, must eat to survive. Their concerns about food, however, expand and assume considerably more than the biological reality (Maurer & Sobal, 1995).

"Let's Do Lunch," a nonstandardized assessment for adults with developmental disabilities, administered during mealtime, was devised to deal with the challenges of combining quality of care, client satisfaction, and payer acceptance. It is based on structured observation. It addresses the respective influences of the performance components listed in the American Occupational Therapy Association's (AOTA) *Uniform Terminology*: the human abilities that, in a variety of combinations and discrete operations, form the foundations for performance areas. Typically, these components are considered to be

- sensory
- perceptual
- neuromuscular
- motor
- cognitive
- psychosocial.

In addition, "Let's Do Lunch" simultaneously allows for freedom of expression to address the social and cultural issues that can have a profound effect on the client's overall satisfaction. "Interestingly . . . lower levels of functional status are not necessarily related to lower levels of satisfaction" (Wilson & Cleary, 1995). It cannot be overemphasized that the two areas of concern—the performance components and the human experience—must merge at the time of assessment. Both functional status and level of satisfaction must be addressed. "Let's Do Lunch," despite its simplicity in design, is one way to accomplish this objective.

RELATING THE SOCIOLOGY OF FOOD TO THE OCCUPATIONAL THERAPY TREATMENT ARENA

In order to gain a more complete understanding of the "Let's Do Lunch" assessment tool, it is appropriate to explore the sociology of food. The cultivation, preparation, and consumption of food involve thousands of years of culture, custom, attitudes, and values that can be analyzed in terms of division of labor, power, or gender roles, not to mention celebrations, culinary choices, rituals, dietary rules, and so forth. It becomes a very long list.

Performance Components that Emerge at Mealtime

Mealtime behaviors include and are partly driven by sensory, perceptual, neuromuscular, motor, cognitive, and psychosocial components. As Judith Goode writes, "food is both physically manipulated to feed us and intellectually manipulated to refer metaphorically to important aspects of existence. The unique, incorporative nature of eating makes food an important sacred and social symbol" (Goode, 1992). While a person's sensory, cognitive, physical, and emotional state interact with what occurs at mealtime, these individual components are always in a dialogue with tradition and animate and inanimate props in the surrounding environment. These props, with their range of calming to noxious elements, exert their own powerful influences. It is through a discussion of some of the mixtures of these essential ingredients associated with mealtime that "Let's Do Lunch" takes on its significant linkage to functional outcomes and managed care, including the setting of purposeful goals, quality services, and cost containment.

Social Status Demonstrated at Mealtime

One of the areas of interest to sociologists is social status and how it is conveyed in cultures. Of issue here is the awareness that food items can reflect a particular social status and are often selected accordingly. Pheasant under glass or certain wine selections speak to one end of the spectrum, while a soup may represent the opposite. While Goode speaks about certain food items as conveyors of status (Goode, 1992), my experience within facilities serving people with developmental disabilities suggests that status is perhaps marked more frequently by the individual's ability to communicate and exercise opportunities for additional portions or choices. Additionally, there are customs intertwined with pecking order rules that dictate the proper approach for acquiring additional food. It is of interest that "in Denmark, it is customary to ask for more, in Ireland second helpings are a must, in Bulgaria you are warned to take small portions and will be expected to eat several" (Marshall, 1995). In institutional settings, people sometimes grab additional portions when customs, communication, and other problems, such as inability to inhibit or poor impulse control, dominate the moment.

Gender- and Age-related Issues Expressed at Mealtime

Selection is also influenced by gender and age. A study referenced by Goode indicates that, in public settings where food choices were open, men's and women's choices differ distinctly. In family restaurants, food choices reportedly cluster to age (Goode, 1992).

Cognitive Functioning Observed at Mealtime

Level of cognitive functioning, I find, is also a factor in some behavioral responses observed at mealtime. Similarly, more complex levels of food presentation (dishes, meal structures, and cycles) engaged in by "higher level" clients, transmit noteworthy social and cultural messages.

Mealtime exhibits a temporal aspect. One often observes a client whose functioning is punctuated by intrusions from profound problems, who is still able to anticipate an upcoming meal or snack. Ordinary meal cycles mark regular activity and leisure cycles. In *Food Choice and the Consumer* M. Douglas notes: "While there is a broad range of content negotiation within the meal the format remains fixed, and it appears the structure per se is actually more important in the choice process than the contents" (Marshall, 1995). Judith Goode speaks of the significance of special food events that historically mark major breaks in productivity: weekends, harvests, successful hunts. (Goode, 1992). Well-known, too, are get-togethers at Sunday brunch, special parties, banquets, and other events. These and other celebratory temporal markers are certainly present at day programs, residential settings, group homes, sheltered workshops, and in virtually any environment that serves people with or without developmental disabilities.

Organizational Skills—Teasing Out the Scripted Cultural Rules vs. Individualized Choices

How foods and meals are organized, and the individual's involvement in the "doing," provide insight into mealtime activities. There are rules for appropriate compositions of a meal; dishes must be organized in time sequences or spatial arrangements to constitute a meal. Meals and, indeed, feasts follow a scripted sequence. In what order are dishes presented? If presented simultaneously, as in a cafeteria, does that order persist? Soups first and sweets or nuts last finds expression in the cliche: "from soup to nuts." If an individual undergoing evaluation eats dessert first as a deliberate choice, then that may be noteworthy. I have witnessed this many times and noted it as an aberration to convention. Although it is difficult to make conclusions about the causes, some possible reasons warranting further investigation might include sensory preferences (taste), cultural factors (lack of socialization to rules), or cognitive factors (sequencing deficits). The therapist documenting this information might best use it later, when reviewing patterns of scoring, to identify and prioritize areas of concern and decide whether anything, if at all, is necessary for remediation.

Rules About Eating Utensils vs. Using One's Hands

Eating with the hands is generally discouraged in Western society. According to David Marshall, "in cultures where it is practised it becomes an art form in its own right signifying informality and social intimacy." He says later, "these unspoken rules about how food should be eaten are found across cultures and they can be a source of embarrassment for the uninitiated— eating is also about etiquette" (Marshall, 1995).

Social Boundaries Conveyed by Food "Rules"

Relationships between individuals and groups can be viewed as being controlled by rules for food; they have the ability to define inclusion, encourage discipline, and assist with the maintenance of social boundaries. It is the rare adult with developmental disabilities, no matter how low the IQ measures, who does not understand that there is a "staff" breakroom that is "off-limits." Whether the door is locked or not is of little significance; there is an awareness that staff enters freely and clients do not.

Food transactions describe a great deal; the food giving and food receiving relationships are notches of position in the food chain. The "haves" and "have-nots" in a total system are clearly defined by a variety of symbols. This is true for any such system, whether it be an institution serving adults with developmental disabilities, the army, or any other setting that has the capability or responsibility for total care. The holder of the key to the kitchen is in a position of power, while KP duty is interpreted as low status or punishment.

Messages Conveyed Through Diets, Food Consistency, and Preferences

Across cultures, children's food tends to be easy to chew and digest. What messages are imparted when adults are given pureed foods? It cannot be assumed that a person with profound cognitive deficits has no awareness of what another is served. I have witnessed disdain, envy, anger, and agitation when one individual notices and covets another's meal. The recognition of the differences between his or her own and the others' meal carries meaning. Further, the study of food preferences has been well researched, with consistent results showing that food preferences have a distinct foundation in sensory preferences. It is entirely possible that someone with pureed food at a table with another eating a regular diet may begin to demonstrate negative behaviors associated with a) dissatisfaction over the recognition that things are different, and b) the deprivations caused by pureed foods that starve the individual's sensory diet of tactile, olfactory, or gustatory input.

Ethnicity and Food Preparation

While it is almost common knowledge to remark that food items are associated with ethnic groups, it is perhaps more significant and less well known that ethnicity is revealed by the complex rules for how to prepare the items and when to eat. "Many people in the United States eat as many bagels as Jewish-Americans or as much pasta as Italian-Americans, but they do not follow the rules for how to prepare these foods, when and with whom to eat them, and how they should be served" (Goode, 1992). In working with clients in a cooking group, who were born and raised in the mountain culture of eastern Kentucky, I found it was not enough to have eggs and bacon and margarine. To be true to the mountain culture, lard and biscuits were essential ingredients in this "All-American" breakfast meal.

Significance and Power of Timing and Belief Systems Associated with Mealtime

Controlling when one should actually begin eating, the pace of eating, and how much one consumes—all these can communicate messages about personal traits, previous experiences, and group affiliations.

The power of believing can surface in and around mealtime. If one believes that he or she will be healed, be sickened, or find comfort by ingesting certain food items, it may well happen. The following was overheard in Harlan County, KY: "You know, turtles have all kinds of meat in 'em, chicken, duck, fish, cow, hog, and every kind of meat there are, and make awful good eating" (Bronner, 1986). To others from another locale, this diet would be considered inedible or worse! Refusal to eat certain foods or, alternatively, craving for certain foods may be traced to the power of believing. The therapist should consider this during the evaluation stage.

Placement of Food Items as an Indicator

The positioning of food items reflect still more rules. For those who have difficulty in or reluctance to moving their hands across their bodies at midline, customary positioning of foods becomes dysfunctional. Self-styled modifications will give insights into sources of difficulties or demonstrate a level of adaptability.

Mealtime Communications—Verbal and Nonverbal; Subtle Role Definitions

During the act of eating, whether defined as a "power lunch," "tea for two," "dinner dance," or "pot-luck dinner," there is an opportunity to communicate appropriate role behavior. In our roles as participants and therapists, we are able to engage in this communication. We are able to learn through listening and observing and interacting. Nonverbal communication speaks the loudest. In the preface to *Mealtimes for Persons with Severe Handicaps*, the editors (Perske, Clifton, McLean, & Stein, 1986) recount a mealtime during which they were to simulate being "handicapped" for the duration:

> I learned that it's hard eating my meals when I couldn't do it myself. Its harder when I'm not able to speak for myself: to tell others what I want to eat next, what I don't want to eat, and to say, "Slow down!" It could be maddening when a certain movement of hands, arms, lips, jaws, tongue or swallowing mechanism began to trip over itself and mess up what was intended to be a beautifully orchestrated sequence of actions. It ripped at everything I am or could be when the person helping me eat was uptight and rushed. Once I received a little respect from my "feeder." He never knew I didn't respect him either. On the other hand, it might not be an picnic helping me to eat. Mealtimes like this can be tough on everybody (Perske et al., 1986, p. xix).

Relationship of Quality of Life to Mealtime

Of note here is Perske's estimation that in excess of 80 percent of people with severe handicaps do not experience relaxed, human communion types of meals comparable to those described by individuals without handicaps. For each culture, there is an ideal mealtime experience. Many of us could provide a clear description of one that incorporates our own values, rules, customs, and parameters for sensory equilibrium. While Perske's statistics describe an alarming percentage of people who represent deviation from the ideal, it is perhaps incumbent upon us, as occupational therapists, to offer the managed care health market a wake-up call about what we can offer to quality of life issues. Mealtime, in particular, is laden with issues that directly relate to quality of life or client satisfaction. Occupational therapists have the professional training to examine a mealtime and to modify it to achieve desired outcomes, to look at variations from the norm and to analyze those differences in terms of a person's handicapping condition. The functional status, therefore, can be jeopardized by either internal or external challenges, or both; the everpresent social overlays influence outcome as well.

"LET'S DO LUNCH"—A TOOL TO STUDY THE INTERACTION BETWEEN SOCIAL, PSYCHOLOGICAL, AND BIOLOGICAL DETERMINANTS

"To study a person's food-related behavior is to study the interaction of a person's social, psychological, and biological needs" (Axelson & Brinberg, 1989). They continue with a discussion of how a social psychologist views the *effect of culture* on behavior (the beliefs, preferences, and attitudes of the individual), whereas an anthropologist views culture as a *direct determinant* or explanation of an individual's behavior.

An occupational therapist, with the "Let's Do Lunch" assessment, is able to merge the two positions, to see people as expressing their individual histories and narratives, as well as reflecting a cultural legacy through their behavior. At mealtime, the therapist is able to observe behaviors, rules, gender, age, and other issues that are passed down from previous generations or significant others. This is what the sociologist and social psychologist address. Paradoxically, to observe and study environment and culture as *determinants* of behavior is what the anthropologist views as important. The expression "institutionalized behaviors" is an example of the anthropological frame of reference.

Another dimension is created by the occupational therapists's unique training with underlying performance components, as described in *Uniform Terminology for Occupational Therapy, 3rd ed.* (AOTA, 1994). This enables an expansion of the notion of culture as a determinant for individual and group behavior; it introduces the dimension of physiological determinants. "Let's Do Lunch" is a tool that structures observations and quickly permits the therapist to tease out, within the evaluation process, the individual's unique presentation as both a cause for and result of behavior, as well as to understand the significant influences of underlying performance components. What comes to mind is a recipe that might read as follows:

▮ mix an individual's unique presentation that is the sum of interactions from his or her physical and psychological history

▮ place this into a mold in the shape of current surroundings

▮ position it in living space and leave at room temperature, to enable a pattern of synergies to occur

▮ meanwhile, set the table for a dialogue between therapist and client

▮ when ready, subject the product to a "taste test"

▮ decide what would improve the ingredients, conditions, process, and taste, articulating some functional outcomes.

Context in Which "Let's Do Lunch" Was Developed

Adults with developmental disabilities come in all textures and, while all have needs and wants, only some are able to effectively express them. If all could find the words to relate their vestibular needs, their visual deficits, and their wonderment at the ramifications of cause and effect, assessments would indeed be a "piece of cake." Yet, the reality is that many juggle components of physical, emotional, motor, visual, and other sensory deficits that are, in part, not self-comprehended nor offered to the team in a neat package. The kaleidoscopic patterns of presentations require a professional to properly identify the contours and significance of the various performance components. The occupational therapists's eye, having been structured and trained to observe both the individual elements and the gestalt, is able to simultaneously assess the participant's strengths and needs, and establish functional outcomes with enduring capabilities.

"Let's Do Lunch" captures the client's strengths and needs in perceptual, neuromuscular, sensorimotor, psychosocial, and physical areas. The surrounding mealtime issues—already described—provide the stage on which the occupational therapy performance and contextual components present themselves and interact.

In his preface to *Mealtimes for Persons With Severe Handicaps*, Perske notes:

> It had to be written, this book on mealtime experiences for seriously handicapped persons. Too many voices across the nation have said so. This may come as a surprise to those who wouldn't expect such a subject to be interesting reading. ... They [the contributors to his book—SB] recalled that mealtimes weren't seen as heroic or interesting at institutions where they worked. That was the time when almost all of the institution's staff left the grounds to fill the community's restaurants, leaving 'the ignoble task of feeding' to a few aides. Or it was the time when the community professionals stayed away from the homes because, as one nurse stated, "There wasn't anything therapeutic about that hectic time." But a new interest in these mealtimes is emerging. There is an upsurge in training opportunities that can lead to increased mealtime sensitivities and skills" (Perske et al., 1986).

While in complete agreement with Perske's insights regarding training opportunities at mealtime, "Let's Do Lunch" is based on the expanded belief that *evaluation* opportunities exist at mealtime. These evaluation opportunities are as varied and satisfying as an extravagant smorgasbord. Sensory development, social and emotional growth, self-help skills, fine and gross motor development, and decision making, flavored by culture, values, and all the other elements of a sociological perspective, offer a feast of material that meets the criteria associated with managed care, functional outcome, and quality care within a time-specific period.

Why Mealtime is the Perfect Activity for Evaluation Purposes

> For the occupational therapist, mealtime is one of those "perfect" activities— everything needed in a comprehensive evaluation is available to the trained eye and ear. For the client, the evaluation is synonymous with the everyday activity of lunch. Any anxieties associated with testing or assessment situations are rare or nonexistent. The client usually views the interaction as a social one—after all, we're "doing lunch!"

> There are times, nonetheless, when a therapist may choose to remain outside of direct interaction with the client, because the individual, so starved for

attention, processes the contact in an all consuming manner. The client's riveting reaction can skew and overshadow the usual behaviors available for observation and could easily become counter-productive to the ultimate goal of the assessment. The therapist would do well to borrow the "participant-observation" methodology from the anthropologist's repertoire.

Participant-Observation Methodology

Participant-observation is rooted in an 18th century technique that assumes it is possible for a person to be able to enter into, explore, and understand the distinctive experiences of others. The investigator participates as a member of the group being studied. Participant observers are sometimes known by the group members to be observers, though they join in the activity as well as assume the obligations of a member. In other situations, the observer is thought to be an ordinary member and the group members are simply not aware that they are being observed. This concept was introduced in 1925 by E.C. Lindeman in his book, *Social Discovery* (Lindeman, 1925).

Because we cannot truly enter into the mind or body of another person, the observer must bring to the encounter a skill level and focused inquiry that differentiates him or her from the casual observer; that is to say that the therapist-observer must have the perspective and capability to ask the significant question(s). "Let's Do Lunch" is an example of this approach.

■ It structures and prompts the therapist to be an observer.
■ It enables the therapist to ask the significant questions relating to performance components and environment.
■ It enables the therapist to enter into a nonverbal dialogue.
■ It enables the therapist to move from total participation to separation, in a wax-and-wane pattern, in order to find the "just-right" distance that allows for both an empathic and objective position.

In other words, the therapist must assume a position as close to center stage as possible, without a disruption of the authenticity of the environment. The environment, rules, and expectations are certainly familiar; a meal is something that the clients know they can count on. It is the rare resident who does not know how to find the dining room or is unaware that food is available if certain sequences can be mastered. Variations on the theme of food procurement are what becomes "food for thought" to the observing therapist.

In defining food-related behaviors, it can be described simply as what people do; their actions towards food. "People can consume food, sell food, buy food, throw food, use food as a weapon, and perform a host of other actions toward foods" (Axelson & Brinberg, 1989).

The Application of Clinical Reasoning

Observing client behaviors becomes the basis of a chain of critical reasoning steps. The therapist's trained eye begins to analyze, make inferences, checks them out for their reproducibility, and begins to understand which circumstances result in which behaviors. The therapist gathers evidence to identify and record what influences (biological or social) configure with the observations noted as significant. Throughout the entire process of the "Let's Do Lunch" assessment, the underlying concern of the therapist is to attempt to determine what it takes to facilitate optimal functioning in each of the performance components. What type of cueing or "seasoning" will it take to produce in an individual an outcome showing less restriction or a higher level of performance? As discussed at the outset of this chapter, in a managed care environment, the social science or quality of life model operates with attributes of functioning—the little things that constitute a foundation for higher levels—and our value, as clinicians, is to quickly ascertain for the record what those attributes are for each client in our care. Under what circumstances will the client be less at risk for injury and more likely to achieve health? What information can be passed along to others in this person's support system that describe the personal textures as well as needs and wants? Delegating routine and nonskilled treatment strategies to others is cost-effective, but plans must be clearly presented.

Changing the Conditions to Improve Performance

Joan Toglia discusses "The Dynamic Interactional Approach" and assessment in her *AOTA Self-Study Chapter on Cognitive Rehabilitation* (Toglia, 1993). She describes the approach as seeking "to examine the extent to which task performance can be changed by determining which conditions increase or decrease symptoms." Further, she "emphasizes how the individual goes about performing the task rather than the task itself. In contrast, conventional standardized tests are designed to identify and quantify the deficit" (Toglia, 1993). During an assessment, the dynamic interactional approach, similar to participant-observation, has attributes of awareness questioning, strategy investigation, task grading, and response to cueing.

These concepts are at the core of "Let's Do Lunch." Because this is a nonstandardized tool, it is perfectly acceptable and indeed desirable to interact, to cue, to suggest, to experiment, to experience pleasure, to find something mutually amusing and, if possible, to laugh. Remember Perkse's statistic that only about 20 percent of people with handicapping conditions find mealtime at all pleasurable! Besides, with defenses down, reliable information flows.

A Description of "Let's Do Lunch"

The residential facility where I work and where I developed the "Let's Do Lunch" tool, serves 180 adults with developmental disabilities. Their diagnoses range from mild to severe retardation and many carry dual diagnoses. Everyone is ambulatory some with mobility aids, and no one is on feeding tubes. "Let's Do Lunch" is a task analysis of 60 steps that follows a person from the starting point of entering the dining room to the end point of locating the exit in order to leave. Most everyone exhibits a variety of conditions; no one has challenges limited to only cognitive deficits. The 60 steps track mealtime at this facility. The task analysis, if it is to be of value to others in different environments, can be constructed to reflect alternative settings.

Scoring the Assessment

In addition to the "personalized" task analysis, there is a rating system of 0 to 3, where 0 signifies independence, while 1–3 indicates the type of cueing or assist required:

- 1 for verbal
- 2 for physical
- 3 for total assist.

Not applicable, NA, is always an option. If used, however, a clarifying statement is appropriate. For instance, "9. Sees Food Items," may score NA, if the client is blind or has marked visual deficits.

"Lets Do Lunch" is scored subjectively by the therapist, who uses observational skills to examine and note an individual's responses to each subskill. It is a time to comment on the individual's functional status and quality of life issues.

Each of the six scoring codes represents a performance component:

■ sensory
■ perceptual
■ neuromuscular
■ motor
■ cognitive
■ psychosocial.

Performance components are checked selectively and reflect, in the final analysis, an assessment of strengths and needs. It is entirely possible that summary recommendations from the assessment may lead to referrals for services with *others* on the team, such as an ophthalmologist, physical therapist, or neurologist. A therapist's comments on any item can be noted in the space below the action, and therapists are urged to use this space to describe how a client performs. If a client displays some dysfunction, whether or not the task is completed, a score is given. There are situations when performance components need not be marked, such as if the task item is completed or the functional outcome achieved. However, narrative comments entered below the item are often helpful and are factored into the final summary.

Sometimes, I have paused in a deliberation over the significance of an observation. Should it be recorded? Is it part of an unfolding pattern, or simply an insignificant aberration? Is it merely a quirk that has no ultimate significance? It is a hard call until all the data are in. Sometimes, the entry of a question mark is used, instead of a check under a performance component. This simply reflects that the therapist feels uncertain about the area that underlies the difficulty or inability to perform the task. All these notations and marks contribute to the picture that comes together at the end.

My overall experience suggests that it is far easier to disregard superfluous information in the final analysis than it is to try to reconstruct subtle points that occurred along the way. There should be adequate information to allow the therapist to synthesize and summarize. Checks in the performance component columns are summarized to indicate specific areas in which the client shows both strengths and needs. Patterns of strengths, deficits, and question marks are noted, and these contribute to the analysis of the patterns of scoring. The component(s) that received the most checks, because of difficulty in execution, may become a ready-made "functional outcome" for needs-driven goal setting. Question marks may be factored into the final analysis and carry weight as well. Notations in the form of "0" scores, indicating independence, or narrative comments about strengths are extremely helpful when the time comes to identify strengths onto which treatment strategies are built.

It is important to reiterate that, in almost each of the 60 items listed, there are elements of *all* performance components. The therapist needs to note those task items that are problem areas so that further investigation and outcome formulations may be initiated. Clarifications are always helpful in the execution of the recording. For example, if a client had difficulty entering the dining room, it might be helpful to indicate whether it was

- a cognitive problem, where the client was new to the facility and did not know where to enter
- a visual perceptual problem, where the client could not locate the door handle
- a neuromuscular problem such as inadequate strength to open the heavy door
- a psychosocial issue that the dining room was very crowded and the client expressed a preference to return when it was less congested.

Patterns of deficits and strengths are of great importance. There is really no rule that says that a certain number of checkmarks is required in a column for the component to gain significance. Patterns are the key to understanding the generalized ripple effect on a person's functional status by a performance component.

The case examples that follow illustrate only some of the infinite permutations inherent in the "Let's Do Lunch" tool. In these examples, the reader also will see how it is possible for someone to complete the tasks independently but still demonstrate problem areas that require a critical pathway to prevent injury. In deciding whether it is appropriate to pursue a critical pathway or not, the therapist may ask some questions. Will the problem have an impact on health? Safety? Relationships? Quality of life? The presence of affirmative answers suggests that intervention should follow and, in turn, the functional outcomes be negotiated and defined by the client and therapist. Treatment strategies will build on the client's strengths, noted during the observation. The strengths become the foundations to support the bridges leading to the desired outcomes.

Case Example 1: Julie—Using "Let's Do Lunch" as an Assessment Tool and Blueprint for Low-cost Interventions

To illustrate the point, review these findings. When a client, who shall be referred to as Julie, and I did the "Let's Do Lunch" assessment, the following information was obtained: each time she entered the crowded dining room, she dropped to the floor. This behavior was recorded in items 2 through 15. It was my opinion that she essentially shut down when confronted with a sensory bombardment; sitting on the floor was her way of expressing this overload. Julie is nonverbal. Other interpretations among team members included "attention-seeking motivations" and wanting food brought to her rather than obtaining it herself. While items 16 through 60 further corroborated the assumption regarding a dysfunctional sensory processing system, the items also highlighted problems with performance. It also became obvious that a desirable and functional occupational therapy performance outcome would have to revolve around sensory modulation strategies, because whatever strengths she exhibited, they quickly seemed to become nonfunctional as a result of a sensory system overload. With the intention of increasing her ability to handle the dining room stimulation, therapy should enable her to locate the end of the line (item 2) and, moreover, *stand on line* (item 3). In turn, she should be able to make her own food choices and let go of the seeming negative behaviors, so as to enjoy and participate more fully in the mealtime process. These are quality of life issues. There are cost factors here as well. Items 4 through 15 would bring her to a position of greater independence, freeing a staff person from dealing with Julie's obstructive positioning on the floor, as well as another staff person who customarily brings a meal to the table where she is brought by staff upon getting up from the floor.

The particular "flavor" of Julie's therapy should reflect the therapist's ability to assume the participant-observer's role and all that is implicit in that. Because I viewed her dysfunctional behavior of dropping to the ground when on overload, I checked "S" for sensory issues and tackled the outcomes based on a sensory-modulation approach. The most practical and immediate intervention was to arrange for Julie to come to the dining area when the line was about to open, reducing the visual and auditory stimulation, which only grew as mealtime progressed. She was positioned and ready to obtain her meal prior to the others. After getting through the line, during which she made her food selections, she was provided with a tactile and proprioceptive focus for attention, that is, she was given a trolley that could substitute as a walker and tray-holder to carry and roll her meal. Julie was taught how

Resident: _JULIE_   Therapist: _S. BACHNER, OTR/L_ Date: _1/29/97_

"Let's Do Lunch" Assessment Tool
Task Analysis: Eating in the Lodge

Scoring Codes:
S=Sensory= tactile, proprioceptive, vestibular, visual, auditory, gustatory, olfactory
P=Perceptual=stereognosis, pain response, body scheme, visual perceptual, visual acuity
N=Neuromuscular=reflex, ROM, muscle tone, endurance, postural control
M=Motor=gross coordination, crosses midline, laterality, praxis, oral motor control
C=Cognitive Integration=level of arousal, attention span, initiation, problem-solving
p=Psychosocial=social conduct, self-expression, self-management

TASK 0=independent, 1=verbal cue, 2=physical assist, 3=total assist	S	P	N	M	C	p
1. Enters Dining Room ⓪1 2 3 ELBOWS & KNEES FLEXED – HOLDING WASH CLOTH IN Ⓛ HAND	?		?			
2. Locates End of Line 0 1 2 3 DROPS TO FLOOR BEFORE LOCATING END OF LINE	✓					
3. Stands on Line 0 1 2 3 REFUSES TO STAND. SITS ON FLOOR ; BODY IN FLEXION	✓					
4. Collects a Tray N.A. 0 1 2 3 STARTS TO SCREAM	✓					✓
5. Puts Tray on Counter 0 1 2 3 N.A.						
6. Faces Correct Direction 0 1 2 3 N.A.						
7. Moves "Forward" 0 1 2 3 N.A.						
8. Balances on Two Feet 0 1 2 3 N.A.						
9. Sees Food Items 0 1 2 3 N.A.						
10. Reaches for Food Items 0 1 2 3 N.A.						
11. Inhibits Impulse to Take All Food 0 1 2 3 N.A.						
12. Makes Food Choice Decisions 0 1 2 3 N.A.						

		S	P	N	M	C	p
13. Holds Loaded Tray with Two Hands *N.A.*	0 1 2 3						
14. Navigates Turn Off of Line to Seating Area *N.A.*	0 1 2 3						
15. Ambulates Efficiently with Tray and Contents *N.A.*	0 1 2 3						
16. Visually Scans Room *APPEARS TO LIMIT SCANNING TO APPROX. 5 FOOT RADIUS*	0 1 2 ③						
17. Visually Targets an Available Seat *GUIDED TO TABLE*	0 1 ② 3	✓	✓				
18. Visually Targets and Available Seat with Friends *N.A.*	0 1 2 3						
19. Gets to a Targeted Seat	0 1 2 ③						
20. Puts Tray on Table *STAFF DID THIS*	0 1 2 ③						
21. Pulls Chair Out	⓪ 1 2 3						
22. Sits Down and Positions Legs Under the Table	⓪ 1 2 3						
23. Achieves Good Upper Body Posture in Seat	⓪ 1 2 3						
24. Achieves Good Lower Body Posture in Seat	⓪ 1 2 3						
25. Aligns Self with Tray at Midline *DONE BY STAFF AS TRAY PLACED ON TABLE. UNCLEAR IF SHE HAS 'SHUT DOWN'*	0 1 2 ③	?				?	
26. Acknowledges Peers at Table (or nearby) *JUST LOOKS*	⓪ 1 2 3	?	?			?	
27. Visually Attends to Tray /Contents	0 ① 2 3						
28. Reaches for Utensils (Wrapped in napkin)	0 ① 2 3						

	S	P	N	M	C	p
29. Uses Two Hands to Unwrap Utensils *CONTINUES TO* 0 1 2 3 *HOLD CLOTH IN (L) HAND ; USES (R) TO SEARCH FOR* *UTENSILS*	✓					
30. Places Napkins in Lap – *NO* 0 1 2 3						
31. Uses Bilateral Hand Movements to Open Packets 0 1 2 (3) *WON'T RELEASE WASH CLOTH*	✓					
32. Seasons Food with Salt and Pepper 0 1 2 (3)						
33. Holds Knife by the Handle 0 1 2 3 *DOESN'T USE KNIFE*						
34. Spreads Butter with Knife 0 1 2 3						
35. Cuts Food with Knife 0 1 2 3						
36. Grasps Eating Utensils with Functional Grip (R) or L) 0 1 2 3 *RAG /CLOTH IN (L)*						
37. Visually Targets Desired Food Items 0 (1) 2 3						
38. Initiates Movement of Utensils Toward Food Item 0 1 2 3						
39. Loads (Spoon) Pieces with Fork (0) 1 2 3 *SEEMS TO SPOON FOOD 3 EYE-HAND COORDINATION* *(? DEVELOPMENTAL)*						
40. Contains Food Items on Plate/Bowl 0 1 2 3 *HAS DIFFICULTY. GIVEN HI-SIDED DISH. RESULTS BETTER*						
41. Brings Food to Mouth with Utensil (0) 1 2 3						
42. Closes Lips to Contain Food in Mouth 0 (1) 2 3 *FOOD SPILLING ONTO CLOTHES*			✓			
43. Chews Bolus with Teeth (0) 1 2 3						
44. Swallows Bolus (0) 1 2 3						
45. Safe Chewing and Swallowing (0) 1 2 3						

		S	P	N	M	C	p
46. Wipes Mouth as Needed	0 (1) 2 3		✓				
47. Targets Drinking Glass	(0) 1 2 3						
48. Crosses Midline (R/L) with Hands as Needed NO	0 1 2 3						
49. Reaches/Grasps/Lifts Glass to Mouth	(0) 1 2 3						
50. Drinks Liquid with a Safe Pace and Adequate Swallow	(0) 1 2 3						
51. Finishes all Food Items on Plate	(0) 1 2 3						
52. Pushes Chair Back	0 (1) 2 3						
53. Sitting to Standing with Adequate Balance ARMS RETURNED TO TOTAL ELBOW FLEXION. FLEXED POSTURE	0 1 (2)(3)	✓		✓			
54. Reaches To Table and Picks Up Tray REFUSES	0 1 2 3						
55. Re-Aligns Body for Ambulation FLEXED BODY. FEET HIT FLOOR HARD, eg. MARCHING	0 1 2 (3)	✓					
56. Carries Tray without Spilling N.A. REFUSES. SEEMS TO NOT WANT TO ASSUME NEEDED BODY POSTURE	0 1 2 3	✓					
57. Determines Where to Return Tray SEEMS TO FOCUS ON IMMEDIATE SURROUNDINGS; WANTS TO PROTECT SELF	0 1 2 3	✓					
58. Reaches Location for Tray Deposit NO – WANTS TO GO TO EXIT DOOR	0 1 2 3						
59. Deposits Tray in Return Window N.A.	0 1 2 3						
60. Locates Exit Door from Dining Room LEAVES	(0) 1 2 3						

Summary of Components:

	S	P	N	M	C	p
Needs (Least Functional)	✓	?	?		✓	
Strengths (Most Functional)				✓		✓

Item Numbers Identified for TX: #2–15

COMMENTS: SAFE AMBULATION. GOOD STRENGTH. "P" & "N" NOT YET DETERMINED (LITTLE EVIDENCE OF EYE-HAND COORDIN.) "N" BREAKS DOWN FROM PROTECTIVE BODY POSTURE. DOESN'T CROSS MID-LINE. "C" SEEMS NOT TO IMPACT POSIT/NEGAT ON OUTCOMES to hold onto the handlebars and push the trolley to her seat of choice, without concern for spills on the tray, loss of balance, or colliding with another individual. This simple intervention, the trolley and tray-holder, at an approximate cost of $130.00, has been successful. Training was minimal and her comfort level clearly improved. Further, in an attempt to facilitate sensory processing changes, her direct care service provider, at the programming site, was empowered by the OTR to begin a series of sensory-based activities that graded the amount of stimulation deemed acceptable by the client. This work continues and is monitored, upgraded, adjusted, and documented on a routine basis by the OTR. Because the OTR operates in a consultative model, the professional costs are minimized.

Case Example 2: Steve—An Example of How the Tool May Be Used to Identify Additional Areas for Examination

"Let's Do Lunch" may also be used to flag problem areas requiring additional examination. For example, when a young man, Steve, stood in line facing the servers, he was observed touching and holding the wall above his head with his left hand. This was noted on steps 6 and 7, and later step 14. Even as he reached for the food from the servers with his right dominant hand, he maintained contact with the wall. After moving forward along the line, he again caught my attention by giving himself extra proprioceptive feedback, as he leaned the left side of his body into the room divider, while navigating the turn to the left off the line to the seating area. Later, after he was seated, it was noted that he unconsciously positioned his body so that his tray was mostly to the right of his midline (item 25). While there were other noteworthy items, those points formed a cluster and indicated that further assessment of his left-sided sensory responsiveness was indicted. This extra attention showed that his visual response time to stimuli on his left was significantly slower (or nonexistent) than the visual response time to the same stimuli on his right. One might ask: "So what!" After a review of previous accident reports, it was discovered that he had sustained an injury at his programming site when he tripped over an object on the ground that was to his left as he was running. "Let's Do Lunch" highlighted a functional vision problem. A further clinical assessment pinpointed the problem and his injury history demonstrated the need to teach compensatory skills, in order to prevent or reduce risk of further injuries. This information was imparted to Steve and his team. While he had learned to compensate well in obtaining his food and other self-care activities, it was evident that he needed additional training

Resident: *STEVE*   Therapist: *S. BACHNER OTR/L* Date: *6/12/96*

"Let's Do Lunch" Assessment Tool
Task Analysis: Eating in the Lodge

Scoring Codes:
S=Sensory= tactile, proprioceptive, vestibular, visual, auditory, gustatory, olfactory
P=Perceptual=stereognosis, pain response, body scheme, visual perceptual, visual acuity
N=Neuromuscular=reflex, ROM, muscle tone, endurance, postural control
M=Motor=gross coordination, crosses midline, laterality, praxis, oral motor control
C=Cognitive Integration=level of arousal, attention span, initiation, problem-solving
p=Psychosocial=social conduct, self-expression, self-management

TASK 0=independent, 1=verbal cue, 2=physical assist, 3=total assist	S	P	N	M	C	p
1. Enters Dining Room (0) 1 2 3						
2. Locates End of Line (0) 1 2 3						
3. Stands on Line (0) 1 2 3						
4. Collects a Tray (0) 1 2 3						
5. Puts Tray on Counter (0) 1 2 3						
6. Faces Correct Direction (0) 1 2 3 USES (L) HAND TO HOLD WALL ABOVE HEAD	✓	✓				
7. Moves "Forward" (0) 1 2 3 CONTINUES TO USE (L) HAND FOR TACTILE INPUT	✓	✓				
8. Balances on Two Feet (0) 1 2 3 HOLDS ONTO WALL c̄ (L) HAND	✓	✓				
9. Sees Food Items (0) 1 2 3						
10. Reaches for Food Items (R) HAND (0) 1 2 3 (L) HAND MAINTAINS CONTACT c̄ WALL	✓	✓				
11. Inhibits Impulse to Take All Food (0) 1 2 3						
12. Makes Food Choice Decisions (0) 1 2 3						

	S	P	N	M	C	p
13. Holds Loaded Tray with Two Hands　(0) 1 2 3						
14. Navigates Turn Off of Line to Seating Area　(0) 1 2 3 LEANS (L) SIDE OF BODY INTO PARTITION AS TURNS	✓	✓				
15. Ambulates Efficiently with Tray and Contents　(0) 1 2 3						
16. Visually Scans Room　(0) 1 2 3						
17. Visually Targets an Available Seat - STRAIGHT AHEAD　(0) 1 2 3		✓				
18. Visually Targets and Available Seat with Friends　0 1 2 3 ?						
19. Gets to a Targeted Seat　(0) 1 2 3						
20. Puts Tray on Table　(0) 1 2 3						
21. Pulls Chair Out　(0) 1 2 3						
22. Sits Down and Positions Legs Under the Table　(0) 1 2 3						
23. Achieves Good Upper Body Posture in Seat　(0) 1 2 3 FUNCTIONAL						
24. Achieves Good Lower Body Posture in Seat　(0) 1 2 3						
25. Aligns Self with Tray at Midline　(0) 1 2 3 TRAY POSITIONED MOSTLY TO (R) OF MIDLINE		✓				
26. Acknowledges Peers at Table (or nearby)　(0) 1 2 3						
27. Visually Attends to Tray /Contents　(0) 1 2 3						
28. Reaches for Utensils (Wrapped in napkin)　(0) 1 2 3						

		S	P	N	M	C	p
29. Uses Two Hands to Unwrap Utensils	⓪ 1 2 3						
30. Places Napkins in Lap	0 ① 2 3						
31. Uses Bilateral Hand Movements to Open Packets	⓪ 1 2 3						
32. Seasons Food with Salt and Pepper N.A.	0 1 2 3						
33. Holds Knife by the Handle	⓪ 1 2 3						
34. Spreads Butter with Knife N.A.	0 1 2 3						
35. Cuts Food with Knife	⓪ 1 2 3						
36. Grasps Eating Utensils with Functional Grip Ⓡ or L)	⓪ 1 2 3						
37. Visually Targets Desired Food Items TRAY REMAINS POSITIONED Ⓡ OF MIDLINE	0 1 2 3		✓				
38. Initiates Movement of Utensils Toward Food Item	⓪ 1 2 3						
39. Loads Spoon/Pieces with Fork	⓪ 1 2 3						
40. Contains Food Items on Plate/Bowl	⓪ 1 2 3						
41. Brings Food to Mouth with Utensil	⓪ 1 2 3						
42. Closes Lips to Contain Food in Mouth	⓪ 1 2 3						
43. Chews Bolus with Teeth	⓪ 1 2 3						
44. Swallows Bolus	⓪ 1 2 3						
45. Safe Chewing and Swallowing	⓪ 1 2 3						

		S	P	N	M	C	p
46. Wipes Mouth as Needed	(0) 1 2 3						
47. Targets Drinking Glass	(0) 1 2 3						
48. Crosses Midline (R/L) with Hands as Needed	(0) 1 2 3						
49. Reaches/Grasps/Lifts Glass to Mouth	(0) 1 2 3						
50. Drinks Liquid with a Safe Pace and Adequate Swallow	(0) 1 2 3						
51. Finishes all Food Items on Plate	(0) 1 2 3						
52. Pushes Chair Back *TURNS TO (R)*	(0) 1 2 3		? ✓				
53. Sitting to Standing with Adequate Balance *?APPEARS TO TAKE RAPID, SMALL STEPS IN PLACE TO BALANCE SELF*	0 1 2 3	? ✓	? ✓				
54. Reaches To Table and Picks Up (Tray) = (R) OF MIDLINE	(0) 1 2 3						
55. Re-Aligns Body for Ambulation	(0) 1 2 3						
56. Carries Tray without Spilling	(0) 1 2 3						
57. Determines Where to Return Tray	(0) 1 2 3						
58. Reaches Location for Tray Deposit	(0) 1 2 3						
59. Deposits Tray in Return Window	(0) 1 2 3						
60. Locates Exit Door from Dining Room	(0) 1 2 3						

Summary of Components:

	S	P	N	M	C	p
Needs (Least Functional)	✓	✓				
Strengths (Most Functional)			✓	✓	✓	✓

Item Numbers Identified for TX: _____

COMMENTS: *INVESTIGATE & RULE-OUT (L) SIDED VISUAL RESPONSE DEFICITS*
CLIENT'S (L)-SIDED SENSORY-IN-PUT NOTEWORTHY.

to compensate for visual-perceptual and processing deficits peculiar to his left side.

Case Example 3: Helen—Discovering her Narrative over Lunch

Helen further illustrates the evaluation potential in "Let's Do Lunch." Helen was admitted to the facility with multiple problems, including mental retardation and physical anomalies (the extent or etiology of which were not known at admission), and a minimal amount of background information, because she had been "discovered" by a county social service working living in a sibling's shack with no amenities or regard for developmental needs. Because she was nonverbal, glimpses into her preadmission world were obtained only through current observations.

By using "Let's Do Lunch," it was possible to identify a serious visual deficit and further appreciate the impact of her pervious deprivations. For instance, she clearly had difficulty with items 16 to 18:

- visually scans room
- visually targets an available seat
- visually targets an available seat with friends.

Here, a differentiating question was whether this inability could be attributed to the newness of her arrival and absence of friends, or whether it was perhaps visually based. Things became more revealing when Helen refused to sit down in the chair at the table. She was visibly agitated when staff efforts to have her sit persisted. Therefore, items 21 through 24 recorded these behaviors. Problems with utilizing the chair at the dinner table were reproducible at all meals. With further investigation, it became evident that Helen also resisted lying in her bed. Helen's narrative was being told; her responses to table, chairs, and even her bed provided much needed messages to staff about her previous existence. Her story of extreme deprivation was coming through loud and clear, as she communicated nonverbally about her early impoverished environment, one in which she never had available for her use any furniture for sitting or sleeping. While eating—and she was indeed very hungry—she placed the bowl or dish within 4 inches of her eyes and only showed visual attention to items in her central vision (approximately 20 to 30 central). Peers at the table who were in her peripheral fields were not acknowledged. This observation was juxtaposed to Helen's outgoing personality. While she demonstrated awareness of how to use a spoon, other utensils such as a knife and fork seemed unfamiliar (items 26 and 37). In

Resident: _HELEN_   Therapist: _S. BACHNER, OTR/L_ Date: _11/13/96_

"Let's Do Lunch" Assessment Tool
Task Analysis: Eating in the Lodge

Scoring Codes:
S=Sensory= tactile, proprioceptive, vestibular, visual, auditory, gustatory, olfactory
P=Perceptual=stereognosis, pain response, body scheme, visual perceptual, visual acuity
N=Neuromuscular=reflex, ROM, muscle tone, endurance, postural control
M=Motor=gross coordination, crosses midline, laterality, praxis, oral motor control
C=Cognitive Integration=level of arousal, attention span, initiation, problem-solving
p=Psychosocial=social conduct, self-expression, self-management

TASK 0=independent, 1=verbal cue, 2=physical assist, 3=total assist	S	P	N	M	C	p
1. Enters Dining Room 0 1 (2) 3	✓	✓				
2. Locates End of Line 0 1 2 (3)	✓	✓				
3. Stands on Line (0) 1 2 3						
4. Collects a Tray 0 1 2 (3)		✓		✓		
5. Puts Tray on Counter 0 1 2 (3)		✓		✓		
6. Faces Correct Direction 0 1 2 (3)						
7. Moves "Forward" 0 (1) 2 3						
8. Balances on Two Feet (0) 1 2 3						
9. Sees Food Items ? 0 1 2 (3)		✓				
10. Reaches for Food Items 0 1 2 (3)		✓		✓		
11. Inhibits Impulse to Take All Food (0) 1 2 3						
12. Makes Food Choice Decisions _N.A._ 0 1 2 (3)					✓	

		S	P	N	M	C	p
13. Holds Loaded Tray with Two Hands	0 1 2 ③					✓	
14. Navigates Turn Off of Line to Seating Area	0 1 2 ③		✓			✓	
15. Ambulates Efficiently with Tray and Contents	0 1 2 ③	✓	✓				
16. Visually Scans Room ONLY RESPONDS TO STIMULI IN CENTRAL VISUAL FIELD	0 1 2 ③		✓				
17. Visually Targets an Available Seat GUIDED TO TABLE c̄ AVAILABLE SEAT	0 1 ② 3						
18. Visually Targets and Available Seat with Friends STANDS BESIDE CHAIR PER ESCORT #17	0 1 ② 3						
19. Gets to a Targeted Seat	0 1 ② 3						
20. Puts Tray on Table	0 1 2 ③						
21. Pulls Chair Out REFUSES	0 1 2 3						
22. Sits Down and Positions Legs Under the Table REFUSES TO SIT	0 1 2 3						
23. Achieves Good Upper Body Posture in Seat N.A.	0 1 2 3						
24. Achieves Good Lower Body Posture in Seat WANTS TO EAT WHILE STANDING	0 1 2 3						
25. Aligns Self with Tray at Midline CONTINUES TO RESIST SITTING IN CHAIR	0 1 2 3						
26. Acknowledges Peers at Table (or nearby) SMILES AT PEERS IF IN HER CENTRAL VISION (20°-30° CENTRAL)	0 1 2 3		✓				
27. Visually Attends to Tray /Contents MOVES VISUAL TARGET TO 4" FROM EYES	0 1 2 ③						
28. Reaches for Utensils (Wrapped in napkin)	0 1 2 ③						

	S	P	N	M	C	p
29. Uses Two Hands to Unwrap Utensils (0) 1 2 3 *IF GIVEN TO HER*						
30. Places Napkins in Lap 0 1 2 3 *STILL STANDING — N.A.*						
31. Uses Bilateral Hand Movements to Open Packets 0 1 (2) 3 *FINE-MOTOR O.K. —DOESN'T COORDINATE c̄ EYES*						
32. Seasons Food with Salt and Pepper 0 1 2 3 *N.A.*						
33. Holds Knife by the Handle (0) 1 2 3 *ONLY USES SPOON*						
34. Spreads Butter with Knife 0 1 2 3 *N.A.*						
35. Cuts Food with Knife 0 1 2 3 *N.A.*						
36. Grasps Eating Utensils with Functional Grip (R) or L) (0) 1 2 3 *ONLY BRIEFLY —PREFERS TO USE FINGERS*						
37. Visually Targets Desired Food Items 0 1 2 3 *SEEMS TO NEED HIGH CONTRAST, CENTRAL 20°-30°, 4" FROM EYES*						
38. Initiates Movement of Utensils Toward Food Item (0) 1 2 3 *PREFERS FINGERS FOR FOOD EXPLORATION*						
39. Loads Spoon/Pieces with Fork (0) 1 2 3 *CAN USE SPOON BUT LIKES FINGERS*						
40. Contains Food Items on Plate/Bowl 0 1 (2) 3 *GIVEN HI-SIDED PLATE TO ASSIST c̄ CONTAINMENT — DID BETTER*		✓				
41. Brings Food to Mouth with Utensil (0) 1 2 3 *HOLDS BOWL AT 4" FROM FACE c̄ (L) HAND*		✓				
42. Closes Lips to Contain Food in Mouth (0) 1 2 3						
43. Chews Bolus with Teeth 0 1 2 3 *NEEDS MECHANICAL-SOFT/GROUND MEAT FOR SAFETY*						
44. Swallows Bolus (0) 1 2 3						
45. Safe Chewing and Swallowing - *NOT WHEN* 0 1 2 3 *EATING REGULAR DIET (CONSISTENCY)*						

Item	Score	S	P	N	M	C	p
46. Wipes Mouth as Needed	(0) 1 2 3					✓	
47. Targets Drinking Glass *HAVING TROUBLE LOCATING IT*	0 1 2 (3)		✓				
48. Crosses Midline (R/L) with Hands as Needed	(0) 1 2 3						
49. Reaches/Grasps/Lifts Glass to Mouth *NEEDS TO PLACED IN HER HAND*	0 1 2 (3)		✓				
50. Drinks Liquid with a Safe Pace and Adequate Swallow *DOESN'T TIP HEAD BACK. ?WHY*	(0) 1 2 3						
51. Finishes all Food Items on Plate *REQUIRED VERBAL & PHYSICAL PROMPTS TO LOCATE FOOD*	0 1 2 (3)		✓				
52. Pushes Chair Back *N.A.*	0 1 2 3						
53. Sitting to Standing with Adequate Balance	(0) 1 2 3						
54. Reaches To Table and Picks Up Tray	0 1 2 (3)						
55. Re-Aligns Body for Ambulation	(0) 1 2 3						
56. Carries Tray without Spilling	0 1 2 (3)						
57. Determines Where to Return Tray	0 1 2 (3)		✓		✓		
58. Reaches Location for Tray Deposit	0 1 2 (3)						
59. Deposits Tray in Return Window	0 1 2 (3)						
60. Locates Exit Door from Dining Room	0 1 2 (3)						

LACK OF FAMILIARITY ✓ ... ✓

Summary of Components:

Needs (Least Functional) ✓ ✓

Strengths (Most Functional) ✓ | ✓ ✓ | ✓

Item Numbers Identified for TX: ―――――――――――――――

COMMENTS: *IF BOWL REMAINS ON TRAY, CLIENT STRETCHES HEAD FORWARD - OBVIOUS MUSCLE STRAIN, TENSION. TENSION DISAPPEARED WHEN BOWL LIFTED 4" FROM EYES/MOUTH. NEEDS EYE EXAM. ? PREVIOUS SOCIALIZATION TO PEOPLE/OBJECTS* fact, Helen had a distinct preference for using her fingers to get food from her dish to her mouth. This information was recorded in items 38 though 41.

Helen had some teeth for chewing but not a full set. She had problems with item 43, chewing bolus with teeth, and item 45, safe chewing and swallowing. This evidence enabled the occupational therapist to contact both the facility physician and dietician to arrange for a mechanical soft or ground diet to ensure Helen's safety. She had no problem crossing her midline (item 48), but demonstrated a unique pattern for drinking liquids (item 50): she would not tip her head back. Through further observation, this drinking style appeared to be rooted in a reluctance to move her eyes, rather than a dysfunctional swallowing pattern. Diminutive Helen had the appetite of a lumberjack, and yet she would leave food on her plate. If she were directed to the food with verbal prompts, however, she quickly went after it for consumption!

Based on the highlighted items, I was able to submit a report that spoke to Helen's needs with limited visual fields:

▮ her seeming inability to perceive anything in her periphery, up or down
▮ her need to hold items for viewing within four inches of her eyes
▮ her need for chewing and swallowing precautions
▮ her need for assistance with safe ambulation, due to apparent low vision
▮ her impoverished cultural and experiential background, as reenacted through her unfamiliarity with common eating tools and furniture.

Similarly, strengths were noted in neuromuscular and psychosocial areas, comfort with sensory input, ease with gross and fine motor tasks, and potential for cognitive growth through familiarization and cultural assimilation. Based on this input to the team, she was sent for an ophthalmological consult and found to have bilateral cataracts. Plans for surgery were made. Occupational therapy functional outcomes were delayed until the surgery was completed.

"Let's Do Lunch" as a Template

If one chooses, "Let's Do Lunch" may serve as a template for "Let's Do *Anything*." All that is needed is a detailed task analysis. In fact, the task analysis format lends itself to infinite settings, situations, and tasks. The same principle of providing a structured observation is the key. Yet, I am hard pressed to come up with another activity that enables a therapist and client to meet under such motivating conditions, an activity that is part of everyday living, an activity that is so culturally laden, so critical to survival, and one that has the potential to elevate the quality of life for someone with handicapping conditions.

Value in Using the Technique

From occupational therapy students to senior clinical staff, the technique works. Students at the facility like the simplicity of following the course of action step-by-step. It minimizes writing and allows for additional time to focus attention on the observations.

Senior clinicians report the same ease as well but place a greater value on the results. For the experienced clinician, there are the memories of those early days of practice, where one's mission was to juggle all the events and somehow triage presenting issues and conditions that, to the neophyte, all look like foreground. The environment, the components, the interactions, the critical questions, the observations, the "so whats"—these are the issues bombarding the therapist. The experienced clinician has digested these ingredients in evaluation settings so many times and knows in the gut the format for a reasonable sequence.

Examining the setting, the client, the deviations, the problem solving, the flavors, the aromas, the culture—it all becomes possible in short order. Wherever the observer is on the experience continuum, the tool has simplicity, logic, and inherent value. It enables the therapist to quickly get a taste of what is happening and to work within the confines of a managed care environment to arrive at functional outcomes critical to daily living, expression of self, and quality of life. It enables the therapist to describe a client's functioning—the levels of significance that are interpreted as strengths and the potentials that can be tapped—as well as definitions of need that will require a clinician's expertise in designing or conducting a program with measurable, functional outcomes. It's all there!

The value of a service delivery, as mentioned at the outset of this chapter, can be determined by the ratio of quality to cost. "Let's Do Lunch," with a menu of performance components available for selection, blends a biomedical model with the social science and quality of life model, and produces the opportunity for measurable outcomes that have relevance and interest to all consumers: the client, the third party payer, the staff. "Let's Do Lunch" is both a process and a facilitating device for the establishment of relevant outcome.

"Much of what we call the art of medicine," states Donabedian, "consists in almost intuitive adaptations to individual requirements in technical care as well as in the management of the interpersonal process. Another element in the art of medicine is the way, still poorly understood, in which practitioners process information to arrive at a correct diagnosis and an appropriate strategy of care. As our understanding of each of these areas of performance improves, we can expect the realm of our science to expand and that of our art to shrink. Yet, I hope that some of the mystery in practice will always remain, since it affirms and celebrates the uniqueness of each individual" (Donabedian, 1988).

ACKNOWLEDGEMENTS

Acknowledging people for the creation of a product is sometimes risky, for the author takes the chance that important people inadvertently remain unmentioned. With that in mind, I would like to thank my friend and colleague Valnere McLean, MA, OTR/L, FAOTA, my coeditor Mildred Ross, MS, OTR/L, FAOTA, and my husband Paul Bachner, MD, FCAP, for their respective patience, clarity in thinking, and willingness to review the chapter yet another time. Ruth Huebner, PhD, OTR/L, and her students from Eastern Kentucky University, individually and collectively, influenced the chapter's outcome, and I am most appreciative. Thank you, too, to those many people who provided encouragement and for those family members—two and four-legged—who often waited for dinners long overdue without complaint.

REFERENCES

American Occupational Therapy Association. (1995). *Uniform terminology for occupational therapy* (3rd ed.) Bethesda, MD: Author.

American Occupational Therapy Association Managed Care Project Team. (1996). *Managed care: An occupational therapy source book* (pp. 91–98) Bethesda, MD: Author.

Axelson, M.L., & Brinberg, D. (1989). *A social-psychological perspective on food-related behavior* (p. 2). New York: Springer-Verlag.

Boakes, R.A., Popplewell, D.A., & Burton, M.J. (1987). *Eating habits: Food, physiology and learned behavior.* New York: John Wiley & Sons.

Bronner, S. (1986). *Grasping things: Folk material culture and mass society in America* (pp. 160–179). Lexington, KY: University Press of Kentucky.

Caplan, B., and Shecter, J. (1995). The role of nonstandard neuropsychological assessment in rehabilitation: History, rationale, and examples. In L. Cushman and M. Scherer (Eds.), *Psychological assessment in medical rehabilitation* (pp. 359–391). Washington, DC: American Psychological Association.

Chassin, M.R. (1996). Improving the quality of care. *New England Journal of Medicine.* 335, 1060–1063.

Donabedian, A. (1988). The quality of care: How can it be assessed. *Journal of the American Medical Association, 260,* 1743–1748.

Eddy, D.M. (1991). Oregon's methods: Did cost-effectiveness analysis fail? *Journal of the American Medical Association, 266,* 2135–2141.

Ellwood, P.M. (1988). Shattuck lecture—Outcomes management: A technology of patient experience. *New England Journal of Medicine 318,* 1549–1556.

Forer, S. (1996). *Resource guide on outcome management & program evaluation for occupational therapy.* Bethesda, MD: American Occupational Therapy Association.

Goode, J. (1992). Food. In R. Bauman (Ed.), *Folklore, cultural performances, and popular entertainments* (pp. 232–245). New York: Oxford University Press.

Inglehart, J. (1994). *Health policy report, 331*(17), 1167–1170.

Joint Commission on Accreditation of Healthcare Organizations (JCAHO). (1994). *A guide to establishing programs for assessing outcomes in clinical settings.* Oakbrook Terrace, IL: Author.

Kautzmann, L. (1997). Health related quality of life status. Unpublished hand-out. Eastern Kentucky University, Department of Occupational Therapy.

Lindeman, E.C. (1925). *Social discovery: An approach to the study of functional groups* (pp. 177–200). New York: Republic Publishing.

Maurer, D., & Sobal, J. (Eds.). (1995). *Eating agendas: Food & nutrition as social problems* (p. ix). New York: Walter de Gruyter, Inc.

Marshall, D. (1995). *Food choice and the consumer* (pp. 266–279). Glascow: Blackie Academic & Professional.

Perske, R., Clifton, A., McLean, B., & Stein, J.I. (Eds.). (1986). *Mealtimes for persons with severe handicaps* (pp. xix–xxi). Baltimore: Paul H. Brooks.

Relman, A.S. (1988). Assessment and accountability: The third revolution in medical care. *New England Journal of Medicine. 319,* 1220–1222.

Rogers, J., & Holm, M. (1994). Accepting the challenge of outcome research: Examining the effectiveness of occupational therapy practice. *American Journal of Occupational Therapy, 48,* 871–876.

Silberman, C. (1991). From the patient's bed. *Health Management Quarterly. Second quarter,* 12–15.

Toglia, J. (1993). Attention and memory. In *AOTA self-study series: Cognitive rehabilitation* (pp. 22–32). Bethesda, MD: American Occupational Therapy Association.

Wennberg, J.E. (1991). The road to guidelines. *Health Management Quarterly. Second quarter,* 2–7.

Wetzler, H. (1994). Outcomes measurement: A way to measure value. *Healthcare Forum Journal.* July/August: Compendium series.

Wilson, J., & Cleary, P.D. (1995). Linking clinical variables with health-related quality of life: A conceptual model of patient outcomes. *Journal of the American Medical Association, 273(1),* 59–65.

APPENDIX A

Resident: _____ Therapist: _____ Date: _____

"Let's Do Lunch" Assessment Tool
Task Analysis: Eating in the Lodge

Scoring Codes:
S=Sensory= tactile, proprioceptive, vestibular, visual, auditory, gustatory, olfactory
P=Perceptual=stereognosis, pain response, body scheme, visual perceptual, visual acuity
N=Neuromuscular=reflex, ROM, muscle tone, endurance, postural control
M=Motor=gross coordination, crosses midline, laterality, praxis, oral motor control
C=Cognitive Integration=level of arousal, attention span, initiation, problem-solving
p=Psychosocial=social conduct, self-expression, self-management

TASK 0=independent, 1=verbal cue, 2=physical assist, 3=total assist	S	P	N	M	C	p
1. Enters Dining Room 0 1 2 3						
2. Locates End of Line 0 1 2 3						
3. Stands on Line 0 1 2 3						
4. Collects a Tray 0 1 2 3						
5. Puts Tray on Counter 0 1 2 3						
6. Faces Correct Direction 0 1 2 3						
7. Moves "Forward" 0 1 2 3						
8. Balances on Two Feet 0 1 2 3						
9. Sees Food Items 0 1 2 3						
10. Reaches for Food Items 0 1 2 3						
11. Inhibits Impulse to Take All Food 0 1 2 3						
12. Makes Food Choice Decisions 0 1 2 3						

		S	P	N	M	C	p
13. Holds Loaded Tray with Two Hands	0 1 2 3						
14. Navigates Turn Off of Line to Seating Area	0 1 2 3						
15. Ambulates Efficiently with Tray and Contents	0 1 2 3						
16. Visually Scans Room	0 1 2 3						
17. Visually Targets an Available Seat	0 1 2 3						
18. Visually Targets and Available Seat with Friends	0 1 2 3						
19. Gets to a Targeted Seat	0 1 2 3						
20. Puts Tray on Table	0 1 2 3						
21. Pulls Chair Out	0 1 2 3						
22. Sits Down and Positions Legs Under the Table	0 1 2 3						
23. Achieves Good Upper Body Posture in Seat	0 1 2 3						
24. Achieves Good Lower Body Posture in Seat	0 1 2 3						
25. Aligns Self with Tray at Midline	0 1 2 3						
26. Acknowledges Peers at Table (or nearby)	0 1 2 3						
27. Visually Attends to Tray /Contents	0 1 2 3						
28. Reaches for Utensils (Wrapped in napkin)	0 1 2 3						

		S	P	N	M	C	p
29. Uses Two Hands to Unwrap Utensils	0 1 2 3						
30. Places Napkins in Lap	0 1 2 3						
31. Uses Bilateral Hand Movements to Open Packets	0 1 2 3						
32. Seasons Food with Salt and Pepper	0 1 2 3						
33. Holds Knife by the Handle	0 1 2 3						
34. Spreads Butter with Knife	0 1 2 3						
35. Cuts Food with Knife	0 1 2 3						
36. Grasps Eating Utensils with Functional Grip (R or L)	0 1 2 3						
37. Visually Targets Desired Food Items	0 1 2 3						
38. Initiates Movement of Utensils Toward Food Item	0 1 2 3						
39. Loads Spoon/Pieces with Fork	0 1 2 3						
40. Contains Food Items on Plate/Bowl	0 1 2 3						
41. Brings Food to Mouth with Utensil	0 1 2 3						
42. Closes Lips to Contain Food in Mouth	0 1 2 3						
43. Chews Bolus with Teeth	0 1 2 3						
44. Swallows Bolus	0 1 2 3						
45. Safe Chewing and Swallowing	0 1 2 3						

		S	P	N	M	C	p
46. Wipes Mouth as Needed	0 1 2 3						
47. Targets Drinking Glass	0 1 2 3						
48. Crosses Midline (R/L) with Hands as Needed	0 1 2 3						
49. Reaches/Grasps/Lifts Glass to Mouth	0 1 2 3						
50. Drinks Liquid with a Safe Pace and Adequate Swallow	0 1 2 3						
51. Finishes all Food Items on Plate	0 1 2 3						
52. Pushes Chair Back	0 1 2 3						
53. Sitting to Standing with Adequate Balance	0 1 2 3						
54. Reaches To Table and Picks Up Tray	0 1 2 3						
55. Re-Aligns Body for Ambulation	0 1 2 3						
56. Carries Tray without Spilling	0 1 2 3						
57. Determines Where to Return Tray	0 1 2 3						
58. Reaches Location for Tray Deposit	0 1 2 3						
59. Deposits Tray in Return Window	0 1 2 3						
60. Locates Exit Door from Dining Room	0 1 2 3						

Summary of Components:

Needs (Least Functional)

Strengths (Most Functional)

Item Numbers Identified for TX: —————————————————————————————

COMMENTS: —————————————————————————————

9

Groups Are Physical, Social, and Emotional Therapy

"A Chance to Tell My Story"

Mildred Ross, OTR/L, FAOTA

"When I talk to you and you listen to me, not only do we see
and hear one another, but, insofar as either of us remembers
the occasion, it is because we produce long-term changes in the
function and structure of the nerve cells in each other's brains."
Eric Kandel, Professor, Columbia University (1992, p. 31)

The purpose of this chapter is to demonstrate how group treatment can be
used for the management and delivery of service to adults with developmental
disabilities. Getting these adults to sit together and meet as a group is an
important intervention, and changes for a better lifestyle may be possible.
The benefits and results from such intervention for this population will be
discussed. The kinds of groups used, the various aspects of the role of the
therapist, and the application of physiological and psychological features
that influence success will be described. The immense diversity existing in
this population, the variety of topics and activities to offer to groups, and
the similarity in needs of this population with all other populations will
be detailed.

GROUP MEMBERSHIP ENABLES AND ENRICHES
SOCIAL DEVELOPMENT

Feeling comfortable in a variety of group settings is an acquired skill for
most people and a very important one. To assume that those who cannot

talk, are slow in thinking, and are limited in verbal expression cannot benefit from a group experience is simply wrong. A person must be in a group to learn how to be in one. Social skills, like other human skills, are acquired chiefly through engagement and practice. Social skills must be experienced with other peers who can offer a challenge not too great yet not too comfortable so that learning occurs. No one should be excluded. Some memberships even have life-saving properties.

AN INDIVIDUAL NEEDS TO BELONG TO MANY KINDS OF GROUPS

In general, group experiences in addition to family are presented naturally as one encounters diverse peer gatherings in school, and joins social, religious, athletic, or other kinds of groups. Such associations provide the advantages of learning how to play, to struggle, to share with others, to be praised, to express hurt, to find redress, to help others, and to accept help, until, finally, the person develops a good identity and rewarding relationships. Through these memorable events, the necessary shaping of advantageous long-term changes in the personality occurs (Kandel, 1992).

These different kinds of group opportunities are not accessed readily by the individual born with a disability, or by the individual who becomes disabled, traumatized, or diseased early in life and may have been institutionalized for long periods. Disability often creates so many demands that even with in the family the need for normal socialization can be overlooked and never achieved. When attention is turned to these needs, therapeutic groups are a proven benefit.

WE LEARN THROUGH OUR NERVOUS SYSTEM

There is a persisting perception that groups are purely psychological events, perhaps because "feelings" are so much discussed. However, it is simultaneously a physiological event due to the chemical exchange that accompanies the action that takes place in the group (Kandel, 1992). This chemical exchange is the communication code that is transmitted from neuron to neuron throughout the nervous system. The motor and behavioral responses are put together from the summation of the interpretation of the communication message. Among the cortical structures involved, the limbic system (the limbic lobe is considered the emotional brain) especially registers the event. The amygdala collects and processes the responses from other lobes, coordinating emotion with memory association, and reports via chemical discharge to the hypothalamus, which regulates the autonomic nervous system (ANS). The ANS influences brain stem regulation of the internal organs. The immune system via hypothalamus and pituitary gland is informed and responds by supplying stress hormones appropriately. The relatively new field of psychoneuroimmunology (PNI) informs us "that the immune system is not an autonomous agency of defense, but part of an integrated network of regulatory mechanisms serving homeostatic functions" (Ader, 1992, pg. 6). "Recent research demonstrates that there are bidirectional communication pathways between the immune system and central nervous system (NS), with each providing important regulatory control over the other" (Maier, Watkins, & Fleshner, 1994, pg. 1004). When members demonstrate the ability to concentrate and participate during a group session, it can be assumed that therapists, discussions, activities, plus myriad other factors are influencing the immune and central nervous systems of members. Internal balance (homeostasis) is the result of the satisfying stimulation provided in the group session. When members seen in the group setting are unable to participate and override their symptoms, therapists then have elements to evaluate for their behaviors. Therapists can assess the acuteness of the person's illness or lack of readiness for the particular group, the depletion of the individual's immune system, or the flawed stimulation presented in the session (Ross, 1997).

Depending on the intensity of the input of the event to each person, cardiovascular, respiratory, sensory, and motor behaviors will be critically affected. Pupils may widen and respiration and heart rate slow in a learning mode. There will be observed outward changes to information heard or to conflict seen. The group members will smile or laugh, relax visibly, and straighten up in their postures. Some participants will stand up and pace, move vigorously or even ominously, in some way. Anxiety, envy, fear, and other negative feelings can be expressed by a rush of words, loss of attention, sweaty palms, yawns, sleepiness, or a flushed face. If you introduce the subject of a forest fire or the suicide death of an individual, and the changes in body behavior may become very evident. As they receive and process sensation, each person exhibits a seamless melding of their total physical, emotional, mental, and spiritual self all at once. Josephine C. Moore says, "We are our nervous system. It's our behavior: it's who we are. You cannot separate neuroscience from behavior" (Royeen, 1990, pg. 10).

APPLICATION OF NERVOUS-SYSTEM LEARNING AND MEANINGFUL STIMULATION TO OCCUPATIONAL THERAPY GROUPS

When conducting a group with persons with chronic disabilities, this writer suggests two guiding principles. The first principle is to consider *when* and *how* the planned activities are to be introduced. The knowledge of how different kinds of stimulation affect the nervous system is a crucial tool in the acquisition of skill that must be acquired to conduct groups of adults who are developmentally disabled. The skilled therapist must learn—through knowledge of neuroscience, through careful observation, and through experimentation—how and when to change activities.

Some operational principles may be stated simply:

- Whatever is novel, alerts.
- Whatever is fast, excites.
- Whatever is routine or familiar, soothes and composes.
- Whatever is slow, relaxes.

The second principle builds on the first, namely, that a moderate approach to arousal achieves longer-lasting results. Group events should not become too exciting or too dull. Consider that if you use novelty too soon or too much with anxious group members, you will lose their attention because too much stimulation is disorganizing. Overfiring of one system can make it difficult for the complementary system to recover, such as keeping the sympathetic and parasympathetic systems in balance. Relaxation may not be easy to achieve as quickly as it may be required (Lutz & Ramsey, 1975, 1979; Noback, Strominger, & Demarest, 1991). Furthermore, there is the chance that the event may be cancelled out as individuals in the group do not relate the excitement to a realistic plan for follow-up. In a therapeutic group the goal is to obtain a sense of inner control, calm and balance, and flooding the system requires a lot of coping skill and self-management to regroup.

Information-processing deficits exist with mental retardation. Can these be reversed, considering the deficits with which such a nervous system begins? Reduced density of synapses, those important sites over which chemical and electrical communication cross, are reported in fetuses and infants with Down's Syndrome (Neistadt, 1994). This means there is less opportunity for available information to permeate the system. Observed deficits in memory, abstract thinking, learning strategies, and attention spans exist. The question is: Can these be improved substantially? Reviewing the physical, biochemical, and electrical properties of the information-processing system that underlies all human learning, the validity of plasticity assumptions for learning following brain injury after birth is very good in its promise (Neistadt, 1994; Moore, 1990). It is not clear how information processing in a brain that begins with prebirth injury or deficiency can be improved. Reason and observation show that exposure to meaningful stimuli, practice within a context, repetition, innate motivation, and an inner state of satisfaction can bring about learning in the individual with developmental disabilities.

GENERAL BENEFITS OF GROUPS

When individuals become uncomfortable and inappropriate with others, they need a setting where appropriate behaviors and attitudes can be practiced safely. In such a setting, persons with extreme and immoderate behaviors that interfere with the safety and rights of others learn to curb those behaviors. It is also a way for those who are withdrawn to test the waters: there is the opportunity for learning from peers about what to say or do in a group, while preserving a sense of safety and privacy. Skilled facilitators encourage the group to distill both general wisdom and individual skills. Good groups provide consistent feedback, so that members can be stimulated and nurtured to change behaviors and acquire hope. Adults who cannot or do not use language to express themselves, or those with poor comprehension, dementia, or cognitive disturbance, especially benefit from group membership as they continue to learn at their pace and make themselves better understood. In a well-conducted group, each member consistently gets a sense of being respected by and connected to others: participants feel more comfortable about changing their behavior. Here, at least, tension and conflict are able to be voiced, not met with punishment or demeaning coddling. For example:

> Kevin is a male adult, who was discharged, from a state facility for mental retardation, to a group home. From there he was referred to a work-service program. Here he attended my "Five-Stage" group. For about 5 years he displayed minimal independent function and was nonverbal. Then at one session, Kevin and the others were holding on to a stretchy parachute. A sandbag had been placed in the cloth to make it heavier to lift. The weight fell out of the raised stretchy cloth and landed near Kevin. In a very unusual gesture for him, Kevin bent down, picked it up, hesitated, and then placed it back onto the cloth. This was the first time he had initiated an act of involvement with the group. This act made him a part of what was going on and, for the

first time, he did something to stay a part of it. He continued with more acts of involvement and less isolating mannerisms. Kevin's behavior in the workshop gradually changed too, requiring fewer prompts to stay on task.

Another young adult, Sam, frequently stayed out all night in bad neighborhoods and would not accept individual counseling. However, he agreed to attend my occupational therapy group and participated in sharing his issues for about 4 years. In this group, he began to report his unsafe behaviors and eventually heard the message of the group members, so that the extreme nature and frequency of his unsafe actions were greatly reduced. Eventually Sam began to respect and trust his peers sufficiently to be able to evaluate many of his situations with them.

A middle-aged adult, Dolores, presented with unpredictable temper tantrums that interfered with her work. She chiefly attended groups that taught relaxation techniques, such as using tapes, guided imagery, and doing exercise. This appeared to reduce her defensiveness better than a direct confrontation of her escalating behaviors. When Delores joined our verbal-sharing group, she willingly shared those experiences that were either pleasant or aggravating to her but quickly displayed irritation by groaning or withdrawing from the group when others were describing theirs. Dolores demonstrated that not everyone wants to talk things over; exercising, engaging in group activities, and learning to share in this way are preferred by some more than others. Delores joined group sessions that were structured to include less verbal sharing and more movement and relaxation activities, and she was able to redirect her inappropriate behavior. She now continues on a job with a job coach.

Another participant, Louise, has mental retardation with serious neurological deficits in perception and tactile sensation but good verbal skills. Although she displays limitations in understanding world events, she shows good ability to profit from her extensive life experiences. She can reflect on these personal, concrete, and meaningful events and learn from them with the help of others and her own willingness to do so. She benefits greatly from expressing herself in groups which she had attended for more than 10 years. As a member of an occupational therapy group, Louise is able to empathize and to relate how she took on similar problems shared by group members, of fighting, wilfulness, and disrespect to others, by self-control, listening, and self-evaluation. That ability greatly influenced, directed and benefited the group members. She told how she threw plates and had to clean up the mess, and how she lost privileges when she screamed. Louise shared how she began to recognize that certain family members disturbed her, that people taunting her in the street made her feel ashamed, or that a pain or sore so frightened her that it triggered her uncontrolled behavior. She explained how describing these feelings to people who listened was helpful to her. Louise could say, "you have to admit when you are wrong," and she got the message across to members by articulating the steps to take to achieve goals. Louise realizes that, despite her ongoing struggles, she is seen as a role model, and she expresses her pride in this. There is no better learning than that received from peers who can share.

THERAPEUTIC GROUPS AT GOODWILL INDUSTRIES

Therapeutic groups usually consist of five to nine adults. In my groups the members usually chose to be with others of similar abilities and therefore, much of the time group membership could be homogeneous. I facilitated three different groups. One group, consisted of adults of all ages whose cognitive functioning fell below 45 IQ or in the low-moderate to severely impaired. These persons could not use language for a number of different reasons or were limited verbally to a word or phrase with difficulties in articulation. The second group consisted of individuals with moderate cognitive impairment between 45 IQ and 65 IQ, also displaying very limited verbal skills. The third group consisted of persons who possessed verbal skills with varying abilities and degrees of comprehension. These adults were considered in the high range of moderate to mild cognitive impairment, approximately 65 IQ and above. In addition, individuals with average or better cognition and diagnosed with traumatic brain injury, autism, or other psychiatric diagnosis, were referred to this group and chose to attend. In this group, participants chiefly wanted to verbalize and share their experiences. There were some individuals who could float between two and even three of the groups because of their interest and their ability to learn from different kinds of experiences. The "Five-Stage" format (Ross, 1997) was used consistently with the first two groups, and principles from the "Five Stages" were incorporated as much as possible into the third group. Usually, this latter group had two co-leaders, but in the last year of its existence (1997) only one facilitator was present. All examples of verbal responses described in this chapter came from this third group which met once a week. Descriptions of the changes in physical behaviors that occurred are illustrations from all the groups. More information on the structure of the "Five-Stage" format is provided in Chapter 10.

EXAMPLES OF THERAPEUTIC GROUP EXPERIENCES

Members Learn to Realize that They Need Their Peers. During their lives most group members experience the extremely transient contact with persons who are hired and who move in and out of their lives. The peers they meet may be their most enduring contacts, like acquiring an extended family. Group members say this in one way or another. There are so few ways to meet so formally and feel a sense of relatedness to each other. For example, in a special sharing session one member brought pictures of his family. He first insisted that the facilitator must see them. It made him feel important to bequeath this special honor, but it sent the wrong message to group members about their value. The facilitator reminded him that since all members had the same interest she would wait her turn. He still could feel important about what he had to show to the group as members responded with good interest and he, again, saw how they cared for him.

Member Has Her Moment to Receive Attention. Once, when members were asked to give their reasons for coming to the group session, Mary, answered that it was "a chance to tell my story." She does recite the same scenario over and over many times, but it is a grand way to say that we all need to relieve the burden on ourselves by reciting our chores, our grievances, our unnoticed victories, all of which make us feel recognized and acknowledged. This population is at risk for the stifling of this very human need.

Members Learn to Listen to Others and Gain Various Advantages. One member reported that she learned about giving and getting "respect" when she began to listen to others without interrupting them before they were finished speaking and, conversely, could assert her right to be listened to in this way. Another person demonstrated that in listening and learning from each other different solutions can be gathered to solve a problem. This occurred when one member related her frustration and difficulty at being required to pack up all her winter clothes and take them to another area for storage. How to do this and how to carry it all loomed as an immense obstacle for her to overcome. The group members attended to this concern with numerous practical suggestions. The discussion diminished her need to be dependent and helped her to learn to do for herself.

ATTENDING TO GROUP PROCESS

Between and among groups of people, there are walls, such as developmental disabilities, that separate one from the other. These walls need to be breached and weakened. A lack of experience and information, an inability to read and pursue continuing education, and inequality in relationships with members from other populations exist. Group process in the hands of a skilled practitioner can facilitate communication among members to ameliorate these serious deficiencies. As group members experience the rules regarding attacking, shaming, or blaming others, as in any other group, they begin to examine issues, learn more factual information, and begin to see where they can take responsibility for their actions and consequences.

Group member Mary, describing her discomfort with a vaginal rash, attempted to better clarify this by beginning to expose herself. A broad range of social know-how existed in the group, and several members registered distress. The facilitator seized on this occasion to teach members to notice how others are listening to them. Rarely are issues of such sensitivity explained, developed, reinforced, and rewarded with this population.

> The therapist interrupted Mary and requested that she look at the faces around her. Most of these faces were expressing some degree of discomfort. One young man was half way out of his seat about to leave but sat back down when Mary was interrupted. Mary, however, could not interpret what the expressions meant, and another member who could explain it did so very simply. One member was very contemptuous of Mary. However, this presented the opportunity to discuss the difference between private and public self-touching. An issue like this illustrated exactly the kind of help members can give to each other. The member who showed contempt relented in her strong feelings, as she saw the incident worthwhile through the eyes of the therapist. Others also learned their right to express their discomfort instead of rolling their eyes and trying to leave when "touchy" subjects arise. In addition, members learned how to get help. In this instance, a nurse was able to help Mary. The members learned that they can go to different people and places to get help; with their problems and that a variety of outcomes are available from many sources. They began to understand what subjects can be discussed in groups and when to protect their privacy.

Many adults with developmental disabilities have no experience with group membership. Therefore, the evolution of the group through the usual stages of development in which members struggle for control or leadership may not happen. Role development—such as of leader, arbiter, or role model—even when it occurs is tenuous and depends greatly on the facilitator to help it flourish. Just the hint of an energizing connectedness among members may be all that happens for a long time.

During an activity group with seven young adults with moderate to severe cognitive impairment, the time "to talk" had arrived. They were asked to talk about something good or kind that had happened to them recently. In this group about half of the members could not produce sound. It sometimes required another member to volunteer to speak for a member; sometimes a member had to explain the request in "code" words to the other member; or the group members would make guesses. This is how it worked. When it was Vivian's turn, to show she understood she thrust her hands forward. Though considered to have very low cognition and to be deaf and without speech, she persisted until the group understood she was proud of her newly-painted fingernails. Vivian then began to untie her shoes. This was a puzzle at first, but, when asked if her toenails had been painted as well, she nodded affirmatively and stopped untying her shoes. It took time, but she was able to reveal that her mother was responsible. All this time group cohesion was building and it was intense as members enveloped her. They could be happy for her—with maybe a tinge of envy—that made this occurrence so human.

Good reasons exist for creating groups with a mixture of different diagnoses so the advantages each population brings can be shared. At times, individuals with traumatic brain injury or psychiatric problems have joined the group of adults with developmental disabilities. These individuals with other diagnoses bring the capacity to verbalize and generalize, which may be lacking with persons with developmental disabilities. This ability promoted greater understanding as everyone contributed to explanations from different levels; everyone growing by helping or being helped. Ben, a young man with a history of autism and psychiatric problems who demonstrated good intelligence, attended the group for 2 years. Ben joined because he "felt so empty inside." At one session, near the end of his stay, he turned to Jenifer, (an adult with developmental disabilities) who was venting her aggravation at taking a bus to work that carried noisy teenagers, and said: "You are not alone, I feel that way too on that bus!" With the help of Jenifer Ben was able to recognize and connect with his feelings. The facilitators knew he had graduated. He, in turn, provided a model for Jenifer of how she might offer a meaningful response when she connected with others.

CONTENT AND CONDUCT OF THE GROUP

Therapists can introduce a rhythm to the group to maintain a sense of balance or to promote the return to homeostasis that is the desired goal. This rhythm consists of increasing or decreasing the degree of excitement by using selected activity and discussion to achieve a balance, so that the members' available energy will be sustained throughout group.

When conducting the group:

> A welcoming smile, a pleasant environment, comfortable seating, and a very brief activity such as a handshake or passing an object will start any kind of group momentarily. Experience showed that when the therapist attended to each individual member very briefly, general focus was achieved. However, an activity must follow quickly to maintain the attention.

Movement or some novel theme creates additional motivation:

> To maintain this focus the next step is to create more energy and interest. To do this, novelty in subject matter or movement that is fast paced can excite and alert.

Consider how touch tracts and their pathways to certain structures like the cerebellum can be effective. Stimulating these pathways initially with an alerting kind of touch, followed up with more moderate-pressure touch, helps to reduce emotion and invites an interest to learn (Ross, 1987). Providing items to handle or introducing different kinds of movement can accomplish this, also. Examples of this are provided in the following chapter, "The Five-Stage Model for Adults with Developmental Disabilities." Even if a group member does not know the date or cannot articulate many words, the individual can relate very naturally on a sensorimotor level and follow simple movements and good touch (Ross, 1997).

Having the group aroused by the movement activity and successfully interested in what is happening becomes the optimal time for performing a perceptual task or having a meaningful discussion:

> Novelty should be introduced judiciously with an entertaining or exciting question or observation in order to continue the interest. As a moderate amount of interest is sustained, the group becomes able to evaluate the experience or to concentrate on one person's problem or exert more patience while waiting for a response from a slower member.

Nearing the end of a session any immoderate behavior like a build-up of enthusiasm or even the realization of hurt and pain can cause the emotional flooding of the whole nervous system. This is not conducive to calm deliberations in the activities of daily life after the group session is over for the day. Therefore, every group needs a cooling down such as closure activities:

> Focusing again on each one individually, stating plans to meet again, and some formal touch that is beneficial for the group are some ways to signal the nervous system that events have remained safe, the familiar is back in focus, and there is incentive to move on.

ROLE OF THERAPISTS AS GROUP LEADERS

Therapists need to call on members and ask: "What did Mary just say?" When it cannot be repeated it might mean that its significance is not understood. The facilitator cues to encourage Mary's continuing contribution. The leader seeks clarification when the adult who is explaining uses the same words over and over again. John may offer an interpretation that is still unintelligible. At this time another member can be asked: "What did you hear John say, Susan?" Susan may be familiar with the code that one word may symbolize, can help interpret John's message, and then get his verification. Mary can be asked again, "if we are all talking about the same thing" she introduced. The leader is in charge of following the ping pong ball of this communication as it flies back and forth, and keeps the discussion focused.

All explanations must be very brief. Two or three sentences that are descriptively concrete are all that is necessary from the facilitator. The group members can do a lot of the work. The leader steers the group members to teach. To a young adult male who insisted that his age of 30 years entitled him to make his own rules about curfews, the group members provided examples about establishing trust, demonstrating responsibility, and simply stating what one expects from others. He was convinced eventually to change his actions. The facilitator started this discussion by stating that "behavior, not age, makes people believe in someone." Attention spans are not experienced sufficiently to stay too long on any one person or topic and need constant spurts of brief redirecting remarks. Memories seem to disappear at times. However, repetition, practice, and the human desire to learn lurk in all populations. The opportunity to be listened to strikes a responsive chord.

With other populations facilitators might use more neutral comments. However, with this population frequent and extravagant, but sincere, praise supplies, supports, and maintains interest. This reinforces members' growth and good decisions.

The ease with which issues of control can be aroused in therapists working with adults with developmental disabilities has to be recognized. Control issues can be a pitfall. In a group of adults of very low function, everyone was requested to bring his own chair to make the usual circle. Some needed to have help initiating the action, but all completed it alone. When this was done a picture was taken followed shortly by a second picture. On viewing the pictures later, the facilitator was amazed. In comparing the first picture of the group (completing the circle on their own) with the next picture of the group as it began, the scene was very altered. The first picture showed an uneven and more oval space between members. In the second picture, group members were evenly spaced in a precise circle. Obviously, in the second picture the need "to control" by rearrangement could not be resisted by the therapist. Therapists need to be very mindful of allowing flexibility, extending patience, and continuing to grow in understanding.

Leadership is ever alert to "fading out" whenever the group demonstrates that it is finding its own voice: leadership can never consider itself as purely directive. The leader serves as a facilitator, keeping members focused and dropping the reins when it is possible. Groups demonstrate they have found their own voice when members make suggestions and these are followed up. All members are called on for answers, definitions, and reactions even if they are unwilling to contribute at a particular time and refusal is accepted. As stated previously, a more active facilitator may be required with some populations than with others, but as soon as possible all learned dependent behavior is deflected using the same group dynamic skills regulating all groups.

A sense of superficiality may appear to exist at times; therapists may also feel discouraged about the direction a session may take. However, it is the accumulation of group sessions that yield results and a quick fix cannot be expected. Under any circumstances, these cannot be short-term groups: the usual short-term verbal group is not effective with this population.

The group format is very applicable to the issues that concern adults with developmental disabilities, like self-respect and conflict resolution. Gaining self-respect can be guided by helping this population use more assertive interactions. Learning rights and expressing them assertively, however, must be done in stages. To this population assertiveness can be construed as showing a range of behavior from bad manners to civil disobedience for which there will be reprisals. Fear of reprisal from caregivers can be very real and confounds the learning process.

As in any group management, conflict occurs and needs to be addressed. This allows the group leader to guide the group toward the practice of assertive behavior, and appropriately expressing what one wants. Conflicts between members are handled at the moment of occurrence and in a direct and clear manner. Many sessions are required to recognize rights and learn appropriate requests. This mastered the therapist then can introduce a variety of ways to reduce frustration, anger and rage, before these feelings escalate. Gradually, it becomes possible to teach members to use relaxation techniques to reduce their quick emotional responses and increase more reasonable behavior. Learning mantras, using mental pictures, tapes, and music, inner strength can build to reinforce the new practice of meeting needs with more effective behaviors. Some adult members tell of the restraints that belittling caregivers may offer when they see them using relaxation techniques, and these are very real obstacles to address with everyone. Some quickly learn how to hide their new growth and understanding when they perceive it to be threatened. For example, Jeanie, a member with Down's Syndrome, described how she made sure her bedroom door was locked when she retired to do the meditation she was taught in the group. She knew her parents would laugh at her because they would not understand. She had had no success in keeping them from checking out her tied boxes in her dresser drawers. Jeanie also could describe her improved relationships with her stepfather as a result of sharing her issues in the group. She began to understand over several years attendance in the group that she had a right to privacy, that she had a right to do what was required, in the context of her situation, and the difference between being "fresh" and being assertive. Therapists learn to proceed at a slower pace to achieve new learning and explore with the group members a variety of means to arrive at desired goals.

When it is appropriate that a decision be based on majority agreement, all members are helped to understand what this means and that it must be respected. Group members could be blunt with another member. For example, Betty, a member with dual diagnoses, often would not talk about herself but referred repeatedly to vague and off-topic issues like "the meaning of boundless" or "belief in heaven or in hell." Group members told her they did not understand what she was talking about, and that such words reminded them of death and dying or made them sad. The facilitator would reinforce the group's wishes by reminding Betty that she should not refer to the unwanted topics even though the members were inconsistent in their attempts to do this. With a more able group, peers are expected to take care of their needs and such protection is not rendered by the leader. With this initial support from the leader Betty's group was able eventually to take responsibility for enforcing its majority decision that each person talk about himself or herself, and for deterring Betty from acting upon her obsessive thoughts. When necessary one or another member headed off any "forgetfulness" on Betty's part. This helped Betty, and when she was asked to describe the group to a new member she stated, "we talk about ourselves." The facilitator took advantage of this by asking quickly, "Can you give an example?" Caught by surprise, Betty answered, "I pick out my own clothes." Betty was very pleased with the group's approval. At another time she was asked what she liked about the group, and she stated it was the "good conversation." She appeared to have more difficulty than anyone in conforming appropriately, but she was committed now to change. For many years she had required a special "management program" in the workshop to control inappropriate behaviors. Now with the group experience Betty has successfully appealed to have this behavioral program dropped. She never misses a group session.

There is a receptivity in this population that some may see as a learned compliance or as their inability to think quickly enough to combat a statement. The receptivity also can be a natural tendency to wish to live peaceably, to live in the moment, to accept limits, and to avoid being hurt or hurting others. The adult usually recognizes with an honest poignancy that he or she needs consistent support to do his or her best.

GROUP LANGUAGE

In all cultures, special words are marked for use that may be understood more readily by the majority of members. In this sub-culture group members have to help the facilitator to learn their special language. Also this population gets very little opportunity to have words defined for them so that it cannot be taken for granted that the meanings of even familiar words are understood. Frequently synonyms for words cannot be offered adequately by group members. Some words appear to carry great weight even when members cannot define them.

Respect.　The use of the word "respect" appears to be very well understood by every member. It may be that society in general uses this word so often that everyone "overlearns" it. This word may convey all that needs to be said about anyone's behavior to another or to themselves. It has become the most effective word to be used in the group to bring about instant attention. "Respect her space," "respect his need not to tell us," "respect her point of view," "respect his right to make that choice," "we do not feel respect from you," and so forth, all appear to promote understanding.

Control.   On the other hand, it was seen in one group that, when members were exhorted to "control" a robot to keep it from falling off the table, this was not understood until the request was changed to "let's play with it." To a population that rarely experiences "control" but appreciates "play," the latter word is understood better.

Game.   However, calling an activity a "game" may discourage some group members from participating, because their respective families have told them not "to act like a baby," which they associate with the word "game." Calling it an "activity" may be more acceptable for some members. Therapists must learn each group's sensitivity to certain words since there are no hard and fast rules. At certain levels of higher function, avoiding the word "play" may be necessary; whereas at lower levels it is helpful.

Angry.   Words like feeling "hurt," "upset," or "aggravated," may be more acceptable than being "angry" or "mad" because most members have been told it is bad or wrong to be angry or mad. It is hard for some to separate the feeling from an action. "Angry" may carry with it the intent to do violence and some cannot unlearn this interpretation easily.

Advocate.   An example of an oft-used word requiring definition arose when group members learned of Congressional action being taken to reduce Medicaid at the federal and then the state level. The word "advocate" was heard and required clarification. One person described it as "the person who takes you places," others went further, stating, "they speak for you," "like you," "stand up for you," and, concluded one member with one word, they are your "backup." Members then saw that a sister, a friend, or a state worker acted in this capacity. The group discussion continued as the facilitator inquired: "Can you be your own advocate?" This led to a very lively discussion and indicated how each member was at a different stage in accepting and using this concept.

KINDS OF GROUPS

The adult population with developmental disabilities benefits from groups that meet to

- cook
- reduce stress
- exercise

▮ enhance community involvement (Edgerton & Gaston, 1991)

▮ improve work concepts

▮ teach arts and crafts

▮ dance

▮ advance the understanding of sexuality (Ludwig, 1995)

▮ promote healthy relationships.

All of these groups can enhance self-esteem and self-expression as well as require problem-solving and choice-making. When persons choose their own groups and goals, it is more likely that they will show greater initiative in carrying on what they have learned (Neistadt, 1995). Only lack of available facilitators, lack of transportation, and lack of money to purchase services, supplies, or admission tickets limits the kinds of groups that can be developed for all levels of functioning (Schleien, Meyer, Heyne, & Brandt, 1995).

This population demonstrates the broadest, most diverse range of individual aptitudes and levels of understanding within any one group of same-age persons. In a group of young, mixed male and female adults, on the subject of romance one man exhibits timidity, denying any interest; another man has a special friend but is vehement about his lack of readiness for more than that. One young woman likes having her boyfriend but also wants to play the field without him knowing this, because she is sure her mother will never let her marry. Another accepts attention from one but confides that she really loves another, to whom she has never spoken. Yet another woman wants to concentrate on her boyfriend, taking the relationship seriously and expecting it to offer more physically to her when she feels ready. She hopes that eventually she will marry. In the same group, stages of readiness, maturity, degree of dependence, and comprehension differ when another kind of subject matter is introduced. This makes it possible for peers with more wisdom in one area to help and share and then on another occasion receive enlightenment from others.

The many changes taking place in the approaches toward long-term support for the population with developmental disabilities assist in the exploration of preventive means, the development of new attitudes such as that reflected in the Special Olympics, and the realization that there are universal natural needs. Deinstitutionalization, community involvement, work experience, and the use of purposeful groups will push progress further. In the Midwest as one example, state-wide Associations for Retarded Citizens (ARC) have very vocal members among the adults with developmental disabilities and provide programming that promote the integration of adults into existing groups in the community (Jackson; Johnson, & Olsen, 1982). The ARC is a grass-roots organization, as opposed to a professionally-created organization, that was started by families of people with developmental disabilities and is an important resource for advocacy. The Association on Aging with Developmental Disabilities describes a retirement support group in its newsletter (AADD Newsletter, 1995).

Observations After Providing Groups for 10 Years to Many of the Same Clients:

1. Ninety percent of the consumers like the group. They come as soon as it is announced. Those who are verbal will repeatedly ask for the group, if a group is disbanded.

2. Clients who act out with hostility on many occasions do not do this on the day they attend the occupational-therapy group. Once or twice a year there may be an exception, but adaptive behavior for that day is the norm.

3. Improved motor behavior is seen over a period of 3 to 5 years by participants in the "Five-Stage Group." With the exception of a very few, this change occurred with persons who had been institutionalized for most of their lives. Those starting with a more kindly, individualized environment can expect a faster rate of change in their abilities. For example, everyone improves from her or his initial performance in the ability to follow visual demonstration or verbal directions. These are important gains, because the improved agility affects physical safety and behavior. Persons who cannot bend with stability to pick up or place an item on the floor learn to maintain their balance. Then they are not knocked over so easily when someone brushes against them. Clients who cannot grasp and release, such as when throwing a ball, grading hand movements while filling a bag without ripping it, or crushing paper inserts to put in a box, all improve. The success is first seen in the group and then observed in the workshop, and since both have an impact on the client, it may be that both workshop and group activity have to coexist.

4. In the activity group that consists of activities and verbal processing, there are gains in social behavior. During group sessions, members exhibit greater awareness with respect to each other's space. They consciously consent to sharing attention and items with each other as they begin and continue to watch each other more consistently. How this may generalize into actions outside the group meeting has not been established. Yet, if it is the case that poor behaviors are

learned for general use, then healthier behaviors also can be learned for general use.

One hundred abstracts (PsycLIT, 1/90–6/95) were reviewed on research outcomes for this population using groups as a means of accomplishing change in undesirable behaviors presented by individuals. However, no groups were reported being used for preventive measures or for teaching methods for change. Single case studies were used frequently to report on individual behavioral programs which never included any group attendance. All of the latter studies were concerned with challenging behaviors. Introducing choices of various activities in recreation and meals "produced significant decreases in frequency and severity of challenging behaviors" (Ip & Szymanski, 1994). A good group provides multiple choices in activities and themes for discussion and can be cost effective. Documenting measurable outcomes "of challenging behaviors" as a result of group membership, can be a good subject for research.

5. A clear outcome of the use of activity and discussion/sharing groups with adults with developmental disabilities is that each individual improves in verbal and nonverbal self-expression, when offered the opportunity. Nowhere else is the adult listened to or attended to with the consistent patience shown by the group with a supportive facilitator. Under other circumstances, the adult is often talked to rather than listened to, because it is easy to do this. Solutions appear simple. However, there can be a depth of reasoning for which the adult is not credited nor helped to explore fully. To illustrate, a female adult was assigned the job of breaking down boxes in the workshop. She was a person with severe dyspraxia, and she was accustomed to experiencing a long waiting time between job assignments. When her hands became bruised in the handling of the boxes, and she saw another worker's canvas gloves lying around, she donned them and continued working. She was accused of taking something that did not belong to her. No one allowed her time to explain that she usually had to wait too long for others to solve her problems, that she only was borrowing the gloves, and that she was tired of sitting around, waiting for a job assignment, if she would be taken off this job. In the group she was guaranteed a chance to explain all of this and took the time to do so. Since the matter already had been resolved the opportunity in the group to express all of her feelings provided closure for her.

6. Self-confidence grows as group members: first, acquire the ability to articulate; then to expand on their verbalization; and finally to

take action. As an illustration, a young adult woman Sally said that she came to the group to learn more about herself and others. However, she remained unable to apply the new assertive language that she rehearsed in the group to the conditions she experienced in her group home. After attending sessions for about five years, she was asked what single lesson she had learned in the group. She responded: "Other people's problems are not my responsibility." Indeed, she constantly worried about what she was expected to do when things went wrong around her. Sally described that her roommate who worked in the same workshop was getting up to give kisses to the man sitting next to Sally. She thought this was poor manners and the bosses would not like it. When asked what she would do about it, Sally responded: "Nothing, it's not my responsibility. But it isn't right." Sally demonstrated that she could relate what she learned from the group as she acted on that rationale.

Others show stronger attempts, but still slip back too easily into their old passive behaviors if not constantly supported by group meetings to maintain newly-acquired learning. It may be expected that outcomes evolve naturally from talking to taking action. This only reinforces the need for using groups with this population.

Members of the population considered developmentally disabled often are patronized. The nervous system records it even when the individual cannot articulate it. The fight-or-flight mechanism is triggered frequently in many individuals in this population. Usually the fight idea is stifled in favor of withdrawal and emotional blocking. This frequent stimulus of being kept in one's place can create ongoing, chronic, and unpredictable stress; J.C. Moore describes this scenario (Moore, 1990). Physically and emotionally, endurance is reduced. Eventually when enough toxins are released within the system, the body can shut down completely. A good group can transcend the need for participants to choose fight or flight and become the one place where members are able to relax from their tensions. Groups can do this when respect and caring prevail, dialogues are fair honest, and clear, and activities teach something that is useful. Then the group becomes an occasion to remember and increases the possibility for needed changes to occur (Kandel, 1992).

ACKNOWLEDGEMENTS

Deep gratitude is expressed to scholarly friends who reviewed and reviewed this manuscript for tidy and explicit expression and clarity of thought.

Therefore, great appreciation is extended to Susan Bachner, MA, OTR/L, FAOTA, Marilyn B. Cole, MS, OTR/L, and Valnere McLean, MS, OTR/L, FAOTA. Warm recognition is extended to my co-therapist, Laurie Donovan O'Brien, BS, who is a sensitive and dedicated advocate for persons with developmental disabilities and with whom I enjoyed many pleasurable years of work and discussion.

REFERENCES

Ader, R. (1992). On the clinical relevance of psychoneuroimmunology. *Clinical Immunology and Immunopathology. 64* (1), 6–8.

Association on Aging with Developmental Disabilities. (1995). *Newsletter, 1* (1). St. Louis, MO: Author.

Edgerton, R.B., & Gaston, M.A. (Eds.). (1991). *I've seen it all!: Lives of older persons with mental retardation in the community.* Baltimore, MD: Brookes Publishing.

Ip, S., & Szymanski, E. (1994). Effects of staff implementation of a choice program on challenging behaviors in persons with developmental disabilities. *Rehabilitation-Counseling-Bulletin. 37*(4), 347–357. (PsycLIT Database, 1995).

Johnson, V.M., & Olsen, L.M. (1982). *A guide to alternative programming for older mentally retarded-developmentally disabled adults.* St. Louis, MO: St. Louis Association for Retarded Citizens.

Kandel, E. (1992). *The biology of mind.* New York: Columbia University.

Ludwig, S. (1995). *Sexuality: A curriculum for individuals who have difficulty with traditional learning methods.* Unionville, Ontario: York Region Public Health Department Healthy Sexuality Program.

Lutz, F.W. & Ramsey, M.A. (n.d.). *Complex organizations: The voodoo killer in modern society.* State College, PA: Pennsylvania State University. [Copies of this report may be obtained by requesting it from M. Ross.]

Maier, S.F., Watkins, L.R., & Fleshner, M. (1994). Psychoneuroimmunology. *American Psychologist, 49* (12), 1004–1017.

Moore, J.C. (April 23, 1990). Current concepts in the neurosciences. *American Occupational Therapy Foundation Mini-course in the neurosciences.* Bethesda, MD: AOTA.

Neistadt, M.E. (1994). The Neurobiology of learning: Implications for treatment of adults with brain injury. *American Journal of Occupational Therapy, 48*, 421–430.

Neistadt, M.E. (1995). Methods of assessing clients' priorities: A survey of adult physical dysfunction settings. *American Journal of Occupational Therapy, 49*, 428–436.

Noback, C.R., Strominger, N.L, & Demarest, R.J. (1991). *The human nervous system* (4th ed.). Malvern, PA: Leo & Febiger.

PsycLIT Journal Articles 1/90–6/95, SilverPlatter 3.11 PsycLIT Database Copyright American Psychological Association.

Ross, M. (1987). *Group process: Using therapeutic activities in chronic care.* Thorofare, NJ: Slack.

Ross, M. (1997). *Integrative group therapy: Mobilizing coping abilities with the five-stage group.* Bethesda, MD: American Occupational Therapy Association.

Royeen, C.B. (Ed.). (1990). Neuroscience foundations of human performance. *American Occupational Therapy Association self-study series*, Bethesda, MD: American Occupational Therapy Association.

Schleien, S.J., Meyer, L.H., Heyne, L.A., & Brandt, B.B. (1995). *Lifelong leisure skills and lifestyles for persons with developmental disabilities.* Baltimore, MD: Paul H. Brookes.

ADDITIONAL READING

Toglia, JP. (1985). Use of games in cognitive retraining, *Physical Disabilities: Special interest section newsletter, 8,* 3–8.

Kielhofner, G., & Miyake, S. (1981). The therapeutic use of games with mentally retarded adults. *American Journal of Occupational Therapy 35,* 375–382.

OTHER RESOURCES

Association on Aging with Developmental Disabilities. 1816 Lachland Hill Parkway, Suite 200, St. Louis, MO 63146.

Missouri Centralized Information and Referral Center for Older Persons with Developmental Disabilities. University of Missouri at Kansas City. (800) 444-0821.

The ROM Dance Network. P.O. Box 3332 Madison, Wisconsin 53704-0332.

St. Louis Association for Retarded Citizens. 1816 Lachland Hill Parkway, Suite 200, St. Louis MO, 63146.

10

A Five-Stage Model for Adults With Developmental Disabilities

Mildred Ross, OTR/L, FAOTA

Persons in good health, who feel good about themselves, are able to take control, exercise choice, and know their feelings. It is another story for individuals whose energies are drained by the presence of a chronic disability and the lack of coping skills. For them, extra warmth, support, and structure need to be supplied, so that such individuals can succeed in learning these skills and retain their available energy. The Five-Stage Model serves as a basic group model for those persons who require that extra portion of support and structure. The stages provide activities for:

- orientation and welcome
- movement and energizing
- perceptual tasks and sensorimotor skills
- cognition for expressing feelings and reflections
- closure and preparing to take control (Ross & Burdick, 1981; Ross, 1987, 1991, 1997).

The Five-Stage Group is a systematic and sequential method for organizing the presentation of activities in a group format. It is developmental, as each stage is dependent on the stage before it to enhance its acceptance. It is hierarchical, in that each stage makes incremental demands on group members to respond to challenges as one stage flows into the next. Tasks chosen for each stage must be able to be graded up or down according to the functional and developmental level of group members. No two groups can ever be alike, as they take the group process from the "here and now" situation as that is presented by members during each session. Observations from peers and therapists are processed throughout the session, as a reflection of what is happening. Its greatest advantage, for those who do not learn particularly well from language, is that these observations relate more to the action and behavior displayed at the present moment by the participants, as they respond to a task and to others engaged in a task, rather than to personal stories or the feelings expressed by participants.

Activities, used in the Five Stages, refer to all the physical actions and to all the verbal exchanges that happen during the group session. Therefore, the initial handshake, a bell that members ring and pass, exercises they follow, an anxious member exiting, any interruption occurring, a concern voiced, two items matched in a perceptual task, or the members describing what they are learning can be considered by the therapist as material to be processed or ignored within the group. When an event is processed, it becomes an activity.

Activity is used to organize behavior. Activities provide the means for eliciting the adaptive responses by doing, moving, shaping, and changing, so that a desired response is achieved, and, "in addition to their active creation, adaptive responses are believed to have an internally organizing and integrative effect on the performance components or subsystems of the human as occupational being" (Wood, 1996, p. 631). It is this internal organizing, within the group session, that is expected to result eventually in behavioral and physical changes. When members become more calm and more alert, it is because the selected activity has organized them. The feeling of being organized helps members to be motivated for change.

Almost all techniques and activities, known to occupational therapists, can be adapted for use in the Five Stages. Therapists can utilize items that provide stimulating sensory qualities, such as sound, texture, color, special touch, joint mobilization, exercise and movement, or introduce the cultural arts, relaxation techniques, and productive discussions. *How* and *when* these techniques and skills are introduced are the key principles of the Five Stages.

The goal of the Five-Stage Group with the adult population that is developmentally disabled is to provide, in a structured framework, the means to practice good social interaction, to experience competencies, and to exercise choice. It accommodates persons who may not speak and may be very cognitively limited but will accept sitting next to another person. It is the quintessential opportunity for peers to learn how to help and be helped by peers. It is a special boon to those persons who like to be with others but are eliminated from the group experience by a flawed criteria that may insist on speech or some level of knowledge.

A Description of the Five Stages

Stage I: Orientation

Purpose. The purpose of this stage is to recognize each member individually, to arouse each member as much as possible, and to review the purpose of the group (Ross, 1997). The therapist can review the purpose with a single statement that covers the intent of the session, such as, "we meet together to work or share time, and to learn from each other."

How an activity is introduced is most important. The previous chapter, "A Chance to Tell My Story," described how information is received by the central nervous system. It is relevant here. Discussions are inappropriate in the orientation stage: emotional issues, especially, are postponed for a later stage, when participants become more organized and focused, moving from self-absorption to greater awareness of others.

Content. Appropriate activities are any 1-minute activity, such as shaking hands, providing a backrub, saying names or hello in a foreign language, or passing a strong smell or lotion, a noisy or musical item, a fuzzy or rough item, or a weight or weighted object. These provide the opportunity to practice using items functionally; for example, using hand lotion mimics the way hands are washed, plucking a musical instrument promotes fine pinch, and handling a weight can correspond to holding a bottle of sauce and pouring it without dropping. Persons can respond to such small demands, and their interest is aroused.

Guidelines for continuing on to the next stage. The allotted time for this stage may take 2 to 10 minutes. The therapist decides when to move onto the next stage. It is usually when most of the members become able to give some degree of attention.

Stage II: Movement

Purpose. The purpose of movement is to increase physical and cognitive readiness for the work of the group (Ross, 1997). Movement increases muscle tone, influences an automatic good postural alignment, and enhances body scheme through involving parts. Physiological changes can take place that will engender a response from the group member. Movement is the quickest way to obtain a response as therapists demonstrate an action, make a request, or require members to reach for objects being passed around.

This stage is not a substitute for individual movement therapy, but it can offer a brief one-on-one to facilitate a better way to move. Individual help is offered when it does not interrupt the group as a whole or distract the individual too much. In this case, movement is meant to energize and to be a way of expressing one's self, as well as interacting with others very naturally. Copying each other, as well as creatively moving to suggest a new way to move, is applauded. Movement generates an increased interest, a good mood, a sense of self and relatedness to others, and this is verifiable on oneself.

Content.   Appropriate movement protocols for cardiovascular improvement, warm-ups, and strengthening can be borrowed from low-impact aerobics, adding weights appropriately for strengthening, and using stretching exercises. Resources for ideas can come from libraries, adult courses, and local state health departments, as well as from the local department for the aging. The ROM Dance on audiotape and videotape is an excellent example of a protocol that mobilizes all joints creatively (Harlowe & Yu, 1981). Placing items in the hands of members promotes novel ways to move. These items can include cans of food, theraband strips, batons, canes, plates, cones, or scarfs. Heavy or lightweight items provide different sensory inputs and may be combined in the same session. Movements used in functional outcomes, such as donning clothes, reaching into closets, or negotiating steps, can be practiced by imagining the action and recreating it with group participants. Each member can lead a movement, work with a partner, and join with others by holding hands or holding on to a large sheet, parachute or rope (Ross, 1997). This is a good time to encourage laughter and other expressions of enjoyment.

Guidelines for Continuing on to the Next Stage.   As members appear more alert, the therapist can inquire, after a period of time, perhaps 10 to 20 minutes, if they want to try another activity.

Stage III: Visual Motor Perceptual Activities

Purpose.   This stage chooses activities that combine sensory motor components and cognitive components to enhance awareness of self and the environment, challenge interpretation of stimuli, and force an adaptive response (Ross, 1997).

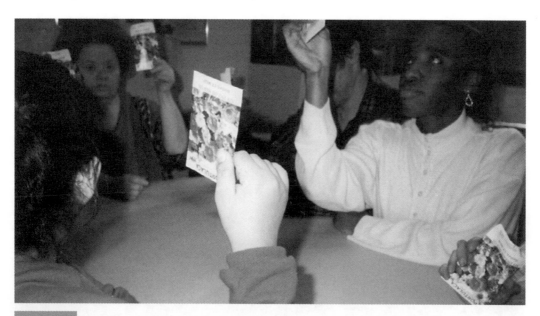

FIGURE 10.1 Problem-solving: "Whatever shall we do with these envelopes?"

In this stage greater demands, of an incremental nature, are placed on the group member. Group action has moved from passive reception to self-directed movement and, now, the requirement is to develop a more constrained, directed and planned response to the selected activities presented.

Content. In this stage, tasks can require less physical exertion, but do require thoughtful action, such as identifying, organizing and interpreting sensory data, and making a more precise, meaningful response. Tasks are selected that will bring successful outcomes for most members within two to four attempts. Therefore, grading activities (making them more or less difficult to perform) is an important concept in presentation. Tone of voice, pace of presentation, and deciding whether to show a complete example or one step at a time are also ways to grade an activity.

Appropriate occupations can range from learning functional tasks such as how to open and close a tie or ziploc bag, how to use a tool like a reacher to pick up a variety of objects, or how to manipulate any item like a top or Jacob's Ladder that requires starting the action and letting go. Almost all activities carry a message or a lesson and conveying that message through performance can be powerful. Manipulating an item successfully leads to: "Wow, I can do that, although I did not believe I could at first!" A group

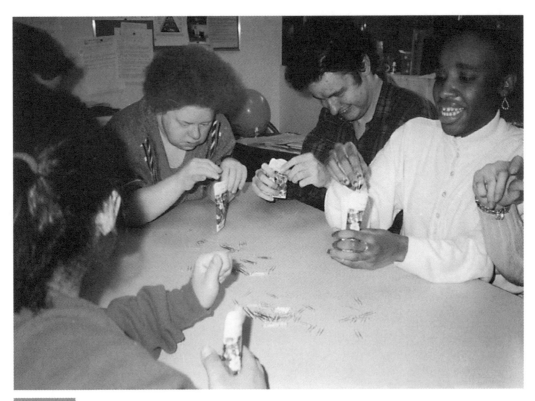

FIGURE 10.2 Decision: "Let's see how fast we can fill them up." (This was not competitive; each person was improving on his or her own past performance).

endeavor can demonstrate how the members work well together as each one, in turn, joins one link to another to make a single design or necklace. Other activities have been found successful:

- identifying tools in a bag
- identifying sounds, smells, or weights
- discriminating between shapes
- judging distances and force by throwing bean bags, aiming golf balls into electric putters, or knocking down plastic bowling pins with a plastic ball.

Sequencing a story from a series of pictures or showing each member's favorite time of the day on a clock with moveable hands invite interest and can be discussed more fully in the next stage.

Relaxation techniques may be introduced here. Guided imagery can be started with the suggestion of a boat floating in water under a blue sky;

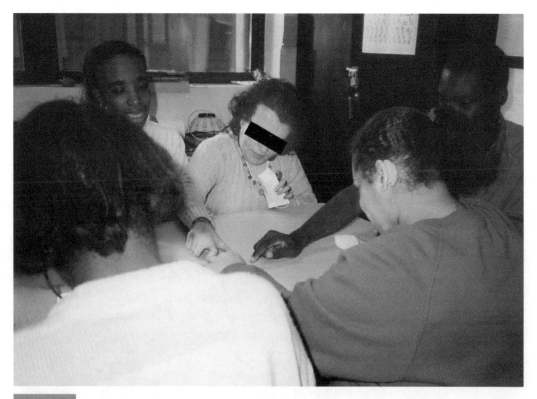

FIGURE 10.3 Carefully spotting and reaching out for supplies without blocking someone else.

each member can then be asked to add to this image. Alternately, the therapist can guide the group with a simple relaxation message, allowing those who want to close their eyes. A member can illustrate a special dance, music, meditation, or the way to massage one's own limbs.

The therapist may pass around heavy items that provide proprioceptive input to joints and can induce calm when members need extra assistance to focus. For example, group members can be asked to hold a weighted mirror and then to select a favorite facial feature on themselves. In the cognition stage this can be used as a memory activity: each group member is required to remember what others have said were their favorite feature.

Guidelines for Continuing on to the Next Stage.   This stage can take up most of the time of the group, if it is a group where world or local current events are discussed, something is being taught like a dance or a game, or where members have stories to share. As suggested, Stage III may merge into Stage IV, as members begin to express feelings and closure to the activity.

However, when the activity presented is quickly accomplished by group members, they can be asked if they want to go on to another one and this becomes Stage IV.

Stage IV: Cognition

Purpose.   This stage crowns all that has gone before as group members have the opportunity to demonstrate organized thought and behavior in their performance and in relating to each other (Ross, 1997). This is the time to remember any issue that was postponed for discussion at the beginning of the group. Emotions are less intense, focused attention is at its height, and resolution of problems appears to happen more easily. Often, the group directs itself and members will assume roles of leadership even if this is temporary. Therapists promote and support these outward signs of civility and inner security by not interfering.

Content.   This stage need not be verbal. Music can be played and clapping to the rhythm encouraged. Questions can be asked and responded to with a recognizable "yes" or "no" from members. Items used in the group can be displayed and each member invited to go and pick up their favorite one and use it again. A discussion can be initiated; if one or two members are able to verbalize, members can guess how others may answer and that can be verified with the member. The therapist can call attention to an item in a picture and ask the others to point out other features. An activity such as catch, holding hands, or moving some object around the room like a marionette can be used to further reinforce the feeling that the time spent has "connected us all" together.

When verbal communication can proceed, invite discussion of a previous activity, such as a description, how it felt to perform, what could be learned or changed in its performance. Therapists can model answers as well.

There can be the introduction of poetry, story-telling, reminiscences, pictures, and birthday or other cards that play a tune as they are opened. The sequence of activities in the group session may be reviewed. Members may introduce the subject of holidays, birthdays, boyfriends, or other situations they want to share. A short slide presentation can be presented with each group member participating by taking a turn in moving slides forward.

However, as closure approaches, too much novelty, alarming news, or the creation of intense feelings should be avoided.

Guidelines for Continuing on to the Next Stage.   The therapist gauges when it is the opportune time to remind the group that it is nearing the time to end.

Stage V: Closure

Purpose.   To provide the use of familiar activities that signal the closing of the session on a positive, affirmative note (Ross, 1997).

Content.   In this stage, brief activities are used so that group members experience the benefits of accomplishment and an inner sense of balance. A repeat of the same activity presented in Stage I can be used. A review or a summation of what has occurred in the session and each individual's contribution or performance is provided (Cole, 1993).

The therapists may decide whether the group members require a closure that contains additional arousal or maintains prevailing mood, or whether members require additional calming.

- Arousal: Some fast routine, clapping to a song, or providing a cold beverage.
- Even flow: Hold hands, repeat some affirmations, or members may express themselves in some way.
- Additional calming: Members hold hands with closed eyes, or may tell the group what they plan to do when the session is over. Some may linger after the session.

Stage V is never omitted.

Anticipated Outcome.   Members feel relaxed and this can be expressed in their facial features, by their postures, or by a statement. They are alert and calm, starting or appearing to have experienced some pleasure or satisfaction.

II SPECIAL OPPORTUNITIES

Suggested Procedures for Specific Problems

The following needs or problems of adults with developmental disabilities may be addressed in an occupational therapy group by introducing the

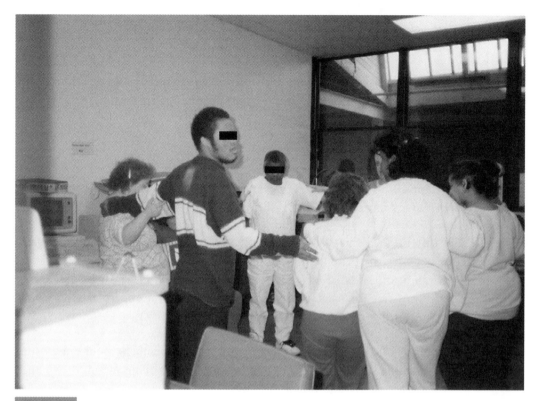

FIGURE 10.4 Stage V: First, we held hands; then, some could reach for elbows, and others made it to the shoulders.

subject for discussion, creating graded activities to practice correction, and reviewing the progress. These are described in relation to *Uniform Terminology, 3rd Ed.* (AOTA, 1994).

Sensorimotor Components

Sensory and Perceptual Processing

Clients bump into each other. A client blocks another's view or gets too close while passing.

It always is a group function for the therapists to emphasize spatial distances that permit safe exercise, and seating where no one's view is blocked. This can promote distances that are appropriate for sitting near each other, talking to each other, or walking around with greater awareness. This has occurred with good success, at least during group sessions.

Clients do not look in all directions and do not scan on either side so that work or other objects, if not placed in front of them, are not seen and not used.

Passing objects around often and turning one's head to watch what is happening can be a frequent activity in the group.

Clients find sorting and matching shapes and objects difficult. They do not recognize mistakes in performing tasks nor take steps to correct.

In the frequent handling of objects being passed around they have opportunities to use them in special ways. Sometimes several trials may be necessary to achieve results. Members build the experience of knowing success while getting to recognize the process of achieving it. Activities like two-piece puzzles that make a picture, or something to squeeze or pump for action are suitable at the very lowest level. Success at this may be limited, but it allows peers to help each other when this is done in a group format. Frequently, members are asked gently during a group activity, "did you do that right?" Adults appear to enjoy it when they either guess or know they did it right.

Clients find it hard to find their own elbows, the calf of their legs, or the middle of the back even with demonstration. Clients do not appear to be familiar with all parts of themselves, as clothes are torn, bunched up, or twisted. They may not recognize where their discomfort is located on their bodies.

Items in movement, such as batons or plates, can be used to touch body parts. Learning to massage arms and legs and pulling sleeves up and down can be done, as well as pantomiming gestures, like sleeping and so forth. While full success may not be achieved, some surprising results are possible.

Clients have excessive needs for touch stimulation or to avoid many forms of touch as in handling textures or being touched.

Use of the vibrator has been seen to neutralize this behavior. Putting a hand-held vibrator into the hand of a group member to use as desired is one option, and offering it on the back, moving slowly, is another.

Very, very rarely is this rejected, but should never be used to surprise. (Ross, 1997, Appendix)

Neuromusculoskeletal

Clients sit slumped in chairs. Clients are unaware of how to choose good chairs in which to sit. Clients complain of backache, pain in legs, neck and shoulder; they may fall out of the chair.

> When group members must look around, attend, and participate, their heads are up, their shoulders braced, and their trunks are stabilized with feet flat on the floor. This is a good feeling that they can get often during group sessions. Rarely are persons slumped in a group session.

Clients lack strength in holding a three-pound bean bag and lack endurance standing and moving in a group for 30 minutes.

> Use bean-bag activities regularly to build endurance. Just passing it around is a proprioceptive activity that influences relaxation. The bean bag can be placed in a stretchy cloth parachute, held, and waved up and down by all members together. It should never be used to throw, as gauging how members will throw is too unpredictable.

While standing, clients cannot shift weight or maintain good standing balance.

> Clients can hold each others' hands or wrists while moving all together. Place a two-by-four in front of each one to step onto and over. Some may need help, but this is a very good activity for persons who lack the experience. However, where poor balance is due to neurological conditions, extreme caution and watchfulness must be used to ensure sufficient support is provided. Also, poor balance may be due to visual problems and this factor needs to be ruled out.

When ambulant, clients demonstrate poor balance, tripping, falling, or bumping into walls, furniture, or each other.

> Clients can stand behind and hold on to chairs to practice balance while moving and swinging legs in different directions. Precautions should be taken that sufficient distance exists between group members doing this exercise. This is another way to teach awareness of others. Neglect of either side can be observed and followed up with help.

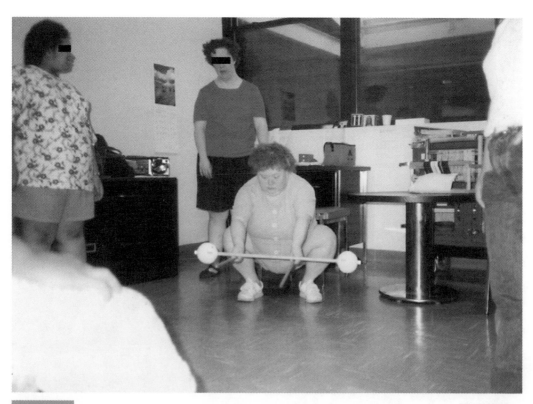

FIGURE
10.5
Learning to squat, to take care of the back, and to coordinate desired movement.

(Author's note: I refer here to unilateral neglect, which means that an individual ignores using one or the other side of the body.)

Bilateral Motor Coordination

Coordinating the carrying of objects with foot movement, alternating limbs in movement, and passing an item from one hand to another hand can be difficult for members in a group. The adult needs to be reminded to use both hands in a task. They also do not know how to handle many familiar objects and explore their use, such as stretching a rubber band around an object, winding up a gadget, cutting off tape from a dispenser, or pouring from a pitcher.

Use Stages II and III as the time to practice these skills. Exercise can be devised, with just these movements in mind, as well. (Ross, 1997, Chapters 2 & 3).

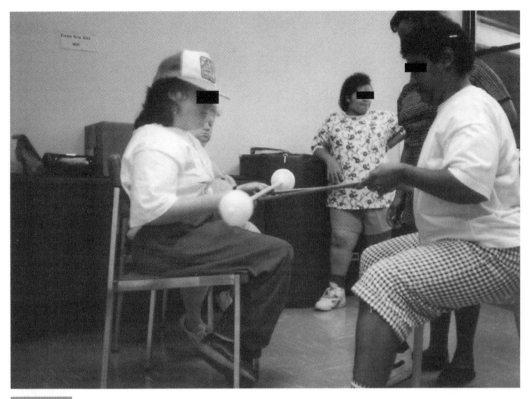

FIGURE 10.6 Working together as partners is important while learning control of movement, direction with coordination, and focus. Even the helpers learn to attend with consideration.

Clients find it hard to grade muscle tension and movement direction. Clients initially find it hard to handle paper without wrinkling or tearing it, or to not break objects by pushing, pressing, or pulling too hard. Grasping, holding, and placing are developmental skills that need much practice. This only can be achieved by doing many similar kinds of activities, repetitively, consistently, and with good humor. Improvements have been observed over 3 to 6 years with very few exceptions.

> Use musical instruments to pluck, strum, press and strike, for example. Carefully undoing sugar-free candies have been useful. Bounce a light wad of paper on a plate, or throw and catch a soft ball.

Cognitive Integration and Cognitive Components

Clients cannot attend to a task without some degree of verbal and/or physical prompts. They never know when it is their turn.

Ask other group members to remind them. Provide group games where this can be practiced often. Recognize that an occasional success may be what can be achieved and praise it (Ross, 1997, Chapters 3–4).

Clients display confusion in understanding environmental cues, such as where to sit in a room, who to watch, how to use and pass an object, and how to use cues such as pathways, aisles, and other guides.

Clients do not ask for help. Clients do not help each other, may hurt another physically, or else may give away their property. Responsibilities of ownership and rights are not understood.

All issues may never be resolved, but finding activities that incorporate these skills can help. (Ross, 1997, Chapters 4–5)

Two adults find it hard to wait their turn or mistreat another.

Adults are required to work this out between themselves, immediately. This has met with success.

Group members demonstrate no comprehension of winning a game, being competitive, or improving their own performance. Alternately, members cannot bear to lose a game or a turn.

Group membership provides these experiences over and over. Regular participation in a group gives these clients a chance to know one another and experience these difficulties in familiar surroundings with familiar people. The experience of group membership can help to lessen these difficulties.

Adults cannot remember the sequence of a task and, if some part of a task is learned, the memory of how it's done suddenly is forgotten. What was learned yesterday may be forgotten by the following day.

Other members are encouraged to wait before helping or to help with only one step at a time. Learning how to help others can be important for peers who are able to grow in this understanding.

Psychosocial Skills and Psychological Components

It is observed that clients can increase their ability to perform motor and perceptual tasks when given the opportunities to practice them. However, it is in the world of feeling that they live and that influences their social behaviors. The interactive skills appear to be the hardest to acquire and depend greatly on internalizing new attitudes through encountering new experiences in the group.

Psychological

Adults may demonstrate unrealistic attitudes developed through the years, such as "all work is exhausting" and "extending themselves in work is benefitting others, rather than themselves." They may believe that either fun is all they should expect or that fun is childish and must be disguised when participated in singly or collectively. Many other examples of lack of establishing one's own values, interests, and self-concepts exist. Sharing, awareness of the needs of others, and awareness of the differences that exist in each individual must become a part of the client's engagement in all activities.

Social

Adults display such self-absorption that a balanced view of their place in the order of things is skewed. For example, discrimination between great wrongs and small ones cannot be made, emotional flare-ups are too frequent, and the efforts of others are not appreciated. This self-absorption impairs role performance, social conduct, interpersonal skills and self-expression. A more balanced view can be learned by many adults, if consistently worked on in group. Role models do emerge in a group setting. Therapists need to praise every good action observed and briefly draw its implication for the group.

Self-Management

Concepts that can be reviewed include:

- being on time
- allowing sufficient time
- planning and making the preparations ahead of time
- assuming responsibility for mistakes and fixing them.

Summary.   The Five-Stage Group sessions have had accomplishments. At the very lowest level, crying and uncontrolled bladder behaviors have become controlled. At the more moderate levels, outbursts both physical and verbal have become better monitored by almost everyone with these problems. At the highest level, these adults have been able to demonstrate leadership behaviors, such as taking charge of a stage in the group. They are able to open the group using the welcoming steps and to lead the movement stage. These adults can be assigned to supervise and assist others with more physical or cognitive problems, setting up their lunch so independent eating is possible, assisting them during the day in removing and donning outer clothes, and keeping an eye out for the needs of those who may not know how to ask for help.

Occupation is defined as "chunks of culturally and personally meaningful activity in which humans engage" (Clark, Parham, et al., 1991). By attending the group, members are thus involved in an occupational act, and anyone who wishes to come (or who simply follows other members as they come to the group) is initiating engagement in an intended personally meaningful activity. Within this major catagory of occupation falls the myriad of tasks or activities selected for use in the Five Stages. These are different from the kinds of general activities used in other groups and may differ in the way they are presented. This is important to understand and is why a variety of activities are suggested as examples under each stage description. Throughout the session, the selected activities involve every member separately in a 1- or 2-minute task. Alternatively, all the members are involved at the same time in an interactive game, discussion or collective project that can take about 10 to 20 minutes. Each member gets a turn, a chance to be singled out, but only briefly, each time it is his or her turn. Activities need to be adapted to fit within that time period. Everyone in the group is working to some degree on the goals of relaxing, experiencing, and connecting with one another. Activities are chosen that can be completed successfully within three attempted trials whether or not these trials require another demonstration, a verbal cue, a physical assist, or a hand-over-hand help from the therapist or from another member.

Advocacy

With the recent advent of managed care and cost containment in areas of chronic care, funding has become less available. As institutions close and class action suits are initiated, new arenas emerge for serving a population that is handicapped: for instance, group homes, supervised apartment living, and day care programs. Even the structure of how the day is to be spent undergoes changes. Whatever those changes, individuals with developmental disabilities continue to need ongoing preventive-care services in addition to

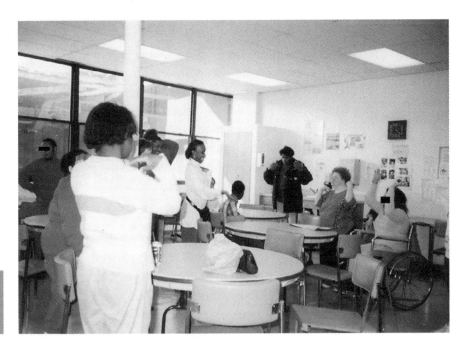

FIGURE 10.7

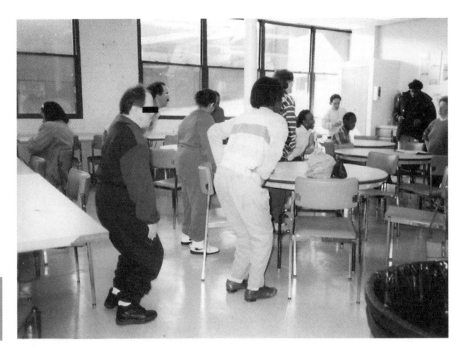

FIGURE 10.8

Alternately, the two female adults, on the extreme right, lead the exercises shown in Figures 10.7 and 10.8.

medical and management care. The Five Stages Model is one of the means whereby behavioral issues can be addressed, social stimulation needs met, and hidden skills tapped in a cost-effective manner. Advocating for a nonintrusive means for instructing this population in stress-reduction methods is also in the mainstream of prevention now. Using a group approach from which the individual's life narrative and needs emerge has historical precedence for other populations with disabilities. In referring to the need to preserve such methods as narrative and life history in the present climate, Burke and Kern write:

> The challenge for our profession is to fit these methods into the lexicon of functional and physically measurable change. Hence, each therapist must accept the responsibility for ensuring that methods such as narrative and life history are preserved regardless of the environments they find themselves in and that the data gathered from using these methods are talked about and documented in useful, outcomes-driven, consumer-oriented packages (Burke & Kern, 1996, p. 392).

Group outcomes for the population that is developmentally disabled can impact peers learning to help each other and can affect management costs by requiring fewer controls as behaviors improve. The message here is that retaining a group approach also can be the challenge for our profession to fit "into the lexicon of functional and physically measurable change" (Burke & Kern, 1996, p. 392).

The group may not be a panacea for the ills that the adult with developmental disabilities acquires. However, there is great advantage to these adults when they know that they belong to a special association of persons, who are interested in them, beyond the need to feed them and keep them clean. Occupational therapists understand that their most impressive asset is advocacy. People who are involved in healthcare, managed care, politics, and insurance want results, but results which include a sense of satisfaction on the part of the consumer. Despite "bottom line" arguments, consumer satisfaction will shape the way new services will be delivered. When therapists believe in the efficacy of groups for treatment, then groups will be done.

REFERENCES

Amerian Occupational Therapy Association. 1994. Uniform Terminology (3rd ed.). *American Journal of Occupational Therapy 48*, 1047–1059.

American Journal of Occupational Therapy (1996). *Special issue on managed care. 50*, 407–471.

Burke, J.P., & Kern, S.B. (1996). Is the use of life history and narrative in clinical practice reimbursable? Is it occupational therapy? The issue is. *American Journal of Occupational Therapy, 50,* 389–392.

Clark, F.A., Parham, D., Carlson, M.E., Frank, Gelya, Jackson, J., Pierce, D., Wolfe, R.J., & Zemke, R. (1991 April). Occupational science: Academic innovation in the service of occupational therapy's future. *American Journal of Occupational Therapy, 45,* 300–310.

Cole, M.B. (1993). *Group dynamics in occupational therapy: The theoretical basis and practice application of group treatment.* Thorofare, NJ: Slack.

Collins, L.F. (1996). Excelling in a managed care environment. *OT Practice, 1,* 20–22.

Harlowe, D., & Yu, P. (1981). The ROM Dance Network, P.O. Box 3332 Madison, WI 53704-0332.

Joe, B.E. (1997). Managed care: Does it measure up? *OT Week, 11,* 14–16.

Kerr, T. (1997, January 6). The numbers game in managed care. *Advance, 3,* 14.

Ross, M. (1987). *Group process.* Thorofare, NJ: Slack.

Ross, M. (1991). *Integrative group therapy* (2nd ed.). Thorofare, NJ: Slack.

Ross, M. (1997). *Integrative group therapy: Mobilizing coping abilities with the Five Stage Group.* Bethesda, MD: American Occupational Therapy Association.

Ross, M., & Burdick, D. (1981). *Sensory integration, a training manual for therapists and teachers for regressed, psychiatric and geriatric patient groups.* Thorofare, NJ: Slack.

Wood, W. (1996). Legitimizing occupational therapy's knowledge. *American Journal of Occupational Therapy 50,* 626–634.

ADDITIONAL READING

Vohs, J.R. (1996). Jumping tracks. *Developmental Disabilities Special Interest Section Newsletter. 19,* 1–3.

Writing about her 23-year-old daughter, born with cerebral palsy and cognitive difficulties, the author of this excellent article described how using a vocabulary of "slots, facilities, placements, coverage, 'day hab,' functional skills, acquisition, resident, consumer" brought limited and frustrating results for her and her daughter throughout many years. When the author began to use a contrasting vocabulary for goals for her daughter consisting of "home, neighborhood and community, friends, job contribution, citizenship, lifelong learning and education, and adventure," her daughter's needs began to represent the needs all people have. This freed up approaches and promoted the achievement of many of her daughter's dreams. We can do the same and reduce the separation between "normal" populations and populations born with disabilities. Set goals for the population that is developmentally disabled, using an effective language of "lifelong learning, education, and adventure," so that they will achieve social integration, continue skill learning, and realize some dreams.

Index